Julia Dalgleish
Stuart Dollery

The Health and Fitness Handbook

Editor: Heather Frankham

Longman

Lifetime

Pearson Education Limited
Edinburgh Gate
Harlow
Essex CM20 2JE, England
and Associated Companies throughout the world

ISBN 0 582 41879-8

British Library Cataloguing-in-Publication Data
A catalogue record for this book is available from the British Library.

Set by 35 in 11/13pt Sabon
Printed and bound in Malaysia

Contents

Introduction

Over the past decade the fitness industry has undergone many changes. Fitness fads have come and gone but the real alteration has occurred in the calibre of instructors sought after today and the number of local authority centres, private health clubs and corporate fitness facilities that are now operational within the United Kingdom.

The first nationally recognized qualification was introduced in 1986 with the RSA certification in exercise to music. Despite an increase in the number of higher education colleges offering sports science and recreation-related degrees and HNDs there was often little similarity between the knowledge covered and practical skills required. Very few courses enabled the student to apply industry-specific skills from the very start of their employment. The training providers within the industry became acutely aware of this and developed a myriad of courses to provide potential instructors with the right skills. However, not all such courses were generally recognized within the industry by fitness and general managers.

Enter the NVQ 2 in Coaching, Teaching and Instructing – introduced in 1998, revised in 1999 and gaining ground and recognition in 2000. Despite a hiccup with the ownership of the National Fitness Register the FIA is now compiling the register of people qualified to this national standard. The NVQ 2 is split into two stages. On successful completion of a training course you are awarded an NVQ 2 Stage 1 certificate. This proves your competence at the end of a training period. To obtain your full NVQ 2 Stage 2 certificate you have to prove your competence within the workplace and apply your newly learnt skills across a wide variety of people and situations.

The Health and Fitness Handbook covers the syllabus for the NVQ 2. The information within the text has been designed to make it easily accessible and user-friendly regardless of which teaching discipline you are investigating out of the five currently available: gym instruction, circuit training, exercise to music, step and aqua.

The Health and Fitness Handbook is aimed at anyone interested in becoming more involved within the fitness industry. This could apply to current instructors looking to expand the variety of classes or programmes that they teach or to refresh their knowledge in line with the new National Vocational Qualifications and standards operating within this field. Alternatively, this text could provide an opportunity for class and club participants who are regularly active to deepen their knowledge or for those who think they might like to be more active but prefer to be armed with some knowledge before committing to it.

As the need became greater for instructors to achieve their NVQ 2, it became obvious that there was no one text on the market that catered for this. There are many good anatomy and physiology texts but none which relates to exercise. There are excellent exercise physiology texts but none which applies it to the variety of disciplines within the gym or studio. *The Health and Fitness Handbook* was born out of the need to provide all this and in addition to touch upon the essential elements of health and safety, customer service and promotion of physical activity necessary in the role of instructors today.

Chapters 1–7 contain all the underpinning knowledge relevant to the NVQ 2 in coaching, teaching and instructing. These chapters contain essential anatomy and physiology in order to meet the NVQ 2 syllabus. Some of the material within these chapters will ring distant bells reminiscent of O-level and GCSE biology and science. Other chapters may be new and challenging, such as kinesiology. Much thought has gone into making this chapter as easy as possible to read and apply to the gym and class environment so that the subject's importance can be appreciated. Only with an understanding of kinesiology can you accurately analyse the safety and effectiveness of an exercise or activity. From Chapter 8 onwards the text relates to the practical application of this knowledge specific to the five NVQ 2 disciplines.

Chapter 8 on health screening introduces ways and means for you to ensure the safety and relevance of every exercise session for your participants, and will go partway towards helping you to provide a good standard of care. The practices in this chapter and in Chapter 16 on health and safety will promote your awareness about your responsibility as an instructor.

Chapter 9 then details how to structure a workout and what is involved within each component, while Chapters 10–14 apply this knowledge to the five disciplines. Chapter 15 covers the essential teaching skills an instructor should possess and implement through every discipline whatever the environment.

Finally, Chapters 16–18 relate to all five disciplines, covering the compulsory three units within the NVQ 2 on health and safety, customer service and promotion of physical activity. In a service industry, customer service skills are essential to understand and implement at all times. Chapter 18 is aimed at increasing awareness of how to encourage individuals or groups to be active outside of the standard gym or studio environment. This may involve outdoor cross-training, utilizing other services within a club or centre or incorporating activities into an individual's daily duties, whether the aim is to improve health-related fitness or to increase an aspect of their physical fitness.

Lifetime Health & Fitness is one of the largest training providers within the UK. We pride ourselves on having a professional and passionate team of tutors who deliver and assess these nationally recognized qualifications. We are now implementing the new NVQ 3 standards in coaching, teaching and instructing that aim to standardize the knowledge and experience of senior instructors and personal trainers within the industry. We hope to continue to increase the level of knowledge and enthusiasm both of instructors new to the industry and those already within it. We hope this text will inspire interest in and understanding of the human body, how activity affects it and how it impacts on our health and quality of life.

About the authors

Julia Dalgleish began on the uncharted road to a career in the fitness industry with a joint honours degree in Physiology and Psychology in 1992. This was followed by a year completing practical and vocational training through a diploma in dance and fitness teaching. Julia's experience in the fitness industry includes many years of teaching aerobics, step, aqua and circuits classes as well as working in a gym, conducting fitness appraisals, planning exercise sessions and writing individualized exercise programmes. This experience was gained in a variety of settings from village halls through to local authority leisure centres, private health clubs and corporate fitness facilities.

Through her roles as studio programme co-ordinator and fitness manager, Julia spent much time recruiting and developing staff and she later chose to make this her primary focus, joining Lifetime Health & Fitness in December 1997. During her time at Lifetime, she has trained many hundreds of fitness instructors, instilling in them her own high professional standards and inspiring them to deliver the highest possible levels of instruction. Now an internal verifier and programme co-ordinator, Julia is responsible for a team of tutors and the quality of training and assessing. She remains determined to have a positive impact on the fitness industry via the experience of the participants and the inspiration and quality of the instructors who now work within it.

Stuart Dollery graduated from West Sussex Institute of Higher Education in 1990 with a BA (Hons) degree in Sport Studies and has spent the past ten years in the fitness industry. He has worked in both the public and the private sector in roles ranging from gym instructor to head of fitness and as owner and director of Reform Personal Training.

Since graduating Stuart has gained accreditation through AFAA, APT and RSA. He has been lecturing for the past five years, both full-time for Lifetime Health & Fitness and as a visiting lecturer for the University of the West of England. He is a qualified assessor, internal verifier and course director for many of the OCR and YMCA-accredited programmes. He has lived in Bristol for the past eight years with his wife, Lisa, and daughter, Josie, and is looking forward to the birth of his second child very soon.

About the editor

Heather Frankham founded Lifetime Health & Fitness in 1993, initially running RSA exercise to music courses and providing consultancy for Country Club Hotels and the Marriott Chain within their leisure division. She gained a BEd (Hons) in Mathematics and Physical Education in 1990 and taught across the 4–18 age range for four years with responsibility for physical education and health education programmes. Later studies included an MSc in Exercise and Health Science at Bristol University and an MBA in Foundations of Senior Management with the Open University.

As managing director of Lifetime Health & Fitness and its London-based subsidiary, Fit to Perform, Heather has overseen the development of courses and materials and was responsible for the initial conception and structuring of this text as a resource for students on Lifetime's courses.

About the illustrator

Duncan Pearson qualified as a chartered physiotherapist in 1991. In 1992 he gained an MSc in Exercise and Health Science from the University of Bristol. He currently practises as a physiotherapist in Bristol.

Duncan started his career in art at the age of 18 when he won a national art competition with one of his drawings. Throughout his years as a student he supplemented his income by illustrating for a number of organizations, including the electricity board. More recently he has provided illustrations and cartoons for the health authority and books published through the University of Bristol. Some of his illustrations have been used by organizations on the world wide web.

Duncan's artistic interests lie in drawing and illustrating for health- and exercise-related areas. He enjoys helping people to understand the field through his cartoons. As a keen sportsman himself, he has represented Great Britain as a member of the British team for triathlon and duathlon in his age group. His cartoons often reflect his own experiences and feelings as an athlete.

About Lifetime Health & Fitness

Lifetime Health & Fitness is the leading national provider of fitness instructor and management training to health and fitness clubs within the UK. With clients including Marriott Hotels, David Lloyd, Cannons, Holmes Place, Tweed Park and Club Haus, Lifetime has designed and implemented training programmes to meet the needs of the ever-changing leisure industry. Certification to national standards is central to Lifetime's mission to increase the skills and professional standing of fitness instructors. *The Health and Fitness Handbook* provides a text for all those looking to get into the fitness industry, covering the syllabus for the Level 2 coaching, teaching and instructing disciplines of gym, exercise to music, circuits, step and aqua. We hope it will inspire you and support you through your entry into the fitness industry.

Acknowledgements

There are so many people who have helped in the writing and development of this text – from Lifetime Health & Fitness tutors who have input their ideas, researched specific subjects and proofread the final text, to our students who have worked with the text at various stages of development and fed back their thoughts and ideas, and our admin team who have helped to pull it all together.

Particular thanks go to:
Sallyann Lynn for her ongoing support throughout the project and for giving up her own time to help the authors meet deadlines;
Lyn Goodliffe for her work in reviewing chapters and providing constructive feedback;
Hannah Dawes for providing administrative support throughout, scheduling tutors to provide time for the authors to write and review each chapter;
Marcus Sanger, Mike Beeney, Tim Holbrook and Rob Linsell for their technical input and support to the authors in writing the text. Their passion for the fitness industry is evident in all that they do and their support and encouragement have helped greatly in bringing this text to print.

For the authors, the writing of *The Health and Fitness Handbook* has been an ongoing project for many months, and has inevitably encroached on their personal lives.

Julia's thanks and acknowledgements are extended to her partner, Mike Yeatman, and to her mother, father and new father. Her father inspired her to put pen to paper, Mike provided the ongoing support and space to write the book, whilst her mother was a constant source of motivation and encouragement.

Stuart's thanks and acknowledgement also go to his family: his wife, Lisa, and daughter, Josie, whose support has enabled him to follow his passion for fitness and educating others.

Concepts of fitness

CHAPTER

1

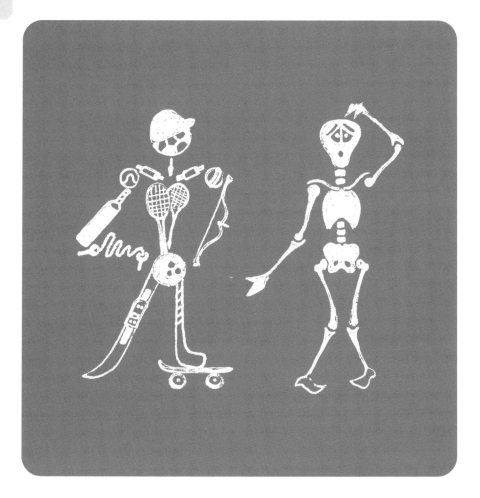

Topics to be covered in this chapter:

- An introduction to fitness
- Components of physical fitness
- Health-related fitness
- The benefits of regular exercise and effects of overtraining
- Factors affecting fitness and barriers to exercise
- The short- and long-term adaptations to exercise
- The wellness concept

An introduction to fitness

Fitness means different things to different people. If someone says their goal is to become 'fit', they will have a very specific and personal image of what this means to them and what they expect to have to do to reach this goal. For some people, fitness represents a highly specific goal such as being able to complete a marathon in less than three hours. For others, it may be managing to get to the gym three times a week, while yet others may suggest it means that they can get through their working days without feeling exhausted and manage to stay awake until the end of *Coronation Street*! The reasons these definitions vary so greatly is due to the altered attitudes of fitness professionals, health education authorities and the services provided by the leisure centres and health clubs that have grown and developed enormously over the last decade.

Our current understanding and objectives about fitness have changed in part due to the **Health of the Nation Report (1994)**. This revealed that a large proportion of our population (around 80 per cent) was inactive. A frighteningly high percentage of these people were then classified as sedentary. The number of obese individuals within our population is on the increase and **coronary heart disease** (CHD) remains the UK's leading cause of death. Both of these conditions can be positively affected by regular activity. However, it was only in 1992 that physical inactivity was recognized as a major independent risk factor for CHD and the government is now attempting to encourage more people to be more active, more often.

The **Allied Dunbar National Fitness Survey (1992)** revealed that 75 per cent of the general public (over the age of 16) understand that exercise confers important health benefits but not what this means. There has therefore been a need to educate the population as to how to gain these benefits.

People may realize that they need to be regularly active to stay healthy but they do not know how often to be active, how intense this activity should be and whether some activities are better than others for conferring health and fitness benefits. The latest guidelines produced by the **American College of Sports Medicine (ACSM) (1998)** have attempted to provide us with some distinctions and answers.

This chapter will attempt to clarify the wide array of definitions on what constitutes fitness and to emphasize the concepts of both health-related fitness and wellness that are now coming to the fore in the fitness industry. The benefits of exercise and the dangers of overtraining will be considered and a realistic look will be taken at the adaptations that we can expect to see within the short and long term with moderate, regular exercise.

Components of physical fitness

Many individuals when thinking about fitness will mention specific aspects that need improvement. For instance, many people wish to become stronger while others want to improve their flexibility.

The definition of **physical fitness** written by the **ACSM (1990)** states that physical fitness is

> a set of attributes that people have or achieve that relates to their ability to perform physical activity.

Physical fitness is considered to be made up of measurable components that enable people to improve their performance across the wide range of sporting activities. Fitness in this sense is usually achieved through a specific training programme that is completed through structured fitness sessions either in a gym or studio environment, outdoors or on an athletic track.

There are five major components of physical fitness that need consideration when assessing fitness and designing exercise programmes.

Cardiovascular fitness

> Cardiovascular fitness represents the ability of the heart and lungs to deliver an adequate supply of oxygen to the exercising muscles.

How hard the heart is working can be revealed through heart rate values. The higher the heart rate, the more intense the activity and the higher the oxygen demand from the working muscles. The heart rate will always rise when the oxygen demand for the muscles increases; this is what is known as a linear relationship.

The aim of any fitness programme is to improve the efficiency of the heart and lungs. These improvements occur in three main ways. Initially, we can maximize the amount of oxygen entering the lungs, secondly, we can improve the uptake and transport of the oxygen into the bloodstream and finally, we can increase the ability of the muscles to take up and utilize this oxygen. If these improvements are made, a reduction to the resting heart rate can usually be seen in the long term. This shows that the heart has to beat fewer times in any one minute to circulate the necessary amount of oxygen. Cardiovascular fitness is beneficial to enable individuals to complete all activities with more ease, with less energy expended.

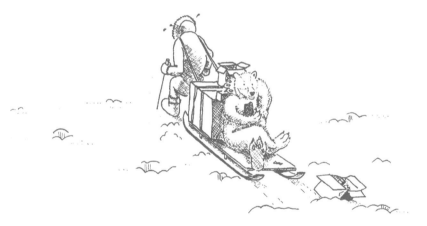

Muscular endurance

> Muscular endurance can be described as the number of repeated contractions a muscle or muscle group can perform against a resistance without fatiguing or the length of time a contraction can be held without fatigue.

Muscular endurance programmes involve large numbers of repetitions with light resistance and can prepare individuals for a variety of long-distance events or continuous daily activities. With this type of training the muscles become very efficient at taking up and utilizing the oxygen delivered to them. The obvious change that an individual will note when they have improved their muscular endurance is that they can continue exercising for longer periods of time with less discomfort.

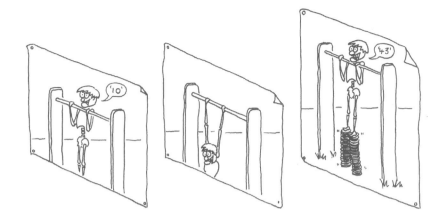

Muscular strength

> Muscular strength is defined as the maximum amount of force a muscle or muscle group can develop during a single contraction.

This may also be thought of as a one-repetition maximum, which is often used as a method of assessing strength. When muscular strength has been achieved, there is usually an obvious increase in size of the trained muscles and noticeably more weight will be lifted within this one-repetition range. Improvements in strength will be beneficial for many daily activities from lifting shopping to moving furniture.

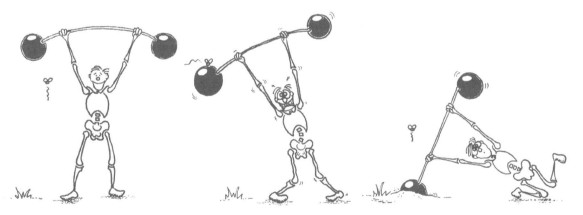

Flexibility

> Flexibility can be considered as the range of movement which can be accomplished at a particular joint.

Flexibility is specific to each joint within the body. Being flexible in one joint, like the hip, does not ensure flexibility at another, say the shoulder. Flexibility is often a neglected aspect of fitness training and can not only confer benefits for specific sporting events, but can also contribute to independence in later life.

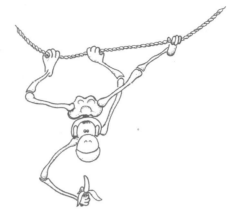

Motor skills

> The umbrella term of motor skills includes the co-ordination, speed, power or agility required to complete an activity.

These skills need to be specific to the activity concerned, as it is the nerve to muscle connection that is being trained.

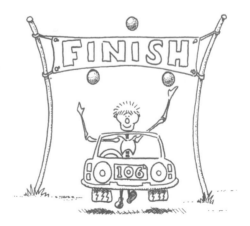

A balanced, individualized exercise programme can affect all of the above aspects. There are, however, genetic factors that can place an individual at an advantage or limit their attainment of these components of fitness.

Health-related fitness

If you choose six people and ask them to define health there is likely to be a range of opinions. It is useful to consider someone you believe to be healthy and attempt to list the characteristics that make this person appear healthy to you. This list may range from characteristics such as shiny hair, a glowing complexion, balanced eating habits, a sense of wellbeing and strong self-esteem coupled to a lack of disease, illness or incapacity.

The definition of health-related fitness places the emphasis on activity improving health and preventing disease states. It is described by the **ACSM (1990)** as:

> a) An ability to perform daily activities with vigour; b) The demonstration of traits and capacities that are associated with low risk of premature development of hypokinetic diseases.

'Hypo' is literally translated as 'under', kinetic as 'movement'. So hypokinetic disease is that associated with lack of sufficient movement. This list of diseases has expanded over the years, with the most obvious conditions including **CHD**, **arthritis** and **osteoporosis**.

It is often difficult to get younger generations to appreciate the benefits of health-related fitness. Whereas people in their twenties and thirties usually work towards more physical fitness goals through structured fitness sessions, older generations are more able to appreciate the benefits of reducing the risk of diseases caused by lack of movement and are looking for regular activity that is not necessarily intense in nature.

The benefits of regular exercise and effects of overtraining

Regular exercise can provide numerous benefits. These benefits should be made clear to anyone who is beginning a regular exercise programme. Often people's understanding of the benefits exercise confers reveals a very limited outlook, or their expectations may be unrealistic given the time, intensity and type of exercise in which the individual is considering taking part. Appropriate exercise programmes and regular activity can yield improvements in:

- any of the five components of physical fitness
- blood pressure
- blood lipid and cholesterol levels

- insulin sensitivity and glucose tolerance
- diabetes
- feeling of wellbeing
- stress release
- obesity
- bone density
- arthritis
- clinical depression

Guidelines that recommend the quality and quantity of activity necessary for fitness and health differ. It is now recognized that positive health benefits can be obtained from regular moderate level activity. The American College of Sports Medicine (ACSM) have released guidelines that suggest how frequently we should exercise, for what duration and to what intensity. These guidelines make a clear distinction between physical fitness and health-related fitness.

According to the **ACSM (1990)**, their position statement on the recommended quality and quantity of exercise for developing and maintaining cardiorespiratory fitness in healthy adults is:

Frequency   3–5 times per week

Intensity   60–90 per cent maximum heart rate (MHR)

Time   20–60 minutes

Type   maintained and rhythmical use of large muscle groups

These guidelines are defining exercise parameters and a distinction needs to be made between what is considered exercise and what is termed physical activity.

The definition provided by the **ACSM (1998)** states that **exercise** is:

> planned, structured, and repetitive bodily movement done to improve or maintain one or more components of physical fitness.

Recently however, for health-related fitness gains, the **ACSM (1998)** have changed these parameters and definitions slightly:

Frequency   5–7 times per week

Intensity   50–90 per cent MHR

Time   30 minutes (accumulative)

Type   maintained and rhythmical use of large muscle groups

There are significant changes to this latest guideline. Firstly, the recognition that individuals need only exercise at 50 per cent of their maximum heart rate to gain health benefits. Secondly, that the benefits are realized if the 30 minutes are split into, say, three 10 minute sessions over the course of the day.

These guidelines are defining what is now referred to as physical activity, to make the distinction that the intensity and frequency are different. The **ACSM (1998)** define **physical activity** as:

> bodily movement that is produced by the contraction of skeletal muscle and that substantially increases energy expenditure.

Any person wanting to become or remain active should be educated to appreciate the benefits that this activity can confer. Individuals should also be made aware that the intensity of this exercise does not have to be great so long as the activity is regular. However, people should also realize that more is not always better.

When prescribing activity and exercise for people, the emphasis is on considering their individual goals. These must be realistic, within their capacity and, most importantly, enjoyable. People are motivated to remain active for a variety of reasons. It is our role as instructors to determine what that particular motivation is for each person. The regularity of the activities is more important than the intensity when considering long-term health benefits.

The question of how much activity is needed for optimal health still needs answering and this is the focus of much of the current research in this area. What we currently do know, is that there is an optimal health graph depicting the levels of activity that confer benefits and those that venture into the realms of **overtraining**.

Exercise can be addictive and is increasingly being recognized as such. When anyone begins an exercise programme they tend to see results over a relatively short timespan. This motivates them to continue training and, in some cases, to increase the intensity and/or frequency of the training sessions. Up to a point, results will continue to be seen, until the amount of training exceeds our body's capacity to adapt to it. If we do not provide sufficient rest for the body to recover following a training session, then the body begins working against itself. Symptoms of overtaining are various and, once again, individual. However, common symptoms would include:

- tiredness
- aching joints and muscles
- nausea
- decreased immune system efficiency (leading to extended colds/infections)
- repetitive loading injuries (knee pain, shin splints)
- excessive weight loss
- reduction in bone density (with excessive aerobic work)
- increased length of time to reach fitness goals (plateau effect)

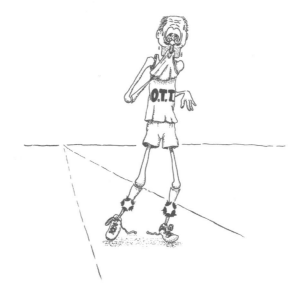

The relationship between training benefits and frequency can be represented as a **dose–response curve**. This depicts how, initially, the more exercise that is done the more benefits will be realized. Then as the level of exercise becomes excessive the body fails to adapt positively to the stress placed on the body. When this optimal level is exceeded, the risks overtake the benefits and overuse injuries and reduced immune system efficiency results in illness.

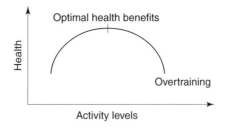

Figure 1.1 The dose–response curve

Factors affecting fitness and barriers to exercise

Aside from the intensity and frequency of activity levels, there are many other factors that affect the speed with which and degree to which adaptations to exercise occur. If you set two individuals off onto the same exercise or activity programme and monitored them over a 12-week period, the results would be different. There is no one programme that can guarantee an identical response in two people. This is due to many factors that we could place under an umbrella term of individual differences, including:

- genetics
- gender
- age
- body type
- nutrition
- lifestyle factors (smoking, alcohol consumption, etc.)

It is, therefore, essential to impress on people the importance of their activities outside of the gym, studio or activity arena and the futility of attempting to work against genetics. Any goal, whatever its size or emphasis, always needs to be grounded in reality. If your genetics means that you have been born a long-distance runner then it is unlikely that you will become a world-class sprinter. If you have been born with the physique of Mr Bean, it will be impossible to attain the sculpted bulk of Arnold Schwarzenegger.

It is worth appreciating the added factor that not everyone will have the desire or ability to devote the time needed to attain his or her fitness or health goals. There are many **barriers** to exercise that prevent or discourage people from maintaining a regular exercise programme, such as:

- time (per week and per session)
- family responsibilities
- work pressures
- cost
- travel
- ignorance of the benefits
- intimidation
- discomfort
- lack of progress towards goals

Fitness professionals today are expected to be able to identify which factors will present the biggest barriers to their client and to programme ways to minimize the likelihood of these barriers affecting their adherence to their chosen lifestyle change.

The short- and long-term adaptations to exercise

We have already described how individuals will respond to any activity to different extents and in different timescales due to a variety of factors. The adaptations that do take place within the body are various and will be experienced at different times. This is important to realize as individuals need to be aware of what progress is expected and to be given a realistic timeframe as to when their goals are likely to be achieved. This may enable them to maintain their motivation for long enough to change their lifestyle positively. In reviewing the benefits of exercise identified earlier in this chapter, we should appreciate that some of these benefits will be seen over the short term of a few months, while others will not be evident for six months or perhaps not even for years. When designing an activity programme participants should not only be made aware of this fact but they should also be given both short- and long-term goals to work towards. This will hopefully maximize their motivation, particularly if the short-term goals are reviewed and updated on a regular basis.

Short-term benefits could include:

- improved posture and body awareness
- improved motor co-ordination skills
- increased feelings of wellbeing
- reduced levels of stress

All of these benefits could be appreciated over the initial eight weeks of an activity programme. Not a conclusive list, these factors alone could make a great difference to someone's enjoyment of life and productivity at work.

The longer-term benefits would then include:

- body composition changes
- improvements in aerobic ability, strength and flexibility
- reduction in the risk of developing diseases

These long-term changes are often more measurable and specific and frequently represent an individual's final goal. However, the short-term benefits should not be underestimated in terms of the positive impact they can have on someone's life.

The wellness concept

Taking all the previous factors into account, the newest emphasis within the health and fitness industry is the **wellness concept.** This too has many definitions dependent on the source quoted. The **World Health Organisation (1984)** defines wellness as:

a state of complete physical, mental and social wellbeing and not merely the absence of disease or infirmity.

Wellness, therefore, takes health-related fitness to a new level. It incorporates the mental and spiritual aspect of the individual. This acknowledges the link between mental and physical health, a link prevalent in Eastern philosophy. This has encouraged health and fitness centres to incorporate relaxation centres and provide a totally **holistic** approach to fitness that is not just centred on the body. To illustrate this shift in emphasis we can see the popularity of yoga, Pilates and t'ai chi.

Each of us will have a different perception of what constitutes 'personal wellbeing'. The wellness concept requires us to be proactive and to focus in on the positive benefits to be gained from adopting a healthy lifestyle. It is this lifestyle change that is considered to be the key to wellness. A proverb says:

Those who think they have no time for bodily exercise will sooner or later have to find time for illness.

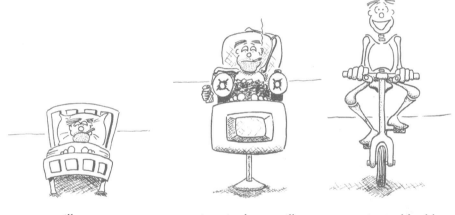

illness   *inactive but not ill*   *proactive and healthy*

Today's population has had the benefit of many health promotion campaigns and general health awareness has never been higher. This is highlighted by the fact that, whereas several decades ago the primary killers in this country were illnesses such as flu, cholera and tuberculosis, awareness about these diseases has meant that mortality rates have plummeted. Now we have to conquer the primary enemy we face today, that of coronary heart disease, through awareness of the possible causes and proactive lifestyle measures that can be adopted to reduce our risk.

Health and leisure clubs have also reflected this changing emphasis on our outlook to life, lifestyles and healthy behaviours. These clubs have metamorphosed from places where people, often grudgingly, attended high-impact workout sessions for the specified three times per week, into more relaxing, stress-releasing multi-activity-centred sites. Nowadays, centres are there to educate and interest those from all walks of life, needing physical, mental, social and even spiritual attention.

CHAPTER SUMMARY

- Fitness and health have different definitions, so an individual can be fit but not healthy and healthy but not fit.

- Physical fitness is represented by five specific components: cardiovascular fitness, muscular strength and endurance, flexibility and motor skills. These components are measurable and easily identified.

- Health-related fitness is represented by an ability to get through daily life with energy while staving off illnesses associated with lack of activity.

- The concept of wellness adopts a more holistic approach to the individual, considering physical, mental and spiritual aspects.

- The benefits of exercise range from increased self-esteem through weight management to reduced risk of many medical conditions such as CHD, osteoporosis, diabetes and arthritis.

- Individual differences mean that people will adapt to an exercise programme in very different ways. Instructors should ensure they are aware of the effects of genetics, gender, age, lifestyle and nutrition on the results of their exercise regime.

- The amount of exercise that confers maximal health benefits is still under review. The current ACSM (1998) guidelines state that, to confer benefits, activity can be of moderate intensity and accumulative, so long as it occurs regularly, preferably on a daily basis.

- It is known that too much exercise can have a detrimental effect on health, reducing the effectiveness of the immune system, reducing bone density and preventing positive adaptations to exercise.

- Individuals will not always understand what amount or type of exercise is suitable for them. They may be ignorant of the benefits and dangers associated with exercise. Education must have a key place within any fitness professional's role.

- Always ensure individuals' fitness or health goals are realistic, achievable and enjoyable. Identify the potential barriers and design both short- and long-term goals into the programme of exercise.

The skeleton

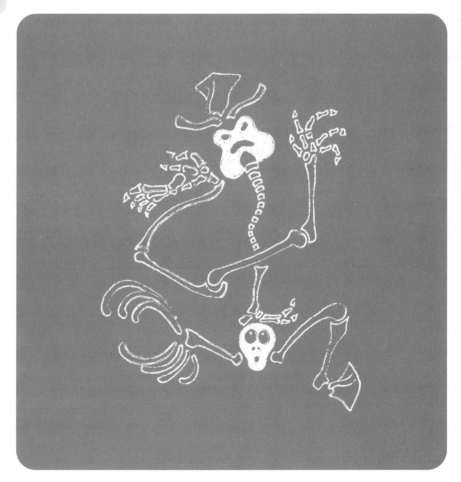

Topics covered in this chapter:

- The skeleton
- Bone
- Cartilage
- The spine
- Joints

The skeleton is our most fundamental structure and without it we cannot stand upright, let alone move. Muscles attach to bones and cross joints to enable movement to occur. The calcium stored within the bone allows muscles to contract and shorten to create this movement.

Our skeleton differentiates us from our primate ancestors. It is the manual dexterity conferred by our thumbs, enabling us to pick up and utilize objects, that is the greatest difference between our skeleton and that of apes. It is important to appreciate the different functions of the skeleton and how these translate into the need for different-shaped bones within our body. The specific ways in which these bones meet to form joints give us the range of movement necessary for various sports and our daily activities.

These joints and their surrounding structures, such as ligaments and tendons, need consideration. Understanding of the structure and function of bones and joints can often be enhanced by looking at diseased states, as in the effects of osteoporosis on bone and arthritis on the joint mobility and movement.

Bones are living tissues that constantly adapt to their environment and respond to the stress placed on them. Exercise is an excellent example of one of these stresses and beautifully reveals our ability to adapt. Observing the difference in bone strength between an athlete and an inactive individual can give us further information on the benefits of regular activity. This chapter should enable you to identify the major bones within the body, their structure and function. Particular attention will be paid to the spine as fitness professionals need a detailed understanding of the many joints that make up this essential backbone. Each type of joint will be considered but their movement potential will be investigated in Chapter 4: kinesiology.

The skeleton

The human skeleton has evolved over millions of years and has had to adapt its structure to deal with very different forces acting through the bones during different activities. Initially our skeletons had to adjust to us standing on two legs, which meant that the amount of stress through the spine increased dramatically. This still proves to be a weak spot in many people today.

Our skeletons provide us with many advantages over those invertebrates with no bony structures and, indeed, even over our closest ancestors. One of the benefits of standing on two legs is that we can use our hands for more tasks. Our manual dexterity (particularly movement of our thumbs) allows us to pick up objects with ease.

Functions of the skeleton

The skeleton is made up of **206 bones**. Not surprisingly, these bones are of very different shapes that suit their function. The skeleton serves many purposes. Certain bones within the skeleton can be seen to serve one principal purpose, but generally each bone serves a variety of functions.

The main functions of the skeleton:

- *It is the supportive framework of the body.*
- *It provides protection for the vital organs.*
- *It acts as an anchor for the muscles to provide movement.*
- *It provides a site for red and white blood cell production.*
- *It represents the site of mineral reserves (e.g. calcium and phosphorus).*

Attempt to identify the predominant function of the following bones:

- skull
- thigh bone
- ribs

The major bones in the human skeleton

Although there are 206 bones in the adult human skeleton, initially you will only need to identify 25 major bones. These are the major bones used for everyday movement and exercise. These will often be referred to in discussing common sports injuries and it will be necessary to recognize them when considering the origin and insertion of the major muscle groups in Chapter 3 and in relation to exercise analysis in Chapter 4.

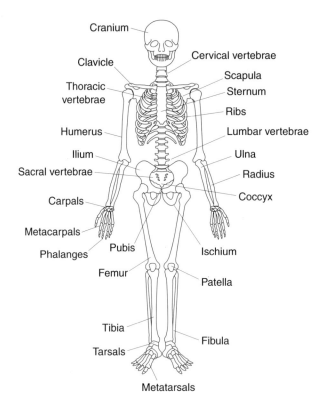

Figure 2.1 The major bones of the human skeleton

Divisions of the skeleton

The entire skeleton is subdivided into two sections. Each section is differentiated through its structure, function and capability for movement.

The **axial skeleton** is the principal supportive structure of the skeleton and consists of the 80 bones of the skull, vertebrae, sternum and ribs. It is considerably more rigid than the other section of the skeleton. Fractures are uncommon in the axial skeleton and, when they do occur, are generally serious in nature.

The **appendicular skeleton** provides the freely moveable frame for the upper and lower limbs. Think of an appendage as one of your arms or legs, this may help you to remember which section contains which bones. This section contains the remaining 126 bones that make up the pectoral and pelvic girdles, arms and legs. Most fractures and dislocations occur in this part of the skeleton.

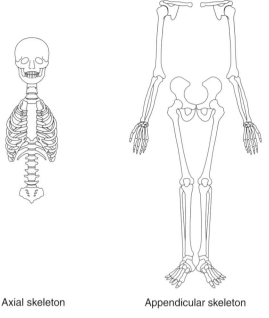

Axial skeleton   Appendicular skeleton

Figure 2.2 Divisions of the skeleton

Bone

Whilst babies are born with over 300 bones, adults have a skeleton comprising 206 individual bones, more than half of which are in our hands and feet.

Bone develops from cartilage. The order and timeframe in which this process occurs is pre-programmed by our genes and happens in a set order. During this hardening process, known as **ossification**, some bones fuse together, thereby reducing the total number of individual bones within the skeleton.

Bone is shaped specifically to fit its function and this process, known as **modelling**, occurs throughout the growth process and afterwards. Bone tissue is continuously broken down and replaced throughout life, with 10 per cent of our bone mass being replaced annually.

Bone is the hardest of all living tissue, being five times stronger than a bar of steel of the same weight. Since bone is specific to its location and function we see a variety of bone structures within the skeleton. In addition to differences between the bones in the same body, there are also gender differences between skeletons. Females have lighter, thinner bones and have a shallower, wider pelvis.

Bone formation and development

During the gestation period (in the womb) the skeleton of the foetus is composed of a rubbery cartilage, called **articular (hyaline) cartilage**. At this initial stage, the cartilage is completely solid, it is not until the later stages of development that bones form hollow centres.

Over the 25 years of the growth process, the articular cartilage is converted to bone, this is the ossification process. Another name for this process is **calcification**, which gives you a clue as to the predominant mineral involved in this hardening procedure.

> *Calcium and phosphorus salts are laid down into the cartilage material and change the cartilage from a rubbery, flexible structure into a material that is the second hardest substance in the body after the enamel found within our teeth.*

The amount of calcium that is laid down, and later withdrawn, is dependent on a number of factors, including dietary intake of calcium, and the subsequent levels of calcium circulating in the blood. The calcium in the blood is there to enable muscles to contract, as will be briefly discussed in Chapter 3. If there is insufficient calcium in the blood, then calcium will be withdrawn from the bones as the bones and teeth contain 99 per cent of the body's calcium stores. If there is excessive calcium in the blood, then more calcium will be laid down in the bone. Hormones circulating within the bloodstream control these deposits and withdrawals.

DID YOU KNOW?

The central hollow cavities within bone structure are the secret of the inordinate strength demonstrated by bone. This centre, known as the medullary cavity, reduces the weight of bone but maintains its strength. It is here that the bone marrow is found, fat is stored and blood cells are produced.

Bones grow at a specific pre-programmed rate, controlled by hormones, into a specific, pre-programmed shape. As with all living tissue, bone has an efficient blood supply to bring all necessary building materials and hormones to it. Each bone is surrounded by a fibrous, cellular and highly sensitive sheath that covers its entire surface apart from the articular cartilage at the bond ends. This sheath is called the **periosteum**. During growth it represents the source of bone-developing cells for growth and repair.

> *The growth of the bone occurs at a specific site, known as the **growth plate**. Once growth is complete, this cartilage plate also ossifies. Once this has happened, growth within the bone stops as the process is irreversible.*

If very young children are exposed to heavy and unsuitable weight training during their formative years, their growth plates can be damaged; this will often limit the height of the child. In some cases, this may result in the growth plate ossifying prematurely. The growth plate is also known as the epiphyseal plate. The end of the bone is known as the **epiphysis**; the shaft (or centre of the bone, that resists bending forces) between the two epiphyses is known as the **diaphysis**. The epiphyseal (growth) plate, therefore, separates these two sections. Development occurs within both the epiphysis and diaphysis and advances towards the intervening cartilage from both ends. The cartilage then thins until the bone centres fuse and growth is complete.

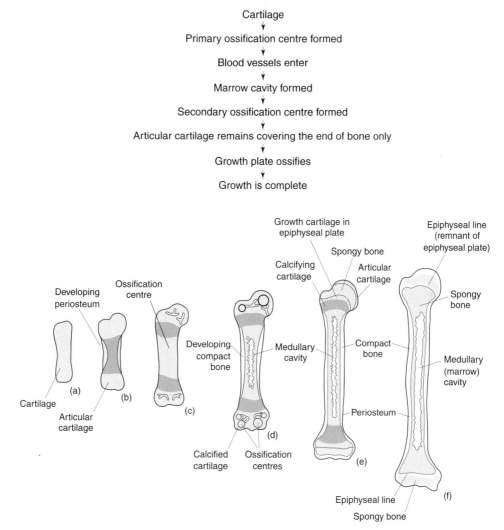

Cartilage
↓
Primary ossification centre formed
↓
Blood vessels enter
↓
Marrow cavity formed
↓
Secondary ossification centre formed
↓
Articular cartilage remains covering the end of bone only
↓
Growth plate ossifies
↓
Growth is complete

Figure 2.3 Bone growth and development

The modelling process continues throughout the lifecycle to ensure bones develop the right shape and respond to the stresses placed through the body as it grows in size and weight. Two main types of cell are responsible for these complex processes: **osteoblasts** and **osteoclasts.** These cells, which lie within the fibrous tissue network of bone, have very distinct roles.

Osteoclasts: These break down and **c**lean old bone.
Osteoblasts: These **b**uild new bone.

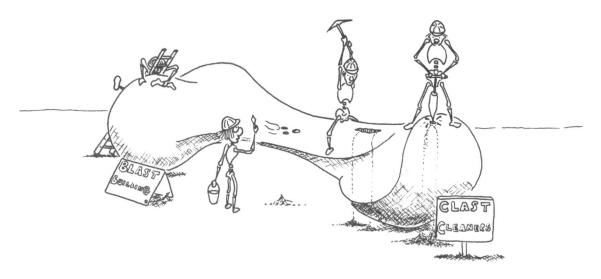

During childhood and growth spurts, the osteoblast cell activity is greater than that of the osteoclasts. This means that the density of the bone should steadily increase along with bone strength. The laying down of calcium salts and the amount of stress placed on the bone by exercise and gravity will also affect this. Beyond the age of 25–30, osteoclast activity increases and can overtake that of the osteoblasts. This means that the bone density and strength can decrease if activity does not compensate for this.

Structure of bone

There are five classifications of bone, as detailed later in this chapter. One of these types is the long bones. These are responsible for stature and reflect the growth process most dramatically. When considering the internal structure of bone and its complex genetically-controlled growth process it is easiest to make reference to the long bones found in the arms and legs.

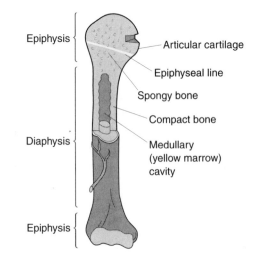

Figure 2.4 The structure of a long bone

Within the two areas of the bone, the epiphysis and diaphysis, there are different types of bone tissue. The different types appear in different quantities in the different bones around the body.

The two bone types are:

● compact
● spongy

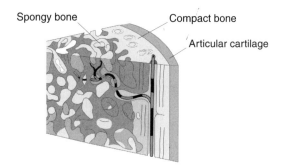

Figure 2.5 Bone tissue types

Compact bone is also known as cortical bone. This is a dense, hard shell that generally makes up the outer layer of the bone. It is composed of tiny tubes of bone called osteons. These are arranged in concentric layers and reveal a regular pattern. Blood reaches these bone cells via an intricate system of integrated canals. Compact bone is the body's second-hardest material after enamel and 75 per cent of bone within the body is of this type.

Spongy bone, also referred to as cancellous or trabeculae bone, is a lattice-like structure resembling a honeycomb, or the inside of a Crunchie bar. It is composed of bony struts, called trabeculae, which are arranged along the lines of greatest stress to confer strength without weight. Within the central space, the **medullary cavity**, the bone marrow packs the spaces between these struts. Red marrow is involved with blood cell production; the yellow marrow stores fat. The remaining 25 per cent of bone is of this spongy type.

Classifications of bone

There are considered to be five different types of bone and their classification is defined by their function:

● long
● short
● flat
● irregular
● sesamoid

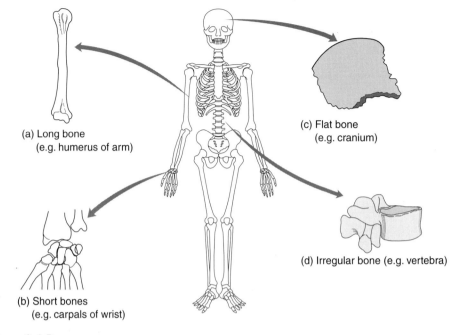

(a) Long bone
(e.g. humerus of arm)

(c) Flat bone
(e.g. cranium)

(b) Short bones
(e.g. carpals of wrist)

(d) Irregular bone (e.g. vertebra)

Figure 2.6 Bone types

Table 2.1 details the structure and function of each type, with examples of where each type can be found within the body.

Table 2.1 Bone types

Bone type	Structure	Main function	Example
Long	Their length is greater than their breadth. They have a tubular shaft with a distinct epiphysis and diaphysis. The epiphysis is covered by articular cartilage.	Lever for movement	Femur, humerus
Short	They mainly consist of spongy bone with outer covering of compact bone.	Great strength but less movement potential	Carpals, tarsals
Flat	This is a sandwich of compact bone with a thin central core of spongy bone.	Attachment for muscles and protection of internal organs	Scull, scapula, ribs
Irregular	They consist of a thin outer covering of compact bone with a spongy bone interior.	Protects and supports internal organs	Facial, vertebrae
Sesamoid	Small nodules of bone located in tendons where they rub over bony surfaces.		Patella

Osteoporosis

Osteoporosis literally means 'porous bones'. The official definition by the **ACSM (1995)** states that this is a disease

> characterised by low bone mass and microarchitectural deterioration of bone tissue leading to enhanced bone fragility and a consequent increase in fracture risk.

It is now considered to affect one in three women and one in twelve men over the age of 65 and is set to reach epidemic proportions over the next decade. **The National Osteoporosis Society** believes that more women will die from osteoporosis than from breast, uterine and cervical cancer combined. The current cost to the NHS is around £750 million per year and is on the increase. Detection of this condition is often difficult, with X-rays only able to detect a deterioration of 30–50 per cent or more of bone mass, at which stage the disease is well advanced. Usually the first suggestion of a problem is when an individual is admitted to hospital with a fracture.

There is much research to determine if there is a specific gene that predisposes an individual to osteoporosis; this work remains inconclusive at present. However, there are many factors that affect the likelihood of contracting the disease, these include:

- *Insufficient calcium intake*
- *Insufficent vitamin D intake – without vitamin D ossification cannot occur.*
- *Poor nutrition and dieting – restrictive, low-calorie diets often contain insufficient calcium and vitamin D. Certain products, like coffee, can decrease absorption of calcium in nutrients.*
- *If peak bone mass was not achieved there is increased risk of reaching the bone's fracture threshold when bone loss continues at a rate of 1–2 per cent per year.*
- *Amenorrhea – loss of periods*
- *Menopause – bone loss can be ten times higher during this process before reverting to the normal loss of 1–2 per cent.*

If the body has insufficient calcium available to it on a daily basis, then it looks to its storage sites. The body leaches the minerals from the bone and in doing so depletes the bone's ability to withstand normal daily stresses and strains placed upon it. This brittleness then leads to fractures. It makes sense, therefore, to prevent or treat osteoporosis by increasing bone density. Exercise is one of these methods.

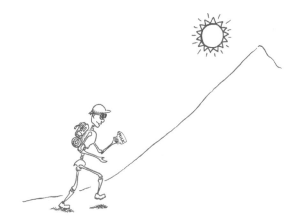

DID YOU KNOW?

The benefits of weight-bearing activity can be best appreciated by looking at the bone density changes in individuals who have had to take bed rest for a number of weeks. Even within the space of a few days the bone density starts to decline. This loss becomes significant after a few weeks. Another interesting case is that of astronauts. If they have been in space for a number of weeks or months, they are generally taken from the space shuttle by wheelchair. Due to the lack of gravitational pull in space there is very much less force acting through the bones and they therefore lose density. A gradual and structured programme is then undertaken to build bone density back up.

Bone density increases are specific to the bone that incurs the stress. This can be seen in professional sports people. Tennis players have significantly higher bone densities in their playing arm by about 30 per cent. Rowers have increased spinal bone densities. However, it must be pointed out that although moderate levels of exercise have a positive effect on bone density, there are adverse effects when we overtrain. Some years ago it was noted that in many top-class triathaletes, the spinal bone densities were lower than expected and continuing to fall in some that were monitored. This was considered to be due to excessive mileage when training for the marathon combined with two activities – swimming and cycling – which were weight-assisted with lesser effects of gravity and impact.

Additionally, if training is taken to excess, calorie-restricted diets are adhered to or psychological stress is incurred, body fat levels drop and hormonal levels can fluctuate. In women a resulting drop in oestrogen and progesterone released from the ovaries causes the menstrual cycle to become irregular, a condition known as amenorrhea. If the protective effect of oestrogen is lost, bone density levels reduce. If the menstrual cycle is lost for 6 months or less the reduced bone density is usually reversible. If it is lost for a period of 2–3 years or more the damage is irreversible.

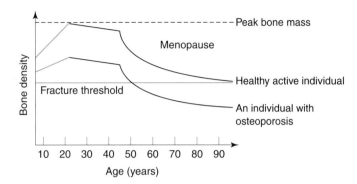

Figure 2.7 Bone density changes over the lifespan

There is some evidence to indicate that excessive training, dieting and stress also cause disruption of male hormones, resulting in lowered blood testosterone concentrations and reduced sperm count. There could be an increased risk of osteoporosis but more research is needed.

The adaptation of bone to exercise

Bone is very active tissue, sensitive to the forces placed through it and capable of growth and regeneration if damaged. If a bone is stressed at a particular point the osteoblast cells respond by migrating to the bone surface and secrete protein to strengthen this area. Over time these proteins become mineralized, with new bone formation occurring on the outer surface of the bone. By increasing its diameter, the bone has successfully increased its surface area. Therefore, any force applied to that bone can be dissipated over a larger area and represents less of a risk of fracture.

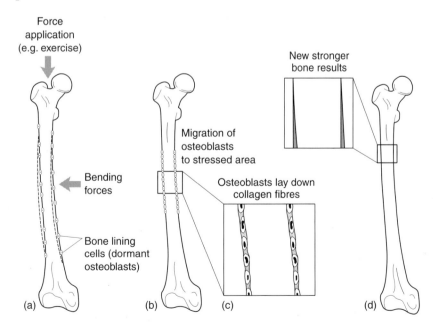

Figure 2.8 Adaptation of bone to exercise

Young bone appears to be more responsive to loading forces than older bone. It is, therefore, essential to attain peak bone mass within these formative years, as it cannot be attained at a later date. However, it must be stressed that bone density can be improved at any age.

Cartilage

As mentioned earlier in the chapter, within the foetus, cartilage represents the main ingredient of the skeleton. In adults it is found in joints and covering the end of bones. There are a variety of different types of cartilage, which have specific roles within the body. The basic structure includes a ground matrix of cells and protein fibres known as collagen and elastin. However, cartilage is devoid of blood vessels and relies upon diffusion of oxygen through the synovial fluid (detailed later in this chapter) for survival. There are three main classifications of cartilage.

Articular cartilage

Articular cartilage (also known as hyaline cartilage) is a bluish-white translucent tissue mainly composed of collagen, with the fewest number of cells and fibres out of the three types. It is this cartilage that makes up the baby's skeleton and allows for the enormous growth from around 45cm up to 1.8m. Once growth is complete, this cartilage can then be found covering the end of the long bones, lining the surfaces of the joints and in many structures of the respiratory tract.

Fibrocartilage

Fibrocartilage is mainly composed of collagen fibres; this tissue is tough and resistant to compression forces. This is essential when you consider it is found primarily between the vertebrae of the spine as the vertebral discs. It also functions as a tough connection between bones and ligaments as found in the hip joint. Here it joins the two parts of the hip together at the joint called the symphysis pubis. This becomes very important in pregnant women when hormones soften it in preparation for the birth process.

Elastic cartilage

The third type is called elastic cartilage and, as the name suggests, the composition of this tissue contains mainly the yellow elastin fibres in addition to those of collagen. This tissue is therefore strong but supple and constitutes the epiglottis and the outer ear.

The spine

The spine is an essential element of the skeleton, being its central axis and main support. It directly or indirectly anchors all the other bones in the body. The spine is often one of the weakest areas of the skeleton, that is prone to injury or range of movement problems. In the majority of cases, spinal pain and discomfort are not due to a specific event when injury occurred, but are due to poor posture causing muscle spasms and tightness that can lead to the spine being pulled out of its natural alignment.

> *The spine consists of 33 irregular bones (if the fused bones are counted individually) that resemble cotton reels and house and protect the spinal cord. The **intervertebral discs**, now known to be made of fibrocartilage, are located between 26 of the vertebrae and act as shock absorbers to prevent damage through impact forces.*

In a growing individual these discs contain a large amount of water. With age this water content decreases and the discs become less compressible and this can lead to problems.

> *Certain areas of the spine are fused. This means that there are no intervertebral discs present and movement potential is limited. This can be seen most clearly at the sacrum and coccyx sections of the spine, as shown in Figure 2.9.*

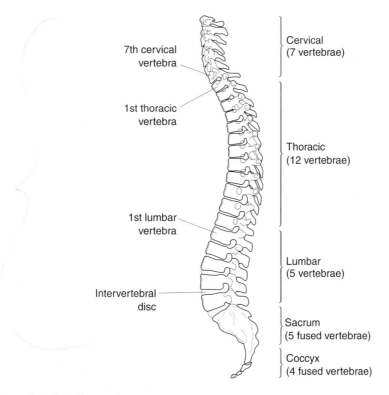

7th cervical vertebra

1st thoracic vertebra

1st lumbar vertebra

Intervertebral disc

Cervical (7 vertebrae)

Thoracic (12 vertebrae)

Lumbar (5 vertebrae)

Sacrum (5 fused vertebrae)

Coccyx (4 fused vertebrae)

Figure 2.9 Spinal curves

Spinal curves

If the spine were a straight rod, the amount of force transmitted through the bones and discs during any impact activity would be huge. The spine therefore has curves to allow a greater absorption of impact as well as increased flexibility and movement potential. There are five distinct sections to the spine that can be identified from top to bottom:

- cervical (7 vertebrae)
- thoracic (12 vertebrae)
- lumbar (5 vertebrae)
- sacrum (5 fused vertebrae)
- coccyx (4 fused vertebrae)

The primary curves are those that are present at birth and include the sacral and thoracic curves. The cervical curve, which develops as the baby lifts its head, and the lumbar curve, which appears as the child begins to walk, are known as secondary curves.

The natural curves should be maintained at all times, whether an individual is lying, seated, or when standing at rest or exercising. It used to be said that, before beginning certain resistance-based exercises, the back should be pressed flat into the floor or seat of the machine. This is no longer advocated because it forces the back out of its natural alignment (known as the neutral spine position).

As suggested earlier, much back pain is due to postural issues that can often be linked to tight muscles or muscle strength imbalances on either side of the spine. Any of the natural spinal curves can become pronounced and lead to distinctive posture-related problems. Looking at the size of the vertebrae within the different curves of the spine, it is obvious that different levels of stress are placed through the bones. The largest bones are found in the lumbar region and indeed the greatest amount of force is placed through this section of the back. This is reflected in the percentage of back problems that affect this area.

There are three known postures that you need to be able to identify and correct through strength and flexibility work:

- lordosis
- kyphosis
- scoliosis

The posture known as **lordosis** is due to an excessive curvature of the lumbar vertebrae and can be seen in pregnant women during the later stages of pregnancy. This is due to the increased weight of the baby altering the mother's centre of gravity and tilting the pelvis forward.

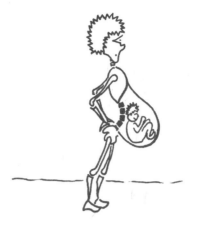

Excessive curvature outwards in the upper thoracic vertebrae is known as **kyphosis** and can be seen in individuals suffering from a 'dowagers' hump' and also in advanced cases of osteoporosis where the spinal bone density has deteriorated.

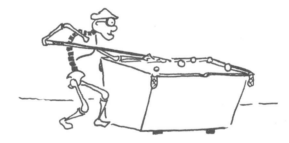

Scoliosis is the final posture and can affect either the thoracic or lumbar curves. It represents excessive curvature to one side of the spine, giving it a distinctive S-shape. This commonly occurs when leg lengths differ or in mothers who favour carrying their children on one hip.

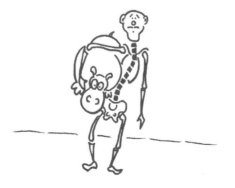

Joints

A joint is where two bones meet, whether or not movement can or does occur.

Movement at any joint is dependent on the type of joint and range of movement available to it and the muscles that cross the joint.

Muscles crossing a joint can produce movement, being linked to the bone via the tendons. The force of the muscle is transmitted through the tendon to the bone. The integrity of the joint is ensured via the ligaments. The joints within our body vary greatly with respect to the amount of movement possible and are, therefore, classified in accordance with their movement potential.

The condition of 'double-jointedness' is a fallacy. What can be seen within individuals making claim to this is hypermobility of the joints generally due to looser ligaments. Care should be taken with individuals with this condition, as they may be prone to joint dislocation. There are three main classifications of joints that will be considered below.

Immovable joint

This type of joint is also known as a **fixed** or **fibrous joint**. There is little or no movement available. Any movement occurring is limited by fibrous tissue, as seen at the sacrum and in the skull.

Semi-movable joint

Also known as a **cartilaginous joint**, this is formed between bone and cartilage, allowing for movement without the need for a joint capsule and synovial fluid as discussed below. There is more movement potential than in a fixed joint, but it is limited, as between the ribs and breastbone.

Freely movable joint

Also and commonly known as a **synovial joint**. This is designed for large ranges of movement and lined with a slippery coating, the synovium, which reduces friction and impact forces. There are many examples within the body, such as the shoulder and hip. This freely movable classification of joints is of most concern to us when considering activity and exercise prescription. As shown in Figure 2.10, there are structures within a synovial joint that are not found in an immovable or semi-movable joint.

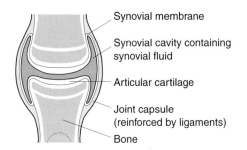

Figure 2.10 Structure of a synovial joint

Synovial joints can be further subdivided into the following categories:

- ball and socket
- hinge
- gliding
- pivot
- saddle
- condyloid
- ellipsoid

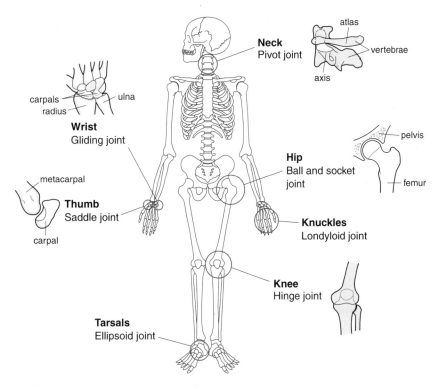

Figure 2.11 Different synovial joints

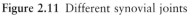

Table 2.2 Synovial joints and their movement potential

Joint name	Movement potential	Example
Ball and socket	Flexion, extension, rotation, circumduction, abduction, adduction	Hip and shoulder
Hinge	Flexion and extension	Knee and elbow
Gliding	Sliding in all directions	Sternoclavicular and carpals
Pivot	Rotation	Atlanto-axial and between radius and ulna
Saddle	All (but with limited rotation)	Thumb
Condyloid	Flexion, extension, adduction, abduction and some rotation	Knuckles
Ellipsoid	Flexion, extension, adduction, abduction	Wrist

Movement within the different synovial joints is made possible by both tendons, which attach the muscles to bone, and by ligaments, which ensure stability of the joint by attaching bone to bone.

Ligaments are another form of connective tissue, composed of mainly white collagen fibres with additional smaller amounts of the flexible yellow elastin fibres. The degree of elastin fibres is specific to the functional requirement of the joint.

> *Ligaments have no ability to contract and are, therefore, static and passive structures dependent on the working muscles. They play an essential role in preventing muscles from being overstretched, supporting joints and holding vital organs in place. Ligaments directly link bone to bone.*

Tendons join muscle to bone and play an important role in a wide variety of movements.

> *The force of the contracting muscle is concentrated and transmitted through the tendon, thereby initiating movement.*

Composed of connective tissue, they represent a tough, inelastic cord, having few nerve endings and little by way of a blood supply. At one end they are formed from the belly of the muscle while at the other they are attached to and embedded within the target bone they wish to move.

Adaptation of joints to exercise

When activity places repeated stresses onto the musculoskeletal system in excess of those incurred during normal daily activities, changes occur within its cartilage components – bone, ligaments and tendons. It is quite usual to experience adaptations in the skeletal muscle before that in the bone or connective tissue. This should be considered when designing a programme, to reduce the potential injury risk.

The connective tissue structures within the joint will adapt to any stress that provides sufficient overload. The cartilage within the joints thickens due to an increase in the number of collagen fibres and an increased number of cells and ground substance. Bone increases in density and strength, while tendons and ligaments can become thicker and stronger.

CHAPTER SUMMARY

- There are 206 bones in the fully grown human skeleton.

- Skeletal functions include providing the body with structure, an attachment point for muscles, the production site for blood cells, a storage site for minerals and protection of the vital organs.

- The process of turning cartilage into bone is ossification. The process of shaping the bone into a specific shape throughout this growth process is modelling. Bone formation and modelling occur throughout life in response to forces applied to our bones.

- There are two types of bone tissue known as compact and spongy bone. Within bone tissue there are bone cells. Osteoblasts build bone cells; osteoclasts clean bone.

- As seen clearly through the structure of long bone, there are clearly defined structures within bone. Growth occurs at the growth plate which separates the bone end (ephiphysis) from the bone shaft (diaphysis). The hollow centre of the bone, the medullary cavity, stores fat and produces blood cells. Surrounding the bone, except covering the bone end, lies the periosteum that feeds and protects the bone.

- There are five types of bones: long, short, flat, irregular and sesamoid. Their shape reflects their function.

- If bones lose strength rapidly, osteoporosis can develop, but this can be positively affected by exercise and dietary intervention.

- The spine consists of 33 irregular bones. The five sections of the spine are: cervical, thoracic, lumbar, sacrum and coccyx. These are nine fused bones making up the sacrum and coccyx.

- The spine is naturally curved. The neutral spine position reveals an inward curve in the cervical and lumbar vertebrae and an outward curve in the thoracic region. Excessive curvatures affect posture and usually cause pain and discomfort.

- The three spinal postures are: lordosis, kyphosis and scoliosis. →

→

- Joints allow our skeleton to move in specific ways. There are many different types of joint, each of which permits only certain types of movement.

- The three major classification of joints are fixed, semi-movable and freely movable.

- Freely movable joints are also known as synovial joints and can further be divided into seven categories: ball and socket, hinge, gliding, pivot, saddle, condyloid and ellipsoid.

- Connective tissue, in the form of ligaments, binds bone to bone. Tendons link bone to muscle. These enable movement to occur in a controlled and smooth way. Cartilage reduces the friction occurring at these sites of movement.

- With regular weight bearing, exercise bones increase in density, cartilage, ligaments and tendons become thicker and stronger.

The muscular system

CHAPTER

3

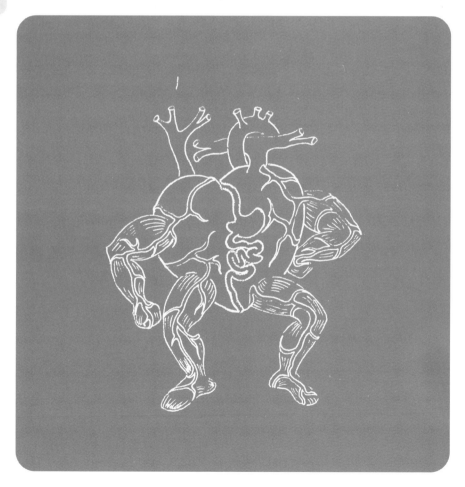

Topics covered in the chapter:

- Types of muscle
- Major muscles of the body
- Muscle structure
- How skeletal muscles enable movement
- Muscle sizes and shapes
- Adaptation of muscle to exercise

There are over 600 muscles in the human body and these are responsible for every voluntary and involuntary movement we make. They convert chemical energy, in the form of food, into mechanical energy, in the form of movement. Muscles in different parts of the body both behave differently and have a different structure. The muscle tissue in the heart is very different from that within the biceps and this is different again from that within the blood vessels. To initiate movement muscles must cross a joint and change length. The way in which a muscle contracts and the force it can generate are dependent on its shape, size and typing. The different types of fibres will predispose individuals to be better at either endurance or explosive activities and goes partway to determining their overall body shape.

It is essential when attempting to analyse movement to be able to identify the major muscle groups, understand how they shorten when placed under stress and the nature of the adaptations that we can expect to see happening within the muscles if they are trained through exercise.

Types of muscle

Muscles, like bones and joints, have a structure that is specific to their function. About 40 per cent of our total body weight is muscle and there are three different types of muscle tissue, found in specific areas of the body, each of which plays a specific role:

- Cardiac muscle
- Smooth (involuntary) muscle
- Skeletal (voluntary) muscle

Cardiac muscle

This is specialist tissue within the **heart**. It is intrinsically innervated, meaning that within the muscle tissue there is a **pacemaker** that controls the beating of the heart. We do not generally have the ability to voluntarily control the heartbeat. The pacemaker within the heart initiates the heartbeat and this electrical signal is then conducted rapidly through the heart muscle tissue. The speed of this conduction is essential and assisted by the branching fibres of cardiac muscle tissue, enabling the heart to contract rhythmically and tirelessly around 72 times every minute for females and 68 beats per minute (bpm) for males. However, the frequency of this beating can be influenced by the nervous system, hormones and medications to accommodate for changes during stress and excitement, exercise and disease states.

Smooth muscle

This muscle is innervated by our nervous system and is rarely under conscious control. Smooth muscle performs **automated tasks** such as dilating (widening) and constricting (narrowing) **blood vessels** for shunting blood to where it is most needed, and propelling food through the stomach and **intestines**.

Skeletal muscle

This muscle type is also known as **striated** muscle because of its stripey appearance. The reason for this will be investigated when muscle structure is looked at in detail later in the chapter. These muscles are under voluntary **conscious control** and are responsible for the stability and movement of the skeleton. They include any of those muscles we train while exercising, such as the **quadriceps** or **triceps**. It is these muscles that form the subject of the remainder of this chapter.

Figures 3.1 and 3.2 show the most commonly used muscles in the human body, that need to be learnt for basic exercise analysis. Whenever labelling muscles on the body it is useful to identify them separately on the anterior (front) and posterior (back) although some muscles can be seen from both aspects.

Skeletal muscle structure

Before scientists could understand exactly how muscles shortened to produce movement they had to turn to the in-depth structure of skeletal muscle. It was obvious in the case of any muscle, such as the biceps, that it did not consist of one single muscle fibre. It was also obvious that, when the biceps caused movement at the elbow, enabling an object to be lifted, the muscle appeared to shorten. What was not obvious was what exactly shortened and how.

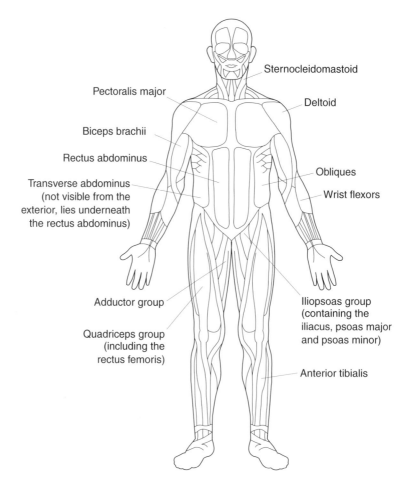

Figure 3.1 Major muscles of the human body (anterior)

Using a variety of techniques and equipment such as microscopes and electrodes, the structure of skeletal muscle was revealed (Figure 3.3).

Each muscle in the body consists of many individual fibres, which, in turn, are made up of even smaller fibres called myofibrils. If a single myofibril is studied it reveals that it is composed of many even smaller elements called myofilaments. There are two distinct myofilaments whose activity has been studied to explain the contraction process. Each myofilament has a specific structure and function. There is a thick filament that is called **myosin** and a thinner one by the name of **actin**.

*Actin and myosin are the contractile element of the muscle. They have a very specific relation to one another and are responsible for the stripey appearance of skeletal muscle. Each repeated unit of actin and myosin is known as the **sarcomere** and it is this that shortens when the muscle is undergoing a contraction.*

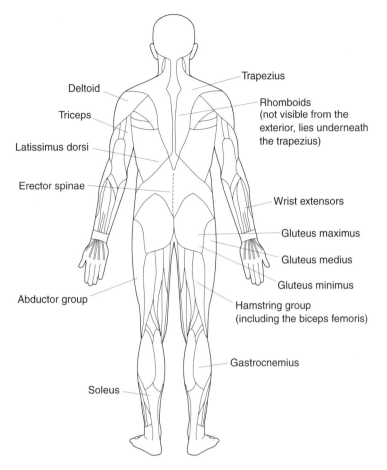

Figure 3.2 Major muscles of the human body (posterior)

All muscles are activated by motor nerves from the spinal cord, which transmit messages sent down the spinal cord from the brain. A branch of the motor nerve innervates a number of muscle fibres – these structures make up the **motor unit** (Figure 3.4).

Some messages activate muscle fibres, while some inhibit muscle activity and prevent muscle fibres from contracting.

> *The strength of the stimuli determines the number of motor units (and, therefore, muscle fibres) active in any one movement and the amount of force they need to develop. With a sufficiently strong stimulus, each muscle fibre within the motor unit contracts maximally. The more motor units are activated, the greater the tension within the muscle. This ability of muscle to engage more muscle fibres when needed is called **recruitment**.*

Most advanced resistance training techniques are built around recruiting as many muscle fibres as possible in any one movement or total exercise session.

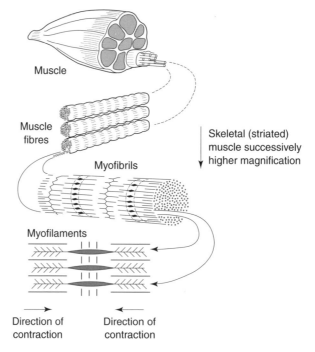

Figure 3.3 Skeletal muscle structure

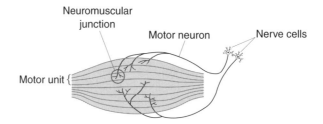

Figure 3.4 The motor unit

Pick up your pen and complete one biceps curl with it. Now do the same with an object that you can only just lift off the table. Feel the difference in the tension generated within the muscle, how much effort it took to lift the heavier object and how many more muscle fibres were recruited as a result.

The body is essentially lazy in that it will expend the minimum amount of energy needed to complete any task. When asked to lift an object it will bring into play the fewest muscle fibres necessary to be successful. If your aim is to produce an adaptation in the muscle through a training programme then you need to ask the muscle to lift a load that it is unaccustomed to lifting, so that it is forced to work harder and become stronger over time. This introduces one of the first principles of fitness: **overload**. Exactly how the muscle fibres overcome a load is discussed next.

How skeletal muscles enable movement

From the detailed study of the intricate structure of skeletal muscle scientists began to understand how a muscle may contract and shorten as it overcomes a load, as in the upward phase of the biceps curl exercise. They suspected that the protein filaments, actin and myosin, held the key and realized that these must form an attachment and move past one another.

For muscle contraction to occur there are three essential ingredients. Firstly, and perhaps most obviously, energy is needed. This **energy** is provided in the form of adenosine triphosphate (ATP) and is the star of Chapter 6, where it will be discussed in detail. A second pre-requisite for successful muscle contraction is **calcium**. This must be present within the muscle tissue and represents the on–off switch for the entire muscle contraction process. Thirdly, and most importantly, there needs to be a **stimulus**. There must be a signal sent from the brain and/or the spinal cord informing the muscle of the need to contract. Once the muscle fibres have received a message from the motor nerve to contract, the process of muscle contraction occurs. This message is sent deep into the muscle tissue to actin and myosin. These two protein filaments **slide** over one another, causing the muscle to shorten but they themselves do not change in length. Exactly how they do this is detailed later in the chapter.

Basic rules

When considering how skeletal muscle contracts to effect movement there are certain facts it is worth remembering.

- *Muscles can only pull on their bony attachment, never push.*
- *All muscles work in pairs. When one muscle within any pair is contracting, the other must be relaxing. This represents the principle of reciprocal innervation.*
- *For tension to be generated within a muscle there must be attachments between actin and myosin.*

Table 3.1 Major muscle pairs

Agonist	Antagonist
Pectoralis major	Rhomboids, trapezius
Latissimus dorsi	Deltoids
Biceps	Triceps
Rectus abdominus	Erector spinae
Gluteus maximus	Hip flexors (illiacus, psoas and rectus femoris)
Gluteus medius/minus	Adductors
Quadriceps	Hamstrings
Gastrocnemius	Anterior tibialis
Soleus	Anterior tibialis

When skeletal muscles contract to initiate movement their fibres can shorten by as much as 30–40 per cent of their original length.

Muscular contraction (the sliding filament theory)

The process begins with **calcium**. This is the muscle on–off switch. Calcium enters the muscle fibres and travels to the protein filaments, actin and myosin. Once the calcium reaches these muscle filaments it interacts with the thin protein actin. The calcium attaches to a component within the actin structure and allows the thicker myosin protein to attach to actin. These attachments are called **cross-bridges**. Without calcium present, the myosin cannot attach to the actin because the attachment site is blocked. Calcium's role is, therefore, to cause a change in the structure of the actin, which reveals the cross-bridge attachment site, to which the myosin can bind.

If there is insufficient calcium within the muscle then there may be fewer attachment sites for myosin to bind to and this will lead to poor, unco-ordinated movement quality. If calcium is totally absent, then no cross-bridges can form and, therefore, no tension can be generated within the muscle and no movement occurs. Excessive amounts of calcium will have the opposite effect and will cause stiffness, leading to an increased risk of injury as the muscle generates too much tension and provides resistance to movement and a different type of lack of co-ordination is seen.

A further look at the structure of actin and myosin reveals the remainder of the story. The myosin myofilaments have long rod-shaped tails, a short neck and two globular heads. The hinge between the tail and neck allows the cross-bridges to attach to and detach from the actin molecule. Actin and

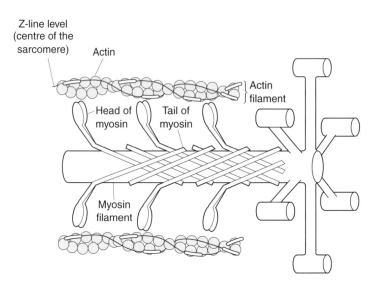

Figure 3.5 Detailed view of actin and myosin

myosin have an extremely regular arrangement within the muscle fibres. In relaxed muscle, there are no cross-bridge formations between actin and myosin.

Once the calcium has revealed the binding site and the muscle needs to contract, the globular myosin heads attach themselves to the now available binding site on actin. It is the structure of myosin that allows the myosin to row the actin towards the centre of the sarcomere.

It is the sarcomere that shortens in length, with the actin and myosin simply crossing over one another to cause the alteration in length. The actin and myosin remain the same length.

The myosin molecules on each side of the central line are orientated in different directions and there are no cross-bridges in the centre of the myosin filaments. The myosin heads always tilt towards the tails, in this way always rowing the actin in the correct direction towards the mid-line (Figure 3.6).

Types of muscular contraction

When any muscle contracts it shortens towards the middle, pulling on its bony attachments. Whether or not the bone moves is dependent on the amount of force of the contraction, the resistance to that movement provided by the object being lifted and the effects of gravity.

There are two main types of muscular contraction to consider:

- Isotonic (dynamic) contractions
- Isometric (static) contractions

Regardless of the type of contraction cross-bridges between actin and myosin will always take place.

Isotonic contractions are dynamic and always involve movement. Literally translated: 'iso' means equal, 'tonic' means tension. Equal tension is exerted throughout the full range of motion of the joint.

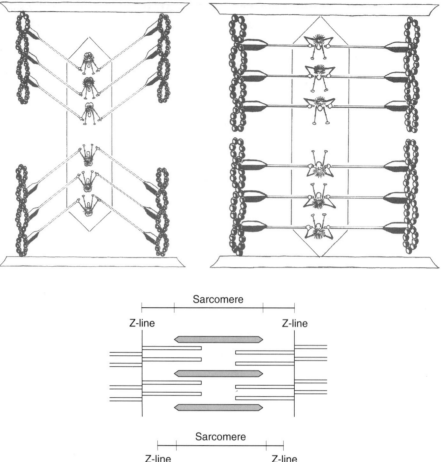

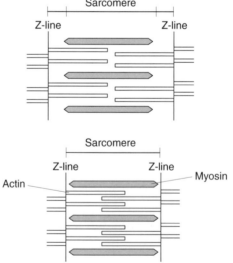

Figure 3.6 Movement of actin and myosin

Under the classification of isotonic contractions there is a division between the two phases of any movement. For example, there is an upward and a downward phase of a biceps curl. The muscular contraction involved in these two phases is different.

The upward phase of the biceps curl, when the hand is being brought closer to the upper arm, is called the **concentric phase**. This is when the muscle shortens following a contraction against a resistance that it overcomes. The angle of the joint is reduced and the origin and insertion of the muscle move closer. This is often referred to as the positive (lifting) phase of a movement. Concentric contraction is necessary if joint movement is to be in the direction opposite to gravity and rapid – regardless of the direction of any other forces.

The downward phase of this biceps curl exercise is called the **eccentric** phase. This is when a muscle lengthens following a contraction against a resistance as external forces overcome the muscle. The angle of the joint is increased, the origin and insertion move further apart and this is often referred to as the negative phase. The muscle tension in eccentric work is insufficient to cause movement, but acts as a brake to control the speed of movement caused by another force and works in the same direction as gravity.

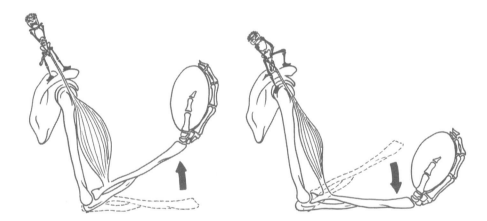

An isometric contraction is one that does not involve movement. Literally translated, 'iso' means equal, 'metric' means length. This means that the muscle stays the same length following a contraction against a resistance.

This could relate to someone attempting to biceps curl a weight that they cannot lift. In an attempt to lift the weight the muscle generates tension, as cross-bridges form, but the muscle strength proves insufficient to overcome the load. The muscle here is exerting a force to counteract an opposing force. The joint position is maintained, the contractile element of the muscle shortens – it is the elastic connective tissue that lengthens proportionately so that there is no overall change in length.

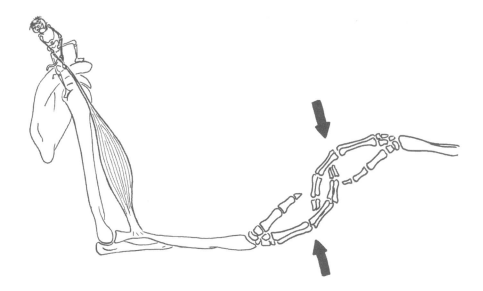

Isometric training is a valid way of training muscles, but care must be taken with individuals with hypertension (high blood pressure) and pregnant women. In these cases, isometric contractions held longer than 10 seconds should certainly be avoided as this can further raise blood pressure levels. This is because, as the muscles are contracted, the blood flow within the working muscles is reduced.

The different roles a muscle can play

Having understood the basics of muscle contraction, we need to cover the different ways in which a muscle can be active during any one exercise. If we consider the biceps curl exercise we know that the target muscle that we are aiming to strengthen is the biceps. This muscle is, therefore, known as the prime mover or the agonist. These are interchangeable terms used to describe the muscle mainly responsible for the exercise being described. As we already know that muscles work in pairs, we should be able to identify that the triceps, being the opposing muscle group, is the antagonist.

At this stage the story becomes a little more complicated as we introduce another two roles that muscle can play. In order to ensure that any exercise is completed with good form, there are muscles that will contract in an isometric way to fix the body position and stabilize nearby joints.

Returning to the biceps curl exercise, for this to be completed effectively the shoulder joint must remain stationary. The deltoid is therefore known as the fixator muscle. Any fixator stabilizes a nearby joint rather than the joint actually performing the movement. Finally, as a muscle nears fatigue during a set of any exercise, other muscles will be recruited to help assist the joint action. These muscles are known as helpers or synergists. In the case of the biceps curl the forearm flexors will play this role. This will be apparent to anyone who has completed heavy strength training using the biceps, as tension is increasingly felt within the forearm as the biceps tires.

Table 3.2 The roles a muscle can play in any exercise

Role	Definition
Agonist (prime mover)	The muscle group responsible for a particular joint action.
Antagonist	The opposing muscle group to the agonist; that is relaxed.
Fixator	The muscle(s) that contract isometrically to fix a nearby or adjacent joint to prevent unwanted movement.
Synergist	Muscle(s) that assist the movement of the agonist.

Table 3.3 Analysis of the biceps curl

Exercise	Dumb-bell biceps curl
Agonist	Biceps
Antagonist	Triceps
Synergist	Wrist flexors
Fixator	Deltoids

Consider the following exercises and identify what role the muscles play by writing the role above each muscle in the table.

Triceps kickback				
	Biceps	Deltoid	Triceps	
Seated leg curl				
	Gastrocnemius	Hamstrings	Rectus abdominus	Quadriceps
Abdominal curl				
	Rectus abdominus	Erector spinae	Obliques	Hip flexors

It is important that at this level you are able to identify the agonist and antagonist within any exercise, making reference to the table of muscle pairings in Table 3.1. It is beyond the scope of this course to ask you to identify the fixators and synergists active in each of these exercises. However, this is useful knowledge to build on as your experience grows.

The best way to balance a programme and appreciate if you are overloading a particular muscle or muscle group in any one workout is to analyse all of the exercises you include in this way.

Having considered how the muscle contracts and the possible roles it can play, it may be useful to consider the specific shape of the muscle.

Muscle sizes and shapes

All the 600+ muscles in the human body are of slightly different shapes and sizes to fit their particular location and, therefore, purpose. Muscles can be classified into four different categories of shapes. These reflect the lines of the fibre direction, the length of these fibres, the speed with which these fibres can contract and the force with which they do so. For example, the obvious difference between the triceps and the pectorals is their size. This difference in size means that the pectorals will be able to generate more force than the triceps.

The four different shapes will be introduced with an example of where each can be found with illustrations to reveal each muscle shape.

All the muscles within the human body can be classified into one of these four categories of muscle shapes. The function of the muscle is related to its shape. When attempting to classify any muscle it can be useful to consider three aspects of the muscle:

- its shape
- the direction of the muscle fibres
- the size of its origin in relation to its insertion.

Table 3.4 Muscle shapes

Muscle shape	Example
Parallel (fusiform)	Biceps
Unipennate	Rhomboid
Bipennate	Rectus femoris, one of the quadricep muscles
Convergent (multipennate)	Deltoids

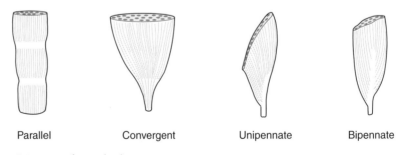

| Parallel | Convergent | Unipennate | Bipennate |

Figure 3.7 Diagram of muscle shapes

The fibres within a **parallel** muscle, such as the biceps, all run in the same direction and are parallel to each other. Parallel muscles are responsible for distinct actions and can contract quickly when necessary. Those belonging to the **convergent** category, such as the deltoid, converge from a large point of origin to a small point of insertion. The latissimus dorsi is another excellent example of this. The fibre directions within these muscles can vary and they are often active in a wide variety of exercises as a result.

Unipennate muscles, such as the rhomboids, generally have fibres that run in the same direction, but the fibre lengths are generally shorter than those within the parallel category. As the name suggests, in **bipennate** muscles the fibres run in two directions, an example is the quadricep muscle, the rectus femoris.

Muscle fibre types

Even within the classification of skeletal muscles and the different shapes of muscles it is acknowledged that not all muscle fibres within any one muscle or muscle group are identical. The different fibre types are classified according to their shortening velocities (speeds) and the principal metabolic pathways used for energy production. Much research has been, and is still being done, in this field. Latest reports have suggested that there are two main types:

- Slow-twitch (Type I)
- Fast-twitch (Type II)

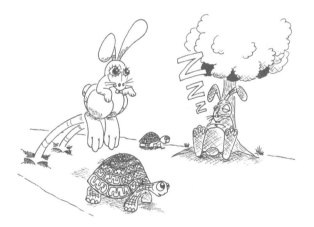

The fast-twitch fibres can be further sub-divided into Types IIa, IIb and possibly IIc. The Type IIa fibres are the most similar to Type I fibres. They are sometimes considered to be the transitional fibres and the ones most likely to adopt the characteristics of Type I fibres with training. Genetics plays a considerable role in determining what percentage of your muscles is made up of which fibres. However, it has now been shown to be possible to train your muscles to develop the characteristics of the fibre type you desire. These characteristics lie on a continuum and can change as the fibre adapts to the function for which it is most recruited. The Type IIb and IIc fibres are more anaerobic and explosive. The Type IIc fibres are the most difficult to activate and are generally only brought into play under the most extreme and maximal workloads.

Table 3.5 Characteristics of muscle fibre types

Characteristic	Slow-twitch	Fast-twitch
Colour	Red	White
Contraction speed	Slow	Fast
Endurance	High	Low
Aerobic capacity	High	Low
Anaerobic capacity	Low	High
Number of mitochondria	Many	Few

Body types

We are all born with muscles of both fibre types; each muscle contains a mixture of each type. As suggested, the type and intensity of our training can further affect the proportions of each characteristic we possess. However, we are born with a natural preponderance of one or the other type of muscle fibre, and this can be appreciated by examining the types of activities we are naturally good at and, therefore, enjoy. Classically, a sprinter will contain a larger percentage of Type II fibres than a marathon runner, whose leg muscles will contain high quantities of Type I.

Our body shape can be seen to fall into one of three types. These body types lie on a continuum and we will show elements of all three.

The first and most athletic of the body types is the **mesomorph**. Typical mesomorphs are muscular, broad-shouldered, thick-chested and narrow-waisted. They display the classic v-shape as seen in a majority of swimmers or to an extreme as displayed by Arnold Schwartzenegger.

A typical **endomorph** is rounder, more pear-shaped. These individuals may often be overweight. A celebrity example might be Robbie Coltrane.

Typical **ectomorphs** are tall, slender and more angular. This type is generally seen in long-distance runners and is characterized by Mr Bean.

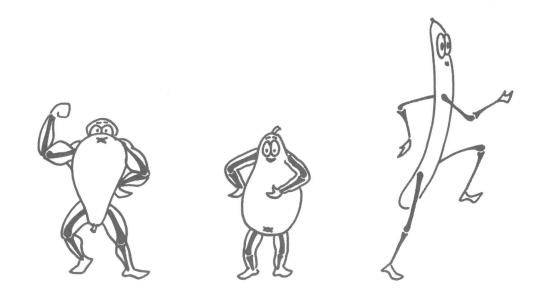

Adaptation of muscle to exercise

As changes to the muscle that occur with training are specific to the type of training undertaken, the adaptations will be considered according to the main three resistance training goals that are further considered in Chapter 9: Workout structure.

- Adaptations to strength training
- Adaptations to hypertrophy training
- Adaptations to endurance training

Adaptations to strength training

This type of training is characterized by near-maximal muscle contractions extended over small numbers of repetitions, with a full recovery between each set. Intensity of this form of training is high, while overall volume is low.

Response

- *An increase in the cross-sectional area of the Type II fibres within the exercised muscles.*
- *A significant increase in muscle glycogen, creatine phosphate and ATP substrate stores explained in Chapter 6.*
- *Elevated levels of glycogen and creatine metabolic enzymes so that the energy stores can be utilized efficiently (see Chapter 6).*

Adaptations to hypertrophy training

This type of training involves lighter loads with more repetitions. The load needs to be sufficiently heavy to elicit concentric and eccentric failure at the end of the set. The rest period is short to moderate.

Response

- *A significant increase in muscle girth – thought to be due to an increase in the number of muscle fibres*
- *Biochemical changes are similar to those for strength as Type II fibres have increased in size.*

Adaptations to endurance training

This type of training results in large numbers of sub-maximal repetitions with little recovery between each set. The relative intensity is low but the duration is high.

Response

- *Increased aerobic potential in both Type I and IIa fibres.*
- *The overall mass of Type II fibres can decrease.*
- *Selective hypertrophy of Type I fibres and an increase in their cross-sectional diameter (although the change is not as great as that in Type II fibres when training for hypertrophy).*
- *Increase in size and number of mitochondria (the powerhouse of the cell responsible for aerobically producing ATP via the oxidation of glycogen). This is explained in Chapter 6.*
- *Greater myoglobin content (the protein responsible for oxygen transport in the cell).*
- *Increased fuel stores of glycogen and triglycerides.*
- *Increase in the level and activity of the enzymes necessary for the aerobic metabolism of glucose.*

The muscular system is another excellent example of how the body's structure intricately defines its function. Each muscle is shaped to produce the necessary amount of force at the correct speed, contains the right blend of fibre types to match the activities of the individual and adaptations that occur within muscle tissue are specific to the training and fibre typing. It is essential to be able to identify the major muscle groups and, in the process of exercise analysis, be able to determine what type of contraction is being undertaken and what other muscles play a role in the exercise.

CHAPTER SUMMARY

- The human body contains cardiac, smooth and skeletal muscle tissues.

- Skeletal muscles contain a mixture of fibres of the slow- and fast-twitch varieties, which have definite characteristics and specific functions.

- The sliding filament theory is the name given to the process of muscular contraction.

- A single muscle is make up of many muscle fibres. These fibres are made up of smaller fibres called myofibrils. Each myofibril is made up of the myofilaments called actin and myosin.

- The smallest unit of contraction is the sarcomere. This contains the actin and myosin filaments that cross over one another to shorten the sarcomere length, after myosin has formed a cross-bridge to action.

- Calcium is the on–off switch and ATP provides the energy needed for contraction.

- There are three different forms of contraction that can occur within in a muscle – concentric, eccentric, and isometric. These are dependent on the length of the muscle fibres when under contraction.

- Muscles are innervated by nerves. A branch of the motor nerve and all the muscle fibres it innervates represents the motor unit. The more tension required by the muscle the more motor units will be activated. This is the process of recruitment.

- Muscles can only pull on their bony attachments. They always work in pairs so when one muscle contracts the other within the pair relaxes (reciprocal innervation).

- Muscles can play a variety of roles, depending on their role in relation to gravity and other muscle groups, their shape and the type of muscle fibres present.

- Muscles can play the role of an agonist, antagonist, synergist or fixator.

- Muscles can be classified in shape as: parallel (fusiform), unipennate, bipennate and multipennate (convergent).

- The fibres within any skeletal muscle are either: slow-twitch (Type I) fibres or fast-twitch (Type II) fibres. These have characteristics that reflect their function.

- Our overall body shape can be categorised as predominantly a mesomorph, ectomorph or endomorph, although we may have characteristics of more than one type.

- Muscles respond to training by increasing in size, due to the fibres enlarging and an alteration to the metabolic activity within the muscle.

Kinesiology

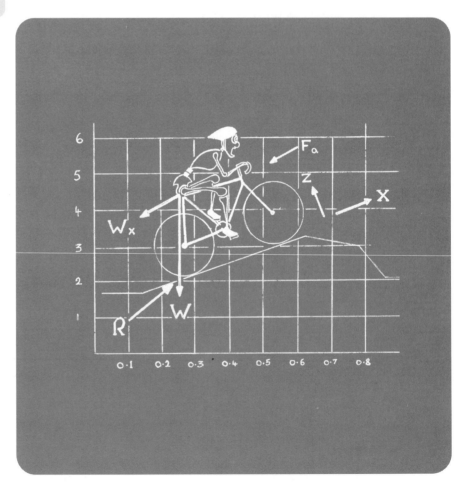

Topics to be covered in this chapter:

○ Introduction to kinesiology

○ Joint action terms

○ Introduction to the origin and insertion of the major muscles

○ Movement analysis tables

Introduction to kinesiology

Kinesiology is the science of human movement. It allows us to explain exactly how our limbs are moving through space in relation to the rest of our body. It requires knowledge of anatomy, physiology and biomechanics and, for this reason, is a subject that takes time to become comfortable and confident with. As with any study of the human body, kinesiology introduces many new, often lengthy, words, so it may take a little time for this subject to make sense. However, once learned, it is an essential skill to have as an instructor, as it allows you to analyse any movement or exercise to gauge whether it is safe, effective or relevant to sports-specific training goals.

In order to understand this subject it is important to review the information contained in earlier chapters of this manual. Initially, you will need to be familiar with the names and movement capabilities of the major joints of the body as detailed in Chapter 2. Then, in order to define which muscles are responsible for these joint movements, the major muscles as detailed in Chapter 3 need to be learnt. There are obviously many more muscles within the body that we could add to this list. However, this is knowledge that you can build on over time and is not necessary at this point. The contraction process and the different types of contraction available to any muscle need to be understood and these are once again covered in Chapter 3. This chapter deals with the origin and insertion of the major muscles.

The best way to commit this knowledge to memory is to practically apply the knowledge as soon as possible once the basics have been grasped. Throughout the chapter there will be references to familiar exercises that are then analysed.

The anatomical position and anatomical terms

All anatomical texts will make reference to what is known as the anatomical position. This is the position when the joints and body segments are in neutral alignment. Weight is evenly distributed between both feet and the arms are resting by the sides of the body with the palms facing forward.

The other important aspect of this position is the location of what is known as the mid-line of the body. This theoretical line is to be found centrally dividing the body into left and right halves. When any limb is moved, it is described with reference to its position from this mid-line.

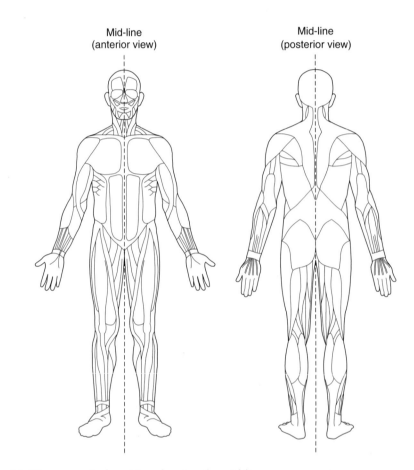

Mid-line
(anterior view)

Mid-line
(posterior view)

Figure 4.1 The anatomical position showing the mid-line

There are a number of positional and directional terms that need introduction here. These are used to describe the aspects of the body and how they relate to the mid-line.

Table 4.1 Positional and directional terms

Anterior	Front
Posterior	Back
Superior	Upper
Inferior	Lower
Medial	Towards the mid-line
Lateral	Away from the mid-line
Proximal	Near to
Distal	Away from
Dorsal	Relating to the back
Prone	Lying face downward
Supine	Lying face upward

Joint action terms

As described in Chapter 2, joints within the human body can be classified as fixed, semi-movable or freely movable. The focus of this chapter will be on the freely movable, synovial joints. Synovial joints can be further classified into seven different categories. These classifications are based on the movement potential of each joint. It is essential to understand the natural movement capability of each joint to ensure the safety and effectiveness of any exercise or activity.

Certain joints in the body are more prone to injury than others. This can be appreciated when considering the shoulder joint. The shoulder has enormous movement potential and the joint has sacrificed stability for movement. This means that the muscles, tendons and ligaments supporting this joint can quite easily be damaged if movement is not controlled, either in terms of speed of movement or in the number of repetitions.

Some movement terms will apply to a variety of joints. Other terms are specific to certain joints. Each joint will be considered in turn. There will be a picture of each joint, the actions possible at each joint and a summary table defining each term used to describe these movements. Unfortunately, as with many areas of anatomy there can be more than one word to describe the same joint action. Wherever possible all the descriptive names are provided so that you will be able to use other reference books without additional confusion.

The shoulder joint

As previously mentioned, the shoulder joint is the most freely movable of all the joints in the body and, as a result, can suffer from a variety of overuse injuries through many sporting activities and exercises. The shoulder is a shallow ball and socket joint and capable of all movements.

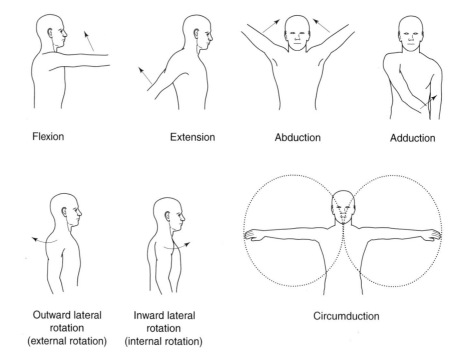

Flexion	Extension	Abduction	Adduction

Outward lateral rotation (external rotation)	Inward lateral rotation (internal rotation)

Circumduction

Figure 4.2 Actions of the shoulder joint

The movement terms 'horizontal adduction' and 'horizontal abduction' could be added to these, meaning, respectively, movement towards the mid-line of the body and movement away from the mid-line of the body in the horizontal plane. Common exercise examples to illustrate all the possible shoulder movements are detailed in the following table.

Table 4.2 Shoulder joint actions and related exercises

Joint action	Exercise
Shoulder flexion	Frontal raise (dumb-bell)
Shoulder extension	Pullover (dumb-bell or machine)
Shoulder abduction	Lateral raise (dumb-bell)
Shoulder adduction	Cable crossover
Shoulder external rotation (outward lateral rotation)	Arnold press
Shoulder internal rotation (inward medial rotation)	Rotator cuff fly
Shoulder circumduction	Not recommended
Shoulder horizontal adduction	Seated chest press
Shoulder horizontal abduction	Seated row

It is important to differentiate the actions of the shoulder joint from those of the shoulder girdle.

The shoulder girdle

The shoulder girdle consists of two bones, the clavicle and the scapula. The only point at which the shoulder girdle attaches to the axial skeleton is via the sternoclavicular joint, which is a gliding joint. It is unusual to get shoulder activity without movement of the scapula, therefore the actions of the shoulder girdle also need to be described in scientific terms. There are essentially four different joint actions relating to the shoulder girdle.

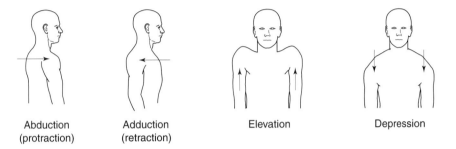

| Abduction (protraction) | Adduction (retraction) | Elevation | Depression |

Figure 4.3 Actions of the shoulder girdle

Table 4.3 Shoulder girdle joint actions and related exercises

Joint action	Exercise
Elevation (upward rotation)	Shoulder shrug (dumb-bell)
Depression (downward rotation)	Eccentric phase of above elevation exercise
Retraction (adduction)	Seated row (machine)
Protraction (abduction)	Not recommended (encourages poor posture)

In case these two joint actions become confusing, Table 4.4 attempts to clarify the relationship between the shoulder joint and shoulder girdle.

Table 4.4 The pairing of shoulder joint and shoulder girdle movements

Shoulder joint movement	Shoulder girdle movement
Flexion	Elevation (upward rotation)
Extension	Depression (downward rotation)
Adduction	Downward rotation
Abduction	Upward rotation
External rotation (outward lateral rotation)	Adduction (retraction)
Internal rotation (inward medial rotation)	Abduction (protraction)
Horizontal adduction	Protraction (abduction)
Horizontal abduction	Retraction (adduction)

The spinal column

There are classically five joint actions available between the numerous joints that make up the spine. However, due to the injuries and the chronic back complaints associated with our current population, it is not always advisable to design exercises to take the spine through its full range of movement. Different areas of the spine are capable of differing amounts of movement and this makes it a rather complex joint to consider. There are 24 separate bones and nine fused bones at the base of the spine. This immovable fused area that includes the sacrum and coccyx is an example of a fixed joint. The first two cervical vertebrae are known as the atlas and axis and represent the pivot joint known as the atlanto-axial joint. Their structure enables rotation of the head to occur. The remainder of the joints between the vertebrae are known as gliding joints. Aside from the atlanto-axial joint there is limited movement potential between any two vertebrae. The movements that are obvious at the spine are due to the combination of several vertebrae, each one only moving slightly. Most of the movement is evident in the cervical and lumbar regions of the spine.

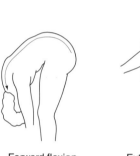

| Forward flexion | Extension and hyperextension | Lateral flexion | Rotation |

Figure 4.4 Actions of the spine

Table 4.5 Actions of the spine and related exercises

Joint action	Exercise
Flexion	Abdominal curl No unsupported forward flexion advised.
Extension	Dead lift (barbell)
Hyperextension	Dorsal raise (not recommended for all) Superman/sand lizards
Lateral flexion	Standing oblique crunch (dumb-bell/machine)
Rotation	Rotary torso (machine) not recommended for all Oblique curl

The elbow joint

The elbow appears at first sight to be a relatively simple hinge joint. This means that, as with the knee, the obvious joint actions will consist only of flexion and extension. The elbow joint is formed by the meeting of the humerus and ulna. However, it must not be forgotten that the ulna and radius also form a pivot joint that allows additional movement that is specific to the elbow. These new joint actions are labelled pronation (palm down) and supination (palm up).

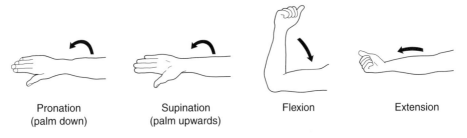

Pronation (palm down) Supination (palm upwards) Flexion Extension

Figure 4.5 Actions of the elbow

Table 4.6 Actions of the elbow joint and related exercises

Joint action	Exercise
Flexion	Biceps/preacher curl (dumb-bell)
	Upright row (barbell)
	Seated row (machine)
	Chins
Extension	Triceps extension/kickback (dumb-bell)
	Triceps press (barbell)
	Triceps/full body dips
	Chest press (machine)
	Press-up

The wrist joint

On detailed inspection, the wrist and hand are a complex joint containing 29 bones and 25 joints. However, in simple terms, when considering the wrist joint on its own, we can classify it as a condyloid joint capable of four main joint actions. Most of the movement occurs between the radius and carpals. Although there are racquet specific exercises that involve the wrist these will not be detailed here.

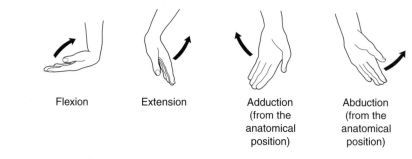

| Flexion | Extension | Adduction (from the anatomical position) | Abduction (from the anatomical position) |

Figure 4.6 Actions of the wrist

The hip joint

The hip is another ball and socket joint. This is a very freely movable joint, but has a deeper socket structure than that of the shoulder joint. The head of the femur links to the pelvic girdle. There are essentially six different joint actions.

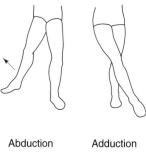
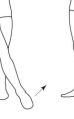
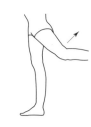

| Abduction | Adduction | Lateral rotation (external rotation) | Medial rotation (internal rotation) | Flexion | Extension |

Figure 4.7 Actions of the hip joint

Table 4.7 Actions of the hip joint and related exercises

Joint action	Exercise
Flexion	Hip flexion (multi-hip machine)
Extension	Leg press (machine)
	Squat
Adduction	Seated adductor (machine)
Abduction	Seated abductor (machine)
Internal (medial) rotation	No specific exercise
External (lateral) rotation	No specific exercise

The knee joint

The knee joint is the largest joint in the human body and is prone to injury through sports such as football, as stresses are applied to the joint against its natural joint action. The two bones that meet to form this joint are the femur and tibia. There is controversy surrounding the exact nature and classification of the knee joint if you consider the potential for rotation when the knee is flexed, and the action of the patella on the femur. However, for the purposes of this discussion, the knee is simply considered as a hinge joint with the potential for flexion and extension.

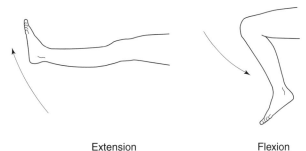

Extension   Flexion

Figure 4.8 Actions of the knee joint

Table 4.8 Actions of the knee joint and related exercises

Joint action	Exercise
Flexion	Seated/lying leg curl (machine) Hamstring curl (machine)
Extension	Seated leg extension (machine) Squats

The ankle joint

The ankle, like the wrist, consists of a multitude of bones and joints within the ankle itself and the foot. This means that there is a larger movement potential than expected. The ankle is actually classified as a hinge joint, with the joint made between the tibia, fibula and a bone known as the talus that links to the tarsals. This means that, as with the knee and elbow, the major joint actions are flexion and extension. However, there are specific terms used to describe these actions at the ankle.

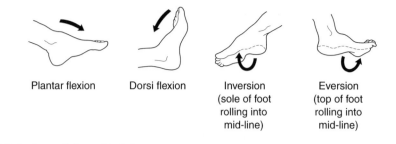

Plantar flexion   Dorsi flexion   Inversion
                                       (sole of foot
                                       rolling into
                                       mid-line)

                                       Eversion
                                       (top of foot
                                       rolling into
                                       mid-line)

Figure 4.9 Actions of the ankle joint

Table 4.9 Actions of the ankle joint and related exercises

Joint action	Exercise
Dorsiflexion	Upward phase of a toe tap
Plantar flexion	Calf raise (dumb-bell)
Eversion	No specific exercise
Inversion	No specific exercise

The specific definitions of each of these joint action terms are detailed in Table 4.10. The joints where each movement is observed are also summarized.

Introduction to the origin and insertion of the major muscles

We know from Chapter 3 that when a muscle concentrically contracts it shortens to cause movement of the two bones to which it attaches. For example, as the biceps muscle contracts concentrically, the radius moves closer to the scapula and, therefore, closer to the humerus. If you know the origin and insertion of a muscle it is possible to analyse any exercise. Only by appreciating the exact joint that each major muscle crosses can you begin to accurately analyse any exercise or movement pattern. It is not essential at this level to be able to quote the exact position of the origin and insertion. The idea is that this section can be used for reference and will allow you to picture the size and shape of muscles.

The origin of the muscle is defined as the point of attachment of the muscle that is closest to the mid-line of the body. The insertion is the point of attachment of a muscle that is furthest away from the mid-line of the body. It is easier to identify the origin and insertion of a muscle such as the triceps. However, in the case of the rectus abdominus this might appear more difficult. A diagram of each muscle is shown and the origin, insertion and the most familiar actions of each muscle are detailed below it. Within the scope of this chapter it has not been possible to detail every joint action each muscle can influence. This depth of understanding is not essential here.

Table 4.10 Summary and definitions of joint action terms

Action	Definition	Joint
Flexion	Decreasing the angle between two bones	Shoulder Elbow Wrist Spine Hip Knee
Extension	Increasing the angle between two bones	Shoulder Elbow Wrist Spine Hip Knee
Hyperextension	Increasing the angle between two bones beyond the anatomical position (beyond neutral)	Spine
Dorsal flexion	Moving the top of the foot towards the anterior tibialis	Ankle
Plantar flexion	Moving the sole of the foot downwards	Ankle
Adduction	Movement towards the mid-line of the body	Shoulder Shoulder girdle Wrist Hip
Abduction	Movement away from the mid-line of the body	Shoulder Shoulder girdle Wrist Hip
Elevation	Moving to a superior position	Shoulder girdle
Depression	Moving to an inferior position	Shoulder girdle
Eversion	Lifting the lateral border of the foot (turning the sole of the foot away from the mid-line)	Ankle
Inversion	Lifting the medial border of the foot (turning the sole of the foot towards the mid-line)	Ankle
Rotation	Medial (inward) or lateral (outward) turning about the vertical axis of the bone	Shoulder Spine Hip
Pronation	Rotating the hand and wrist medially from the elbow	Elbow
Supination	Rotating the hand and wrist laterally from the elbow	Elbow
Circumduction	Motion that in 3D terms would make a cone shape. A combination of flexion, abduction, extension, adduction in sequential order	Shoulder

Deltoid

This is a D-shaped muscle that is responsible for many of the shoulder actions described previously in Table 4.2. The only upper body action that the deltoid is not involved in is shoulder adduction, as seen in a lat pulldown exercise. Therefore, care should be taken not to overload the deltoid. The deltoid has three aspects, known as the anterior, medial and posterior. These are involved in different exercises in differing degrees.

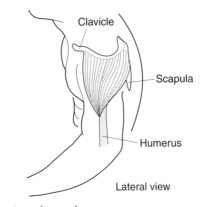

Origin	Clavicle and spine of scapula
Insertion	Humerus
Actions	Shoulder abduction, flexion and extension. Horizontal adduction and abduction in addition to internal and external rotation

Figure 4.10 The deltoid muscle

Pectoralis major

The pectoralis major is the large, fan-shaped chest muscle that enables us to complete exercises like the press-up and pec flyes.

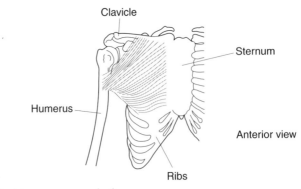

Origin	Clavicle, sternum and ribs
Insertion	Humerus
Actions	Flexion, adduction medial (inward) rotation and horizontal adduction of the shoulder

Figure 4.11 The pectoralis major

Biceps

The biceps muscles are the 'Popeye' muscles of the upper arm and can be very developed in many individuals, sometimes at the expense of the strength in the triceps. These are very active muscles in both everyday life and during exercise programmes.

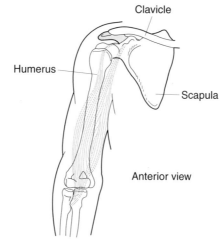

Origin	Scapula
Insertion	Radius and connective tissue of the forearm flexors
Actions	Elbow flexion and supination; assists in shoulder flexion

Figure 4.12 The biceps brachii muscle

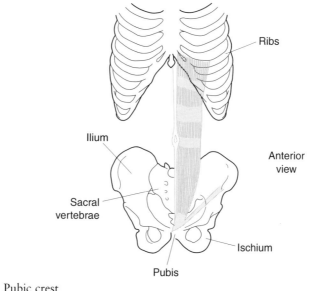

Origin	Pubic crest
Insertion	Ribs and xiphoid process
Actions	Spinal flexion and lateral flexion

Figure 4.13 The rectus abdominus muscle

Rectus abdominus

Literally translated rectus abdominus means 'straight belly'. The rectus abdominus is one flat sheet of muscle with all the muscle fibres running in the same direction. The classic 'six-pack' appearance of this muscle is the result of very low body fat levels to the point where the tendons crossing this muscle can be seen to separate the muscle into six sections (Figure 4.13).

Transverse abdominus

This is the deepest of the abdominal muscles. The muscle fibres run from left to right across the body like a sash. The transverse abdominus is responsible for compressing the abdominal contents and assists in forcing air out of the lungs, particularly during exercise. This muscle is one of the key postural and torso stabilising muscles rather than a movement muscle. When this muscle contracts it does so isometrically and the effect is a flattening of the abdomen.

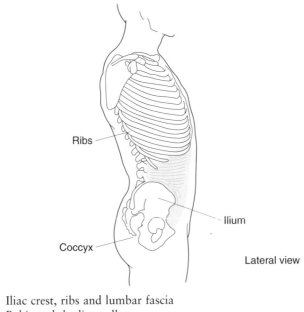

Origin	Iliac crest, ribs and lumbar fascia
Insertion	Pubis and the linea alba
Actions	Pulling abdominal wall inward

Figure 4.14

Obliques

The obliques should be differentiated into two different muscles, namely the internal and external obliques. They are both muscles that run diagonally down the side of the rectus abdominus but in opposing directions.

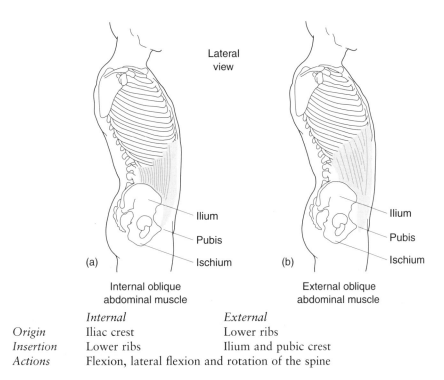

	Internal	External
Origin	Iliac crest	Lower ribs
Insertion	Lower ribs	Ilium and pubic crest
Actions	Flexion, lateral flexion and rotation of the spine	

Figure 4.15 The oblique muscles

Hip flexors

There are a complex array of muscles that assist hip flexion. One of these is the rectus femoris, one of the quadriceps muscles and the only one of the four quadricep muscles to cross the hip joint. This is detailed later in the chapter. For the purposes of this manual the only other hip flexors to be considered are the muscles called the iliopsoas that include the iliacus and psoas muscles.

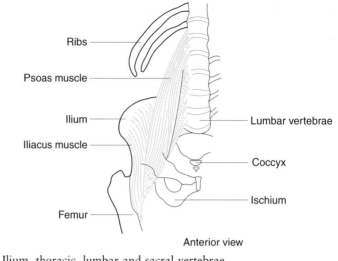

Anterior view

Origin   Ilium, thoracic, lumbar and sacral vertebrae
Insertion   Femur
Actions   Hip flexion and external rotation

Figure 4.16 The hip flexor muscle group

Hip adductors

There are four adductor muscles that make up this group. Situated in the inner thigh, they are responsible for bringing the legs together and for allowing Dorothy to click her heels together in *The Wizard of Oz*. It is not essential to know the names of the separate muscles at this stage.

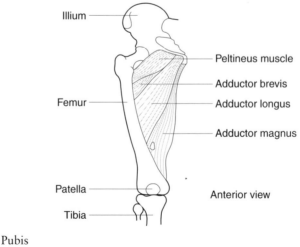

Anterior view

Origin   Pubis
Insertion   Inside of the femur
Actions   Hip adductions, external rotation and assistance in hip flexion

Figure 4.17 The hip adductor muscles

Hip abductors

The hip abductors also consist of a variety of different muscles. The ones to be considered here include the gluteus medius and minimus. These muscles are important to ensure correct running and walking technique.

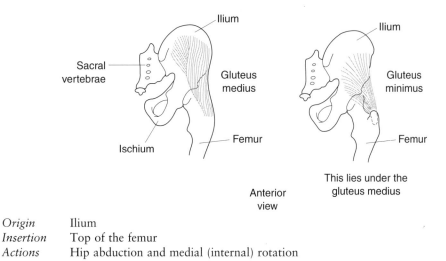

Origin	Ilium
Insertion	Top of the femur
Actions	Hip abduction and medial (internal) rotation

Figure 4.18 The hip abductor group

Quadriceps

As the name suggests, there are four muscles that make up the quadriceps. One of the most powerful muscle groups within the body, they assist in any lower-body activity involving walking, running and climbing.

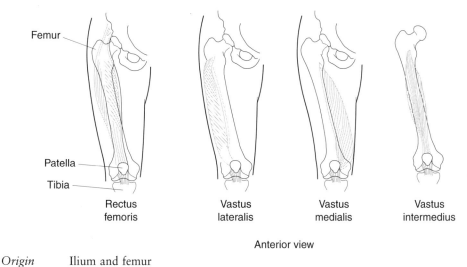

Origin	Ilium and femur
Insertion	Patella and tibia
Actions	Hip flexion and knee extension

Figure 4.19 The quadriceps muscles

Anterior tibialis

An often-forgotten muscle that does not generate much interest when it comes to strength training programmes. It gains importance when cases of shin splits are diagnosed as it is thought the muscle imbalance between the anterior tibialis and the gastrocnemius may play a role here.

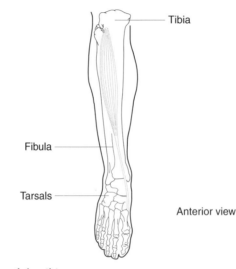

Origin   Outer side of the tibia
Insertion   Inner edge of the foot
Actions   Ankle dorsiflexion and inversion

Figure 4.20 The anterior tibialis muscle

Trapezius

The trapezius is a kite-shaped muscle that has a tendency to be overworked and can build up a lot of tension within it particularly with individuals who have a deskbound or driving job. As the trapezius muscle does not cross the shoulder joint, it is responsible only for actions of the shoulder girdle.

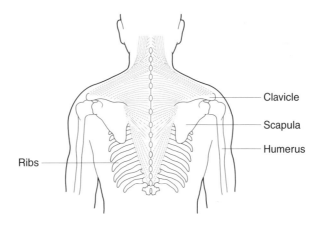

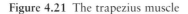

Posterior view

Origin   Base of the skull, cervical and thoracic vertebrae
Insertion   Clavicle and scapula
Actions   Shoulder girdle adduction, rotation and elevation; spinal lateral flexion and
              rotation

Figure 4.21 The trapezius muscle

Rhomboids

These are small rectangular-shaped muscles hidden beneath the trapezius.
There is less publicity about the rhomboids because they are hidden.
The rhomboids are active during exercises that target the trapezius and
often those that involve the latissimus dorsi. They are, however, important
muscles for maintaining a correct, upright posture as they pull the shoulder
blades together.

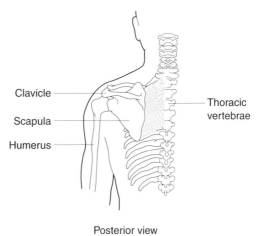

Posterior view

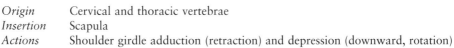

Origin   Cervical and thoracic vertebrae
Insertion   Scapula
Actions   Shoulder girdle adduction (retraction) and depression (downward, rotation)

Figure 4.22 The rhomboid muscle

Latissimus dorsi

This is the largest muscle in the back and, if very developed, gives individuals a 'winged' appearance.

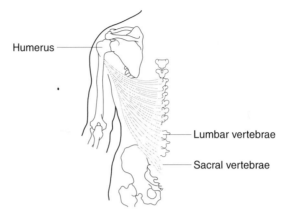

Posterior view

Origin	Thoracic and lumbar vertebrae
Insertion	Humerus
Actions	Shoulder extension, adduction and medial rotation

Figure 4.23 The latissimus dorsi muscle

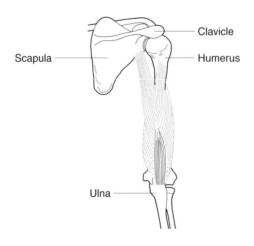

Posterior view

Origin	Scapula and humerus
Insertion	Ulna
Actions	Elbow extension

Figure 4.24 The triceps muscle

Triceps

This is an often neglected and sometimes imbalanced muscle in comparison to its partner, the biceps. It is exceptionally useful for any activity involving straightening the arm (Figure 4.24).

Erector spinae

An essential and confusing array of muscles that span the entire length of the spine. For years in classes and exercise programmes these muscles were neglected in favour of abdominal work. Posture suffered as a result and it is now realized that about 80 per cent of our population suffer back pain at some stage in their life. Problems with the lower back stem from poor posture, bad lifting technique or result from a specific injury. It is important to strengthen these muscles on a regular basis.

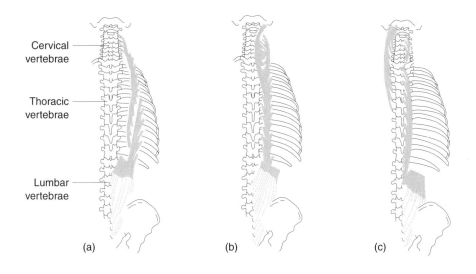

Posterior view

Origin   Iliac crest and sacrum
Insertion   Ribs
Actions   Spinal extensions, hyperextension and lateral flexion

Figure 4.25 The erector spinae muscles

Gluteus maximus

The most powerful single muscle in the human body.

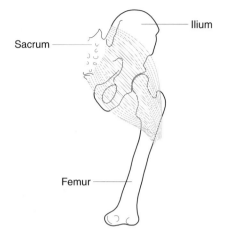

Posterior view

Origin	Ilium
Insertion	Back of femur
Actions	Hip extension and lateral rotation

Figure 4.26 The gluteus maximus muscle

Hamstrings

The hamstrings are made up of three muscles and are notoriously tight in many athletes, particularly footballers, where, once again, many injuries are seen.

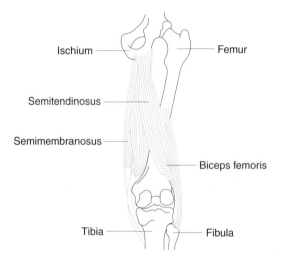

Posterior view

Origin	Ischium
Insertion	Tibia and fibula
Actions	Hip extension and rotation; knee flexion and rotation

Figure 4.27 The hamstrings muscles

Gastrocnemius

This is the largest of the calf muscles and is considered diamond-shaped. These muscle fibres are in constant use whenever you are standing, walking, running, jumping, skipping or stepping. They often need regular stretching as the fibres can get tight and cause discomfort through such constant use. Problems are often associated with wearing high heels as the muscle is then kept in a constantly short, contracted state.

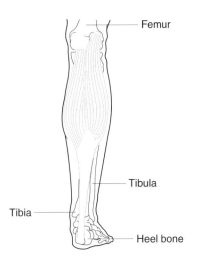

Posterior view

Origin	Femur
Insertion	Via Achilles tendon into heel bone
Actions	Ankle plantar flexion and knee flexion

Figure 4.28 The gastrocnemius muscle

Soleus

This lies underneath the gastrocnemius and is the less famous of the pair, though still active in the same activities as the gastrocnemius and prone to tightness. As this muscle does not cross the knee joint, any stretch that will effectively reach this muscle needs to be done with a bent knee.

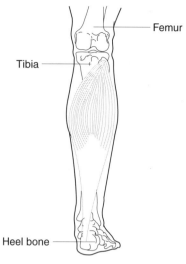

Femur

Tibia

Heel bone

Origin   Tibia and fibula
Insertion   Via Achilles tendon into the heel bone
Actions   Ankle plantar flexion

Figure 4.29 The soleus muscle

MOVEMENT ANALYSIS TABLES

Having considered all the necessary theoretical aspects, it is essential to put this knowledge into practice. The best way to do this is to compile a table as below – write down all the familiar exercises you have worked with and attempt to complete each column. Below are a few examples to start you off. Always begin by completing the movement yourself or observing a partner to help identify the working muscles.

Exercise	Joint(s)	Joint action(s)	Muscle(s)
Lateral raise (dumb-bell)			
Dorsal raise			
Press-up			
Squats			

CHAPTER SUMMARY

- Kinesiology is the study of human movement and incorporates knowledge of anatomy, physiology and biomechanics.

- The anatomical position involves neutral alignment of the body with palms supinated (facing forward).

- The mid-line of the body divides the body into left and right sides.

- Each of the major joints within the body is capable of specific movements. Some joint action terms are only used at certain joints.

- The origin of a muscle is the attachment point nearest the mid-line of the body; the insertion is the point of attachment of the muscle furthest from this mid-line.

- Movement of a joint is caused by a muscle contracting across it. From the origin to the insertion of a muscle it crosses one or more joints.

- To analyse any exercise or movement pattern it is essential to consider the joint moving, the term given to the joint action and the muscles that enable this joint action to occur.

The cardiorespiratory system

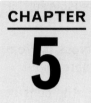

CHAPTER

5

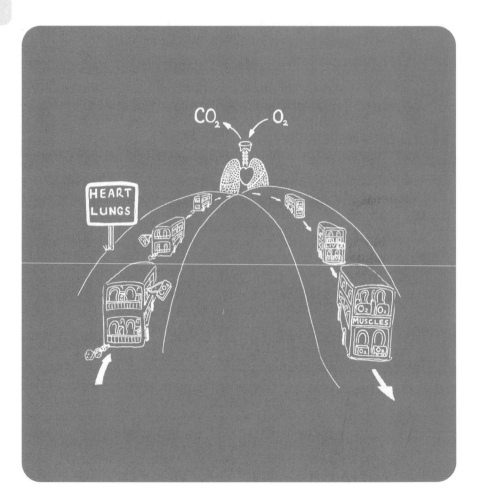

Topics to be covered:

○ An overview of the cardiorespiratory system
○ The respiratory system
○ Breathing
○ Composition of blood
○ The blood vessels
○ The structure of the heart
○ The circulatory system
○ The effects of exercise on the cardiorespiratory system

The cardiorespiratory system is composed of **the heart, lungs** and miles of interconnecting **blood vessels**. It is responsible for the intake, uptake and delivery of oxygen and nutrients to, and excretion of waste products from, all cells of the body. The structure of each component within this system is designed perfectly for the role it performs and will be considered individually in detail. Each aspect responds accurately to the additional demands placed upon it when we exercise. The difference between the systems of an unfit and a fit individual will be highlighted. This will serve to illustrate the body's amazing capacity to adapt to its environment and the training load that we apply.

An overview of the cardiorespiratory system

The cardiorespiratory system is responsible for taking oxygen from the air and transporting it to the working muscles, our internal organs and all other living tissue within the body. It is also responsible for removing carbon dioxide and water from the body – the waste products formed as the muscles and other body organs use oxygen to produce energy.

The cardiorespiratory system can appear confusing at first glance, as there are so many blood vessels and entrances and exits to the heart and lungs to memorize. For the purposes of this chapter the pathways will be simplified to give you an understanding of the major blood vessels involved and the direction of blood flow through these to the relevant body tissues.

The cardiorespiratory system can be likened to many things to gain an understanding of the basic processes involved. The lungs resemble upside-down trees, while the remainder of the heart, blood vessels and molecules that carry the oxygen can be likened to the London red buses. The heart would represent the bus station, the red buses the oxygen-carrying molecule discussed later, the people on the bus the oxygen and carbon dioxide, and the roads the blood vessels. This may be a useful image to refer to if the technical details lose you on first reading!

The respiratory system

The major function of the respiratory system is to bring atmospheric air into the lungs and to allow gaseous exchange to occur between the lung tissues and the neighbouring capillary blood supply. In this way oxygen can be taken in and transported efficiently to the working muscles. However, the system also humidifies and filters the inhaled air, contributes to the acid-base balance of the blood (by elimination of carbon dioxide) and develops sound by passing air through the vocal cords.

The respiratory system consists of more than just the lungs. The structures within the respiratory system direct air through the structures shown in Figure 5.1.

Nasal cavity
↓
Mouth
↓
Trachea (windpipe)
↓
Bronchi
↓
Bronchioles

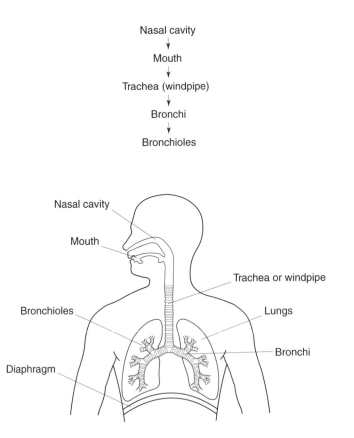

Figure 5.1 Passage of air from the atmosphere to the lungs

Each structure will be considered in detail.

The lungs have a total surface area sufficient to cover a tennis court. They are highly specific in their structure to ensure that they can provide the body with all the gases and nutrients necessary for survival and the demands of the body at any time. Without such lungs, there would not be a great enough surface area for the oxygen to travel across to keep us alive. Considering this, the lungs take up a relatively small space and, together with the heart, are protected by the ribs – a flexible cage that enables the lungs to expand and partially deflate as air is drawn in (**inspired**) and breathed out (**expired**). In order for us to breathe effectively, the air that surrounds us within the atmosphere is drawn into the lungs via a specific process. Initially, however, it is useful to understand the composition of the air that we breathe in.

Composition of air

Essentially, we breathe in to take up and utilize the oxygen in the atmosphere and exhale to rid the body of the toxic build-up of carbon dioxide. It is often surprising to note, therefore, that the composition of air only contains a relatively small percentage of oxygen.

Table 5.1 Composition of air

Gas	Breathed in (%)	Breathed out (%)
Oxygen	20.93	17
Carbon dioxide	0.03	4
Nitrogen	79.04	79

As the table illustrates, we only utilize a small amount of the oxygen that we breathe in. This means that we breathe out a large amount of oxygen with every breath. (It is this fact that enables us to perform cardiopulmonary resuscitation. Here, the oxygen we breathe out is breathed into an unconscious casualty to keep their cells alive and oxygenated.) At rest, only 25 per cent of the blood's total oxygen is released into the tissues, with 75 per cent returning to the heart in the venous blood supply. This represents the body's automatic oxygen reserve, so if oxygen demand increases, the cells can rapidly obtain and utilize the extra oxygen necessary.

It is understandable that we breathe out more carbon dioxide than we breathe in, once we realize that it is a by-product of many of the chemical reactions that occur within the body when at rest and during activity. Nitrogen is breathed both in and out and utilized to a negligible extent.

The lungs

As discussed, the structure of the lungs is often thought of as an upside-down tree. This analogy will be continued as we consider the different structures within the lungs mentioned earlier.

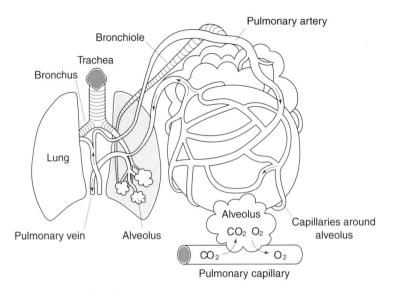

Figure 5.2 The structure of the lungs

Oxygen within the air reaches the lungs via the **trachea**. The trachea and **bronchi** are composed of stiff cartilage and smooth muscle. Their cell lining secretes a mucus shield that serves as a filter for the dust and particles entering the air passages. It also acts as an escalator as it drives particles up and away from the lungs. The trachea represents the main trunk of the upturned tree and the bronchi the major branches.

From the trachea, the air moves into the left and right **bronchi**, which take air to the lungs. Just as the trunk of a tree separates into branches, which separate further into twigs covered with leaves, so the bronchi separate into smaller airways called **bronchioles** which get smaller and smaller until eventually they reach **alveoli** that would represent the leaves of our tree.

Alveoli are tiny air sacs and it is here that oxygen from the air is transferred to the bloodstream. Under a microscope the air sacs look like a bunch of grapes and each air sac is surrounded by tiny blood vessels called capillaries. The walls of the alveoli and the capillaries are so thin that gases such as oxygen and carbon dioxide are able to pass through them. This process is known as **gaseous exchange**.

Gaseous exchange is the name of the process given to the transfer of oxygen and carbon dioxide between the lungs and the blood supply. Oxygen travels from the lungs into the bloodstream. Carbon dioxide takes the reverse journey and travels from the blood into the lungs. The transfer of gases between the alveoli and blood capillaries can take place due to the pressure gradient that is formed. This is because atmospheric air contains more oxygen than the blood that has travelled throughout the body. Oxygen therefore readily diffuses across the alveoli walls into the bloodstream that is deficient in oxygen. This continues until the concentration of oxygen is equalized between the atmosphere and the bloodstream.

DID YOU KNOW?

There are over 300 million alveoli within the lungs. Each minute at rest approximately 250 ml of oxygen leaves the alveoli to enter the blood, while approximately 200 ml of carbon dioxide diffuses into the alveoli to be exhaled. During exercise, these values can increase 25-fold within the lungs of endurance athletes.

Breathing

In order for air to move efficiently into and out of the lungs the rib cage has to expand to accommodate for the increase in lung size and volume. We will now examine in more detail how the lung changes volume.

Inspiration

The lungs themselves contain no muscle. They are dependent on neighbouring muscles to alter their volume. The diaphragm, intercostal and abdominal muscles are responsible for contracting and expanding the thoracic cavity to effect respiration. The lungs are pressed against the chest wall and follow its every movement due to a pressure difference between the air in the lungs and the lung–wall interface. The pleural membranes provide the necessary lubrication and prevent excessive friction of the lungs against the chest wall.

During **inspiration** (inhalation) the diaphragm contracts and flattens, moving downwards by about 10 cm. This causes the entire thoracic cavity to expand. The intercostal muscles contract, causing the ribs to move upward and outward, assisting this increase in volume.

This expansion of the chest cavity causes a reduction in the intrapulmonic pressure (pressure within the lungs). There is now a difference in pressure between the atmospheric air and that within the lungs. There is greater pressure outside of the lungs; therefore, air rushes into the lungs. Inspiration ceases when the atmospheric and intrapulmonic pressure become equal.

Expiration

At rest, this is a passive process. It takes place simply by the recoil of the stretched lung tissue and relaxation of the inspiratory muscles. This returns the thoracic cavity to its original size and pressure, which will be equal to that of the atmospheric pressure once more. During heavy exercise, the internal intercostals and abdominal muscles assist by allowing a greater rate and depth of exhalation.

Following the successful diffusion of oxygen across the alveoli and capillary membranes, the oxygen can then be transported in the bloodstream to the tissues of the body.

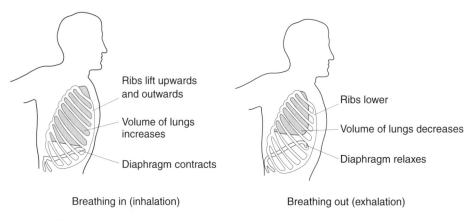

Ribs lift upwards and outwards

Volume of lungs increases

Diaphragm contracts

Breathing in (inhalation)

Ribs lower

Volume of lungs decreases

Diaphragm relaxes

Breathing out (exhalation)

Figure 5.3 The mechanics of breathing

Breathing rates and lung volumes

At rest, an adult breathing rate is around 12 times per minute, in which time we pass about six litres of air through the lungs. This six litres represents the **minute volume** – the total air taken into the lungs during one minute. The minute volume is the product of our breathing rate and the amount of air that is taken in within each breath.

The volume of air that is inspired or expired per breath represents the **tidal volume**. Typical tidal volumes at rest are around 0.5 litres of air.

> Minute volume = Tidal volume × Breathing rate
> 6 litres/min = 0.5 litres   × 12

When we exercise we need to increase our breathing rate to expel the carbon dioxide we have produced and to increase the amount of oxygen we breathe in. A sensor in our brains regulates our breathing rate, which senses the level of carbon dioxide in the blood. As the level of carbon dioxide increases, the brain sends a signal to the diaphragm and intercostal muscles to increase the breathing rate. The intercostal muscles help to force air out of the lungs more quickly, enabling faster oxygen uptake.

 With training, our tidal volume will increase over time to allow more air to be passed through the lungs.

The maximum amount of air we can inhale and exhale in one breath is our **vital capacity**.

 This vital capacity also increases with training to allow a greater and more efficient supply of oxygen to the working muscles. As well as the rate of breathing increasing during exercise, our breaths get deeper, which will increase the vital capacity as well as the tidal volume.

An adult's **total lung capacity** (all the air within the lungs after we have maximally inhaled) equals about 5 litres – roughly the amount of air within a basketball. However, we are never able to exhale all of this air, otherwise our lungs would collapse. We have to retain a small amount of air within the lungs to enable gaseous exchange to occur between breaths. This **residual volume** within the lung equates to about 1 litre of air.

As an individual becomes fitter, their residual volume decreases. This means that, with every breath, a fresher supply of air is being presented to the lungs for more effective gaseous exchange purposes.

The residual volume increases with age and through smoking. This is primarily due to the fact that the breathing becomes shallower. This means the alveoli are presented with less fresh air and gaseous exchange becomes less effective.

Once the oxygen has diffused across the alveoli membrane it enters the bloodstream.

Blood

Blood is the transport system within the body, transferring oxygen, nutrients, waste products and hormonal messages to the sixty billion cells within the body. On top of this essential function the responsibility of the blood cells is to protect the body from infection and increase its immunity. There are about nine pints of blood in the average person. Small increases to this blood volume can be realized through training; significant increases to blood volume are seen during pregnancy, when it is usual for the mother to circulate about 12 pints of blood around her body. Regardless of the size of the change, an increase in blood volume provides the blood with an opportunity to circulate more oxygen.

In order to transport oxygen through the blood a special carrier is needed that holds on to the oxygen until it reaches the muscles and other tissue where it is needed. This carrier is a molecule called **haemoglobin**.

Haemoglobin

Haemoglobin (Hb) plays an essential role in being able to carry about 70 times the amount of oxygen than that simply left to dissolve and drift in the bloodstream. Haemoglobin is found within the red blood cells and is an iron-containing protein. This gives red blood cells their characteristic colour.

Haemoglobin production is dependent on the mineral iron within our diet. People who have an iron deficiency often have less haemoglobin within their blood and hence are unable to transport oxygen as efficiently as others. This can result in feelings of lethargy.

People who exercise often increase their haemoglobin levels, as their body's response to the increased demand for oxygen is to manufacture more haemoglobin to meet these demands. The haemoglobin is also able to carry more oxygen, again increasing the total amount of oxygen that can be transported to the working muscles. These are long-term effects of exercise on the cardiorespiratory system, resulting in decreased resting heart rates and increased recovery rates following exercise.

There are two other situations that cause haemoglobin levels to rise. In response to the increase in blood volume during pregnancy, haemoglobin levels will also increase. High altitude too causes levels to rise. This response is due to the reduced amounts of oxygen present in the air at high altitudes. The body compensates for this by maximizing its ability to pick up the reduced amounts of oxygen on offer with greater concentrations of haemoglobin.

Plasma

This accounts for 55 per cent of the total blood volume and contains dissolved salts, hormones, fats and sugars.

Red blood cells

Otherwise known as erythrocytes, these make up 99 per cent of the total cell volume. These cells are manufactured within the bone marrow where every second 2.5 million die and are replaced. Their primary importance is in the **carriage of haemoglobin** and ultimately the transport of oxygen and carbon dioxide.

White blood cells

Otherwise known as leucocytes, these constitute less than 1 per cent of the cell volume. Also manufactured within the bone marrow, their role is entirely different and concentrated on **immunity**.

Platelets

These are cell fragments (having no nucleus). They act primarily as containers for substances that travel within the bloodstream on their way to sites of injury where they control bleeding and aid the clotting process.

All of these vital activities are taking place within the miles of blood vessels. Structures of these different vessels are representative of their function.

The blood vessels

There are three main types of blood vessel within the circulatory system, each structured to meet the demands placed on it and the specific function it has to play within the body. These vessels are arteries, veins and capillaries.

Arteries

Arteries always carry blood away from the heart. They have thick muscular walls to cope with the high pressure of the blood within them and are elastic to cope with the pulsating flow of the blood as it is ejected from the beating heart. For an explanation of blood pressure turn to Chapter 8.

The blood within arteries is generally bright red, being fully oxygenated. The one exception to this is blood in the **pulmonary artery**, which is deficient in oxygen as it is on its way to the lungs to gather oxygen.

The main arteries, the **aorta** from the left ventricle and the pulmonary artery from the right ventricle, split to form smaller branches. Each time an artery splits to take blood to different parts of the body, it gets smaller and the pressure within the artery decreases. The smallest arteries are called **arterioles** and these lead into capillaries, where the oxygen and other nutrients within the blood can be delivered to the muscles, organs and other living tissue.

Capillaries

These are the essential link between arteries and veins, and represent the site of transfer of the oxygen and nutrients to the cells and collection of carbon dioxide and waste products. They are made of a single layer of cells. A typical capillary is smaller in diameter than a human hair, with special walls called semi-permeable membranes. These membranes allow gases and other small molecules to pass through, while holding on to the larger molecules. Capillaries intermingle with muscle fibres (just as they surround the alveoli in the lungs) to provide the greatest possible surface area where gaseous exchange can occur.

Veins

These always carry blood towards the heart, transporting 75 per cent of the total blood volume. They do not have to withstand the same pressures as arteries. The characteristics of veins are that they are 6–10 times as expandable as arteries, and contain **valves**, to prevent a backward flow of blood.

Most blood is deoxygenated (oxygen-deficient) and of a bluish colour, except the blood within the **pulmonary vein**, which is carrying freshly oxygenated blood from the lungs back to the heart for distribution to the rest of the body.

Once the blood has travelled through the capillaries it enters small veins called **venules** to start its journey back to the heart. The venules gradually join together to form larger veins, eventually taking blood back to the right atrium within the heart. The **vena cava** is the main vein that takes blood back into the right atrium, whilst the pulmonary vein takes blood back into the left atrium.

The heart

This organ is pear-shaped, about the size of a fist, and weighs less than 400g. It beats continuously around 100,000 times per day without the need for conscious involvement. The heart is two functionally distinct pumps. It is divided into right and left sides by a thick muscle wall called the **septum**. The right pump takes blood to the lungs to accept oxygen and release carbon dioxide. The left pump takes blood to the remaining tissues, giving up oxygen and accepting carbon dioxide. There are a total of four chambers within the heart: the two upper **atria** are receiving chambers, able to hold about 45 ml of blood, while the lower, larger **ventricles** represent the pumping chambers and can hold about 60 ml of blood.

The atria

These are the receiving chambers. The right atrium receives blood that has returned from the body, carried in the vena cava (the largest vein in the body). The left atrium receives blood that has been returned from the lungs via the pulmonary vein.

The ventricles

These are the pumping chambers. The muscular walls of the left ventricle are three times thicker than the right as the left is responsible for the **systemic circulation** (to the body tissues), whereas the right ventricle is only responsible for the **pulmonary circulation** (to the lung tissues).

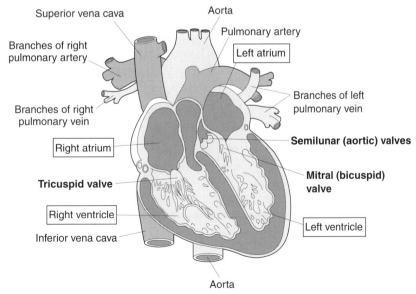

Figure 5.4 The heart

Whilst the right side only has to pump the blood a short distance to the lungs, the left side has to pump the blood up to the brain and out to the muscles in the arms and legs together with all of the living tissue in between! Because of the amount of work the left ventricle has to do to pump blood around the body, it is the largest and most muscular chamber in the heart. It forces blood out at a very high pressure, which is why, if an artery is cut, the blood can travel quite a distance. The closer the artery is to the heart, the higher the pressure – thus, if the **carotid artery** (in the neck) is cut, blood is lost more quickly than if the **radial artery** (in the wrist) is cut.

To ensure that blood only travels in one direction through the heart there are one-way valves that stop blood seeping back the wrong way. There is an important valve between the atrium and the ventricle. This **atrio-ventricular valve** opens as soon as the heart has contracted, to let blood flow from the atria into the ventricle. These atrio-ventricular valves are given different names on each side of the heart. On the right side of the heart the valve is known as the **tricuspid valve**; on the left side of the heart it is known as the **bicuspid** or **mitral valve**.

The other valves are located within the major blood vessels and are collectively known as the **semi-lunar valves**. The semi-lunar valve on the right of the heart lies within the pulmonary vein and is also known as the **pulmonary valve**. This prevents the blood within the right atrium flowing back into the vena cavae. On the left of the heart the semi-lunar valve is called the **aortic valve** and is situated within the aorta to prevent backflow into the left ventricle.

The circulatory system

The circulation is a closed circuit that ensures that every cell within the body receives an adequate blood supply, bringing it essential oxygen and nutrients and taking away waste products. The heart has two sides, the right side sends blood to the lungs to collect the oxygen (**pulmonary circulation**) and the left side pumps blood to the rest of the body (**systemic circulation**). This system acts like a figure of eight with the heart at the centre.

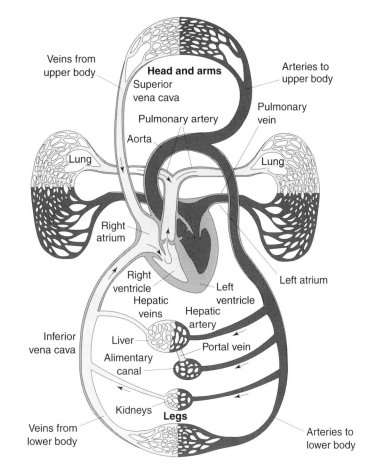

Figure 5.5 The circulatory system

The effects of exercise on the cardiorespiratory system

The main functions of the cardiorespiratory system during exercise are to:

- Deliver oxygen to the active muscles at a rate that matches that used for aerobic metabolism.
- Clear carbon dioxide and metabolic end products at a rate that matches production.
- Assist in the dissipation of metabolically produced heat to the environment by increasing blood flow to the skin.
- Transport regulatory hormones from their production sites to the target tissues.

The cardiovascular response

For more blood to be circulated to the working muscles, three aspects of the heart's contraction can be affected. These will be explained and their individual responses to exercise considered.

Heart rate (HR)

> This is the number of times the heart beats in any one minute (bpm)

Short-term response

There is a strong correlation between heart rate and oxygen consumption. They both rise linearly with increasing exercise intensity. This means that as the exercise becomes more intense, the increase in heart rate directly reflects this.

The average resting rate is 68–72 beats per minute (bpm). Women generally have higher heart rates than men, as their hearts are smaller. The maximum exercising heart rate is dependent on the individual, their age and the activity undertaken. The quickest, rough estimate of a person's maximal heart rate is obtained from taking their age away from a standard heart rate of 220 bpm.

Long-term response

If cardiovascular fitness improves over a period of time, the resting and exercising heart rate will be lower. This indicates the heart has become more efficient at delivering more blood to the tissues in any one minute.

The extent to which the HR is lowered is dependent on the frequency, intensity, duration and type of activities undertaken, though individual differences must be taken into account.

Stroke volume (SV)

> The amount of blood pumped by the heart with each contraction (ml)

The average resting value is thought to be around 70 ml of blood per contraction in sedentary individuals. Those of highly trained individuals have been measured at 100 ml. Once again, women in general have smaller stroke volumes due to their smaller heart size.

Short-term response

During exercise the stroke volume tends to be double that of its resting value. The volume has to rise because the working muscles are demanding a greater oxygen supply, so more blood is delivered for every beat of the heart. As the heart rate has also increased, more blood is delivered and at a faster rate.

Unlike cardiac output and heart rate, stroke volume does *not* linearly increase with exercise intensity and oxygen consumption.

During graded exercise the stroke volume increases until the work rate equates to about 40–50 per cent of the maximal oxygen consumption capacity (**VO$_2$ Max**). Only small increases in stroke volume are seen above this exercise intensity.

Long-term response

As the heart rate decreases with training, the stroke volume has to rise to ensure that sufficient blood flow can be delivered to the cells, whether an individual is at rest or in their active state.

Cardiac output

This is the amount of blood pumped out of the heart in every minute (litres).

Cardiac output is an overall reflection of the functional activity of the heart and is the principal determinant of the rate of oxygen delivery to the peripheral tissues such as our active skeletal muscle.

Short-term response

The average resting value in males is 5 litres per minute. During exercise it can rise to 20–25 litres per minute in healthy males. In women the figure is closer to 15–20 litres per minute. In endurance athletes cardiac output has been known to be nearer 35–40 litres per minute.

This rise makes sense when we consider the relationship between heart rate, stroke volume and cardiac output.

$$\text{Cardiac output} = \text{Heart rate} \times \text{Stroke volume}$$
$$\text{CO} = \text{HR} \times \text{SV}$$

If, in the short term, both heart rate and stroke volume increase, then the amount of blood being ejected from the heart in any one minute must also increase.

Long-term response

When cardiovascular improvements are made and efficiency increased, CO could be higher, to compensate for the reduction to the heart rate. However, as the stroke volume will have increased through training the increase in cardiac output may be small.

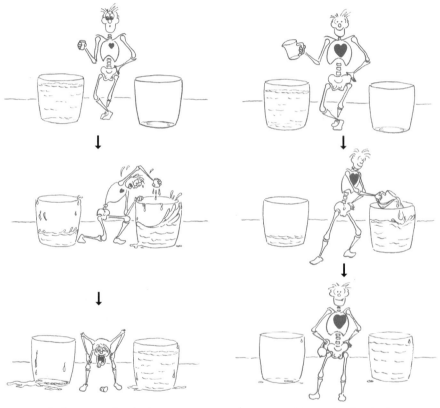

Sedentary individuals   Trained individuals

Table 5.2 Summary of cardiovascular changes with exercise

	At rest	*During exercise*
Heart rate	Av. 72 bpm	Max. 220 − age in years
Cardiac output	Av. 5 l/min	20–25 l/min
Stroke volume	Av. 70ml	140 ml

Most studies use data taken from male subjects. Values for females may differ.

The pulmonary adaptations to exercise

Short-term response

Ventilation rate: this increases to ensure that more air is passed through the lungs and more oxygen is taken up and carbon dioxide excreted. The breathing rate increases linearly with oxygen consumption and carbon dioxide production.

Tidal volume: this increases with exercise and is considered to be the cause of the above change in ventilation rate. For every 1 litre of oxygen to be consumed, we need to have breathed 20–25 litres of air. During heavy exercise breathing frequency takes on a greater role than increases in tidal volume. Our breathing rate can increase to around 80 times per minute.

Long-term response

This is not generally seen to be significant because, if respiration is optimal, the improved efficiency of oxygen delivery becomes the responsibility of the blood transportation system (haemoglobin) and muscle utilization (mitochondria) processes. This has been outlined in the section on cardiovascular changes. However, we do know that training decreases our residual volume to ensure a fresh supply of air and efficient gaseous exchange.

CHAPTER SUMMARY

- The cardiorespiratory system is composed of the airways, lungs, blood vessels and heart and serves to take in oxygen and deliver it efficiently to all the cells in the body.

- Breathing occurs through pressure changes between the air in the atmosphere and that within the lungs.

- Air travels from the atmosphere through the nose and mouth, down the trachea into the bronchi, bronchioles and into the alveoli.

- Inspiration is an active process involving the diaphragm, intercostals and abdominal muscles. Expiration at rest is a passive process brought about by elastic recoil of the above muscles.

- An adult breathes around 12 times every minute. Within each breath about 0.5 litres of air enter and exit the lungs – this is the tidal volume. Therefore, the amount of air passing through the lungs each minute is six litres and represents the minute volume.

- If we maximally inhale, our lungs contain around five litres of air which is our total lung capacity. Our vital capacity is the amount of air we can maximally inhale and exhale in one breath. The air that remains in our lungs after maximal exhalation is the residual volume and is generally one litre. →

- Oxygen diffuses into the blood while carbon dioxide is deposited into the lungs for exhalation; this is the process of gaseous exchange.

- Gaseous exchange is made possible by the thin capillary walls and the oxygen transport capability of the haemoglobin molecule.

- The four main components of blood are: plasma, red and white blood cells and platelets.

- Arteries always carry blood away from the heart; veins carry blood towards the heart; capillaries link the two via arterioles and venules.

- The heart is a pump with four chambers that beats constantly at a set rate determined by a pacemaker. There is a contraction (ejection) phase and a relaxation (refilling) phase.

- The circulation is a closed system that can be considered in two halves. The pulmonary circulation is the blood flow through the lungs; the systemic circulation is the blood flow through the rest of the body.

- In the short term, exercise places additional demands on the body and necessitates a rise in heart rate, stroke volume, cardiac output, ventilation rate and tidal volume.

- In the long term, exercise will cause a reduction to the resting heart rate and residual volume and an increase in the stroke volume and tidal volume.

Energy systems

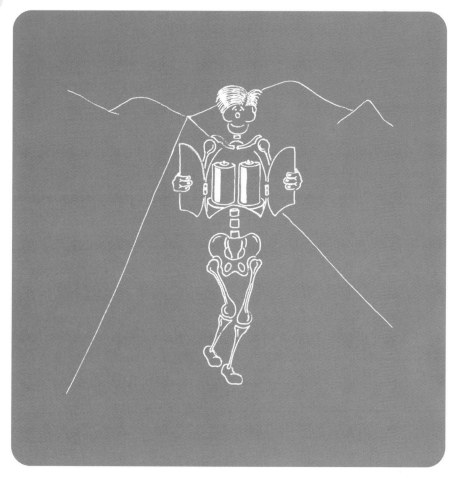

Topics covered in this chapter:

- ○ Understanding energy
- ○ Sources of energy
- ○ ATP – structure and function
- ○ The creatine phosphate system
- ○ The anaerobic system
- ○ The aerobic system
- ○ The energy continuum

Understanding energy

Each cell within our body requires energy to sustain everyday life. The more active we are, the more energy we use. However, we still need energy even when we are asleep. This energy is provided by the food we consume. The food we eat is broken down within our digestive system into smaller, more useful molecules. These molecules enter the bloodstream and are transported throughout the body. Some molecules will be used for immediate energy production whilst others are stored for later use.

Energy is available to us in a variety of different forms:

- Radiant energy
- Chemical energy
- Electrical energy
- Mechanical energy

Energy is not described in terms of the space it takes up, but in terms of the effect it has on other matter within the universe. For instance, the energy derived from the sun can be appreciated by the effect it has on plants in making them grow.

Energy is defined as the ability to do work or to put matter into motion. Energy can, therefore, be actually moving an object and called **kinetic energy**, or stored within it and called **potential energy**. Energy is considered to be the capacity to perform work and is measured in calories (kcal).

Radiant energy

This form of energy would include the energy contained within the electromagnetic spectrum that travels in waves such as light, radio, infrared, ultraviolet and X-rays. The effect of ultraviolet rays is well known because of their role in the tanning properties of the sun. It is the ultraviolet rays that give the skin either a golden brown or a red appearance!

Chemical energy

This is contained within any chemical substances containing **bonds**. The bonds within the structure of any substance contain energy. The amount of energy within these bonds is dependent on what type of bond they are. This information is beyond the scope of this chapter. However, once any bond is broken, energy is released and can be utilized for work. When the energy is held within the bond it is potential energy. When the bond is broken and the energy released it is kinetic energy. An example would be the energy contained and utilized within the food we eat. This process will be a feature of this chapter.

Electrical energy

This energy is the product of the movement of charged particles. This provides us with the electrical power to light and heat our homes in addition to the electrical energy that enables our nerve cells to communicate with each other.

Mechanical energy

This is the energy that enables movement to occur. The bones are moved by the muscles via the contraction process. The muscles shorten to produce the movement necessary for all activities and exercises.

Although we have identified the different forms of energy, this chapter will focus mainly on chemical and mechanical energy and the transfer of energy between the two. It is this conversion of chemical to mechanical energy that enables movement to occur. Once movement has taken place, energy is released as heat generated by the working muscles.

Although we do not need to know the theory behind the **first law of thermodynamics** we should attempt to understand that energy cannot be created or destroyed. This means that plants absorb radiant energy from the sun in order to grow, and when we eat these plants we utilize the chemical energy stored within them to fuel our electrical and mechanical energy needs. Energy conversions are commonplace and occur relatively easily. A product of these conversions is heat. We know, for instance,

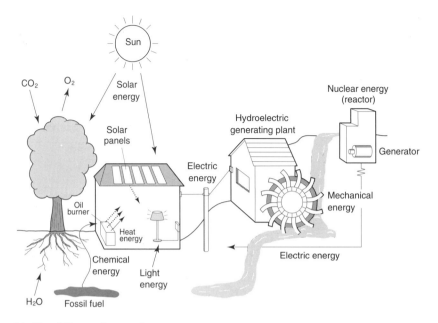

Figure 6.1 The different forms of energy

that in the electric socket of a lamp converting electrical energy into light energy the bulb will become hot. This is evidence of the heat given off through this conversion process. This heat is not lost but utilized elsewhere.

Similarly, when we exercise and convert the chemical energy in foods into the mechanical energy of movement our body temperature rises and we sweat and produce heat as a result.

Sources of energy

In considering the conversion of chemical energy contained within the foods we eat into the mechanical movement of exercise, we need to look at three nutrients that provide us with the necessary energy.

- Carbohydrates
- Fats
- Proteins

These food sources cannot be utilized in the form in which they are eaten. There are many hundreds of complex chemical reactions involved in breaking these foods down into useful molecules. These reactions do not need to be detailed here – however, it is useful to be able to name the transport, storage and smallest molecule that the body deals with within these nutrients.

Carbohydrates

Carbohydrates represent our most ready source of energy. We contain a carbohydrate energy reserve of about 2,000 kcal (units of energy) within the body can fuel about 90 minutes of continuous exercise. Carbohydrates are a vitally important energy source for two main reasons. Firstly, carbohydrates represent the most immediate of the three food sources and, more importantly, they provide most of the glucose required by the brain. The simplest, smallest form of a carbohydrate molecule is **glucose**. All the different types of carbohydrate rely on chains of glucose molecules. This is referred to in more depth in Chapter 7 on nutrition.

Carbohydrates are consumed within our diet in the form of bread, pasta, rice and sugars. These large molecules are then broken down to provide the quantities of glucose required by the brain and within the bloodstream for immediate energy needs. Glucose cannot be stored, so if the brain and blood have sufficient glucose, surplus glucose is converted into a substance called **glycogen**. This glycogen is then stored in the liver and within muscle tissue. Glycogen is then extracted (and broken back down into glucose) when more energy is needed. Any gram of a carbohydrate provides the body with 4 kcal of energy. Carbohydrate is essential for energy production when the intensity of an exercise session is high and the need for energy is rapid.

Fats

Fat provides a substantial reserve of energy. Around 100,000 kcal of energy are stored within the adipose (fat) tissue of an average person. This could fuel over 120 hours of continuous activity. Fat molecules are energy-dense and provide 9 kcal of energy for every gram utilized – twice as much as any gram of carbohydrate. For this reason the body is very efficient at producing energy if it can tap into these large fat supplies.

Eaten in the form of butters, oils, margarine, dairy products and animal fats, the large fat molecules are broken down into **fatty acids** and **glycerol**. These fats circulate within the bloodstream and provide energy if needed. If there is an excess of fats within the diet or bloodstream then the fatty acids and glycerol molecules are converted into **triglycerides**. The majority of fats within the body are in the form of triglycerides. Although fat is an energy-dense nutrient, it requires 15 per cent more oxygen to be present before it is broken down. Fats are the most efficient energy source when the exercise intensity is low and the activity is continuous for a period of time.

Proteins

Proteins have a complex and varied structure. They are made up of chains of small molecules called **amino acids**. Their main function is in the growth and repair of cellular tissue and muscle fibres and they are only used sparingly as a source of energy except under exceptional situations such as starvation and exhaustion.

Proteins are eaten in the form of meat, fish, nuts and seeds and then broken down into amino acids. If excess protein is eaten the body will excrete it. In vast amounts this can place the kidneys under extreme pressure. There is no form in which protein can be stored. If protein is used as a fuel source, it provides the body with about 4 kcal per gram, similar to carbohydrates.

All the nutrients discussed above, even in their smallest forms of glucose, fatty acids and glycerol and amino acids, contain bonds within their chemical structure. It is these molecules that then go into another complex chemical chain of reactions to produce the only substance that can be used by the body to produce energy. The rest of the chapter will focus on the production and regeneration of this substance: **adenosine triphosphate (ATP)**.

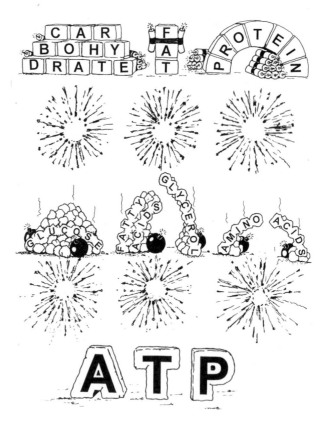

ATP

Our metabolism and survival is dependent on the formation, conservation and resynthesis of ATP. ATP can then be used for all the work necessary within the cells and is, therefore, considered the body's unit of **energy currency**.

The structure of ATP

ATP contains one adenosine molecule and three phosphate groups. Between two of these phosphate groups there is what is known as a **high-energy bond**. This simply means that these bonds contain a great deal of energy, and the way in which the energy can be released is to break the bonds via a chemical reaction.

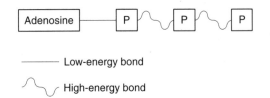

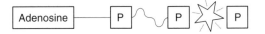

Figure 6.2 ATP structure

If ATP undergoes a reaction where one phosphate group is broken off to release energy, the substance that remains has only two phosphate groups and is known as **adenosine diphosphate (ADP)**.

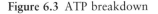

Figure 6.3 ATP breakdown

Stores of ATP are found in most metabolically active cells, but there are sufficient stores to maintain only about 3 seconds of intense activity before resynthesis is necessary. Within the cell there is a sensitive mechanism for detecting concentration levels of both ATP and ADP. Detection of low levels of ATP and a high concentration of ADP stimulates the breakdown of stored nutrients, whether they are carbohydrates, fats or proteins.

The decision as to which nutrient is broken down is dependent on many factors such as:

- the intensity of the exercise being undertaken
- the nutritional status of the individual before and during the activity
- the fitness level of the individual
- genetics

ATP cannot be supplied from the blood or other tissues; it must be resynthesized within the cell. Therefore, the body has ensured several ways of remaking this substance once the natural stores have been depleted. One of the body's major adaptations to any training programme, that cannot be seen, is the increased efficiency of these ATP regeneration pathways.

Resynthesis of ATP

As described above, when energy is released to the muscle for movement, ATP is broken down into ADP and the spare phosphate. To resynthesize the ATP we need to provide energy from another source to join a phosphate back to the ADP to form ATP.

$$ATP \longleftrightarrow ADP + P + energy$$

The energy for the resynthesis of ATP can be provided by three metabolic systems. Each system resynthesizes ATP at a different rate. Whilst all three systems may be used at any one time, the dominant system will depend on the intensity of the activity or exercise.

Each system will be considered in turn, beginning with the most immediate system and progressing to the long-term system. Where possible, all the names given to each system will be introduced.

The creatine phosphate system

(Immediate energy system/Phosphagen system)

Creatine phosphate (CP) is another high-energy compound found in close association with ATP. They are both known as phosphagens. When the high-energy bond in CP is broken, the energy released is used to resynthesize ATP from the available products of ATP breakdown, namely adenosine diphosphate (ADP) and the spare phosphate group (P).

$$ADP + CP \longrightarrow ATP + C$$

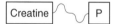

Figure 6.4 CP structure

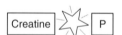

Figure 6.5 CP breakdown

The stores of CP are about 3–5 times greater than that of ATP. There are sufficient CP stores to fuel a further 7 seconds of immediate energy through resynthesis of the stored and broken-down ATP.

The natural stores of ATP and the CP synthesis combined, therefore, can fuel about 10 seconds of activity. This is essential for the onset of exercise, high-energy activities, weight lifting or any explosive moves. Oxygen is not needed for these reactions to occur.

The anaerobic system

(The short-term energy system/Lactic acid system/Anaerobic glycolysis)

Glycolysis is the breakdown of glucose or glycogen so that the bond energy contained within these molecules can be used in the formation of ATP. This metabolic pathway occurs within the main body of the cell and is referred to as the incomplete or partial oxidation of glucose and glycogen into **lactic acid** (LA). It is not the most efficient energy pathway as the lactic acid still contains considerable bond energy.

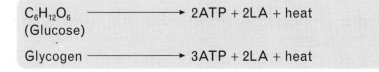

$$C_6H_{12}O_6 \longrightarrow 2ATP + 2LA + heat$$
(Glucose)

$$Glycogen \longrightarrow 3ATP + 2LA + heat$$

The energy released from the bonds within glucose and glycogen is sufficient to restore two or three units of ATP. Glycogen is the body's preferred substrate as an additional unit can be synthesized. Note that neither fat nor protein can be used for fuel via this pathway. This system will provide fuel for large bursts of energy over a longer period of time. However, it is still an anaerobic process, one that does not require oxygen. Therefore, this energy pathway will not be sustainable for long-duration work.

If exercise is continued at high intensity (anaerobically) an **oxygen debt** will accumulate. This represents a state where energy demands and oxygen requirements are in excess of the supply system. This debt needs to be paid back and can only be done when the exercise intensity is significantly lowered or when the activity has been stopped. All the oxygen needs of the body can then be repaid.

The limiting factor of this anaerobic system is the accumulation of lactic acid. When its production is in excess of the amount the circulatory system can remove, this causes muscle fatigue (interfering with the contraction process) and an uncomfortable burning sensation in the muscles. This system is, therefore, only sustainable for up to about 3 minutes.

The aerobic system

(The long-term energy system/Aerobic glycolysis)

This final system requires the presence of oxygen and provides the fuel for sustained, low- to moderate-intensity activity. This is an aerobic process and this pathway has the capacity to utilize all the fuels available – carbohydrate, fats and protein.

$$C_6H_{12}O_6 + 6O_2 \longrightarrow 38ATP + 6CO_2 + 6H_2O + heat \text{ (glucose)}$$

This represents the complete oxidation of glucose, as there is no significant bond energy remaining in the end products water and carbon dioxide.

$$\text{Fatty acid} + O_2 \longrightarrow 129ATP + CO_2 + H_2O + heat \text{ (fat)}$$

This second process is labelled specifically **fatty acid oxidation**. More ATP is produced via this process because fat is an energy-dense substrate, providing 9 kcal of energy for every 1 g of fat used. This process has almost limitless potential. The only limitation would be lack of substrate, either carbohydrate or fat stores.

Mitochondria

Mitochondria are sausage-shaped microscopic organs within the cell which convert oxygen and nutrients into energy. Therefore they are often referred to as the **power houses** of the cell. They provide the energy for all cell work. Although every cell in the body contains ATP, the quantities differ substantially, dependent on which tissue we are considering. The more metabolically active and busy the tissue, the greater the quantity of ATP (and mitochondria) found within it. The liver and muscle tissue, for instance, have hundreds of mitochondria to provide the energy for all their activities.

One of the adaptations of endurance training would include an increased number of mitochondria within the trained muscles. The limitation of this final aerobic energy system would then be the inability of the cardiovascular system to supply the necessary amounts of oxygen to the working muscle cells.

Energy systems in action

To summarize, all three pathways are operational during normal metabolic processes that the body undergoes, day and night. If we decide to place additional physiological demands on the body, as in exercise, the nature of the activity will determine which metabolic system predominates.

Table 6.1 A comparison between the three energy systems

	Rate of ATP production	Substrate	Capacity	Limitations	Activity
CP system	Immediate	Creatine phosphate	Limited – 7 secs	Small supply of CP	Explosive, short-duration activities: 1–10 secs
Anaerobic glycolysis	Rapid	Glucose and glycogen	Limited – 3 mins	Lactic acid accumulation	High-intensity, short duration: 1–3 mins
Aerobic oxidation (glucose)	Slow	Glucose and glycogen	Unlimited	Slow rate of O_2 delivery and glycogen storage	Lower-intensity, long duration: 3+ mins
Fatty acid oxidation	Slow	Fatty acids	Unlimited	Slow rate of O_2 delivery and large amounts of O_2 needed	Lower-intensity, longer duration: best after 20 mins

The more work we perform, the more energy we need to provide for our body. The amount of energy we require during a class or exercise programme equates to the amount of oxygen our cells utilize. A comparison of the amount of oxygen in the atmosphere with the amount of oxygen we expire during an activity reveals how much has been required to sustain the activity. This is a measure of a person's **oxygen consumption**, and a maximum value can be obtained from each individual known as the **VO_2 Max.** figure. This is seen to be an indicator of an individual's aerobic fitness level.

At rest

The body uses mainly glucose and fatty acids for energy pathways via aerobic processes when at rest. The energy required is needed for basic metabolic functions; these are basic cell processes that keep us alive. The speed at which the energy and oxygen are needed is steady and allows time for fat substrates to be utilized efficiently.

During exercise

As activity levels increase, the amount of oxygen needed by the working muscles is also increased. This demand for oxygen is usually around 3–6 litres per minute, whereas at rest it is around 0.3 litres per minute. As exercise intensity increases, it becomes more difficult to provide the required amount of oxygen to the muscles. Once the oxygen demand exceeds our ability to supply it, the body turns to the anaerobic energy systems. The point at which this happens is termed the **anaerobic threshold**.

When the anaerobic / lactic acid energy system dominates at high exercise intensities, the by-product is lactic acid. This builds up within the muscle tissue that is contracting. The lactic acid is then passed into the bloodstream, where it can be transported to the liver. If the exercise intensity is lowered, this lactic acid can be re-utilized. The lactic acid concentration in the blood is representative of the anaerobic threshold and is often sampled to determine an individual's threshold as a percentage of their maximum heart rate. Taking samples of blood from an individual when exercising reveals that there is a distinct point at which the lactic acid concentration on the blood rises sharply and rapidly. Technically, this is known as the **velocity of onset of blood lactic acid concentration (VOBLA)**. Figure 6.6 represents the response to a graded exercise session in which the intensity begins low and raises to maximal levels.

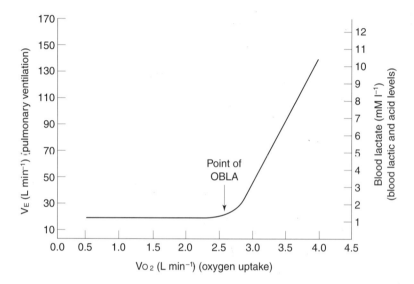

Figure 6.6 A typical VOBLA group

Training adaptations of the energy systems

The VO_2 max. of an individual is used as a benchmark of their aerobic fitness. This represents their maximal ability to take in, transport and utilize oxygen during exercise without reverting to anaerobic energy systems and building up an oxygen debt. As fitness levels increase, so does this VO_2 max. figure. This is a sign that the cardiorespiratory system has become more efficient at taking in, transporting and utilizing oxygen during activity.

With regular cardiovascular training, an individual can tolerate higher levels of lactic acid and can lengthen the time they spend exercising at high intensities before their blood lactic acid levels elevate substantially. The individual will find that it becomes more comfortable training at high intensities because their aerobic energy pathways are operating more efficiently.

A fitter individual will therefore:

- Take in, transport and utilize oxygen more efficiently (increasing their VO_2 max. score)
- Take longer to reach their **anaerobic threshold** (increasing their VOBLA value)
- Train at higher heart rate levels and still continue to use the aerobic energy pathway
- Tap into the aerobic energy pathway earlier

Energy systems in different sports

These three energy systems ensure that every level of energy expenditure can be met as efficiently as possible. All three systems are able to operate on a continuum or simultaneously if energy demands necessitate.

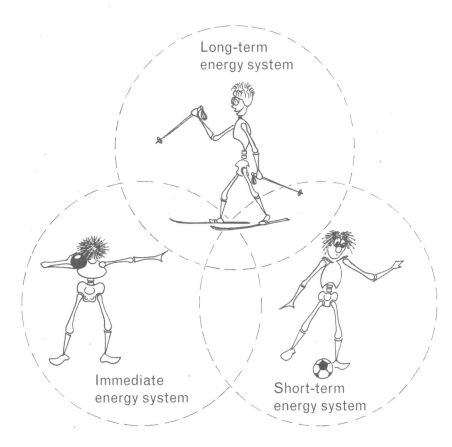

One system will usually dominate during any one activity or sport. This will depend on the nature, speed, intensity and standard of the sport, along with certain factors within the individual.

Individual factors would include:

- the fitness level of the individual
- the type of training adopted by the individual to reach this level of fitness
- the enthusiasm with which he/she plays

For training goals to be realized, sports-specific programmes and classes must consider specific training exercises for the different energy systems within each sport.

Table 6.2 Sports representative of each of the three energy systems

Energy system	Sport
CP system	100 m sprint
Anaerobic system	400 m
Aerobic system	marathon

Whereas these sports are easy to classify, there are others that contain a lot more transitions between the energy systems. Some of the most common sports are analysed below and placed onto the energy continuum. It is important to appreciate that there is a huge amount of interplay between the energy systems and it is not a case of one system switching to the next without overlap.

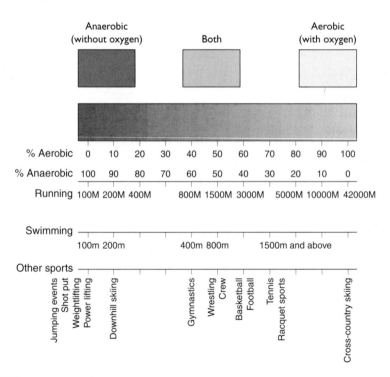

Figure 6.7 The energy continuum

CHAPTER SUMMARY

- All the cells of the body need energy and the molecule ATP provides this. This is the body's energy currency.

- The body has a limited supply of ATP. This will only fuel about 3 seconds of activity.

- The energy from ATP is released through the splitting of a high-energy bond.

- The remaining three energy pathways are designed to produce or resynthesize ATP.

- The CP system provides enough energy for a further 7 seconds of activity.

- The anaerobic system represents the partial breakdown of glucose or glycogen. The by-product is lactic acid, which fuels the body for up to 3 minutes of activity.

- The aerobic system is the most efficient form of energy production. Requiring oxygen, it involves the complete breakdown of glucose or fatty acid. This process has limitless potential.

- Mitochondria within the cells convert oxygen and nutrients into energy. They are the power houses of the cells.

- The three systems can operate at the same time, with one system dominating, depending on the intensity of the activity.

- At rest the body predominantly utilizes the aerobic pathways and uses both carbohydrate and fat substrates.

- During exercise the higher the intensity the less fat is used as a substrate, and the greater the dependence on carbohydrate sources.

- As exercise intensity increases so does the demand for oxygen. The point at which the body turns to anaerobic systems is the anaerobic threshold. Technically, this is known as VOBLA and is found through blood sampling and lactic acid concentrations.

- If anaerobic energy pathways are used, an oxygen debt builds up that has to be replaced. This is corrected by reducing the intensity or stopping the activity.

Nutrition

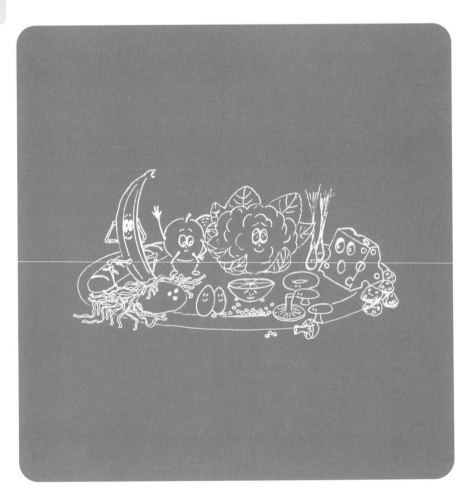

Topics to be covered in this chapter:

- The energy nutrients
- Vitamins, minerals and water
- Obesity
- Common diets, dieting myths and current theories
- A guideline for effective weight management

Food is central to our lives; we cannot survive without it; much of our time is spent buying and preparing it and we are constantly bombarded by advertisements about how food can affect every aspect of our life.

Food alters our body weight, complexion, concentration, energy levels, and our moods; it reduces the likelihood of developing many diseases (CHD, cancer, obesity, and diabetes) and is purported to cure many others. Despite all this positive publicity, we, as a nation, do not eat a healthy and balanced diet. We consume excessive amounts of calories in the form of protein, fat, cholesterol, sodium-loaded processed foods and insufficient quantities of fruits and vegetables and wholesome produce. We all know what we should be eating; yet few of us choose to put this knowledge into practice. Why? Our food choices are dependent on many things that include our religious beliefs, childhood experiences, lifestyles and income. It is, therefore, notoriously difficult to change a person's food choices.

The energy nutrients

This section will consider the three **macronutrients** that are the basis of our diet, namely carbohydrates, fats and proteins. These provide the necessary energy (and ultimately ATP) for all our bodily functions at rest and during activity. Food maintains the structural and functional integrity of our cells and organs.

On a daily basis we require a certain amount of energy to fuel our internal activities at rest. This is known as our **resting metabolic rate (RMR)** and is measured in calories.

This resting metabolic rate will be different for every individual, depending on their overall weight and their ratio of fat-free mass to fat mass. **Fat-free mass (FFM)** is made up of our body fluids, bones and muscle tissue and is more metabolically active (will require more energy) than fat mass.

Regardless of the actual amount of calories necessary to sustain us and our activity levels, we should all consume a balanced diet. This means that we should consume a certain percentage of these calories from each food group.

Table 7.1 Daily nutrient consumption

Nutrient	Recommended daily intake (% total calories)	Actual intake (% total calories)
Carbohydrate	60–65	35–40
Fat	25–30	40–45
Protein	10–15	20–25

The recommended daily intake of each nutrient is illustrated by the food pyramid.

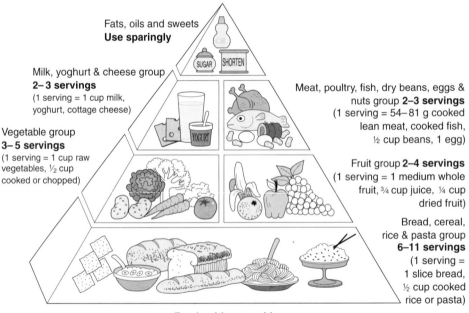

Fats, oils and sweets
Use sparingly

Milk, yoghurt & cheese group
2–3 servings
(1 serving = 1 cup milk, yoghurt, cottage cheese)

Meat, poultry, fish, dry beans, eggs & nuts group **2–3 servings**
(1 serving = 54–81 g cooked lean meat, cooked fish, ½ cup beans, 1 egg)

Vegetable group
3–5 servings
(1 serving = 1 cup raw vegetables, ½ cup cooked or chopped)

Fruit group **2–4 servings**
(1 serving = 1 medium whole fruit, ¾ cup juice, ¼ cup dried fruit)

Bread, cereal, rice & pasta group
6–11 servings
(1 serving = 1 slice bread, ½ cup cooked rice or pasta)

Food guide pyramid

Figure 7.1 The food pyramid

Carbohydrates

All carbohydrates, whether simple or complex, contain three basic elements: carbon, oxygen and hydrogen.

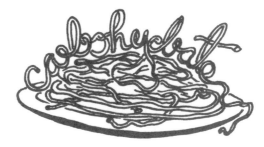

Simple carbohydrates

These are also known as **monosaccharides** and **disaccharides** and are the naturally occurring sugars found in fruits and milk. Table sugar, corn syrup, honey and brown sugar all come into this category.

Simple carbohydrates are also produced in the body as a result of digestion of more **complex carbohydrates** and can be synthesized from carbon skeletons of other compounds, a process known as **gluconeogenesis.**

The simplest of all carbohydrates is glucose, which has the chemical formula $C_6 H_{12} O_6$. It is absorbed in the small intestine and used directly by cells for energy or stored as glycogen in muscles and the liver if energy is not required immediately and glycogen stores are depleted. If all the glycogen stores are full it is converted to fat for storage.

Complex carbohydrates

Also known as **polysaccharides**, these can come from plants or animals.

Plant polysaccharides include the starch found in seeds, corn and grains and the fibre in leaves, stems and roots.

Animal polysaccharides are found as glycogen, the storage form of glucose. This is synthesized from glucose by a process called **glycogenesis.**

Table 7.2 The major sources of carbohydrates

Simple	Complex
Fruit sugar	Wholegrain breads
Milk sugar	Vegetables
Table sugar	Dried peas and beans
Brown sugar	Seeds
Corn syrup	Cereals
Honey	Pasta

Fibre

Fibre is not technically a nutrient as it is generally resistant to human digestive enzymes. It can be classified according to its solubility in water.

Water-soluble fibre is found in citrus fruits and apples and may help to lower blood cholesterol and, therefore, reduce the risk of CHD.

Water-insoluble fibre is found in grain products and bran and is thought to reduce the risk of colon cancer and other digestive disorders by speeding up the passage of food through the colon by absorbing water from the large intestine.

There is research that shows that people with diets high in fibre show lower incidences of:

- obesity
- diabetes
- intestinal disorders
- CHD

Role of carbohydrate

Carbohydrate is the body's most available source of energy. It can be accessed rapidly and in fact glucose is the only fuel source for brain tissue.

1 gram of carbohydrate contains 4 kcal.

The various uses of carbohydrate within the body include:

- It is the primary energy substrate.
- It is the only fuel used by the brain (glucose only).
- It is a metabolic primer – this means it facilitates fat metabolism (without it fat metabolism cannot continue).
- By being a fuel source itself and assisting fat in its role, it limits the need for protein to be used as fuel.

Fats

Fats also consist of purely carbon, hydrogen and oxygen. However, fats contain more carbon than carbohydrates, this means that 1 gram of fat can provide the body with about twice as much energy as 1 gram of carbohydrate.

1 gram of fat contains 9 kcal of energy.

Fats that we consume within food are usually in the form of **triglycerides**. These are made up of a glycerol molecule with three fatty acids attached. It is these triglycerides (known as simple fats) that can then be classified into:

- saturated fats
- unsaturated (mono-unsaturated and polyunsaturated)

Saturated

These fats hold as many hydrogen atoms as possible within their structure. They are generally hard at room temperature and found mainly in animal products such as meat fat, egg yolk, dairy fats of cream, butter, milk and cheese. Plant sources would include palm and coconut oil. There is a strong link between CHD development and large quantities of saturated fats within our diets.

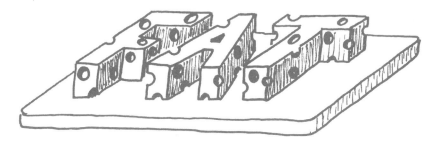

Unsaturated

Mono-unsaturated

This time the fat structure is not fully saturated with hydrogen atoms. They are usually liquid at room temperature but can become hard in the cold. Most are from plants and are associated with the oils of olives, rapeseed, groundnuts, hazelnuts and almonds. They are also to be found in avocados, nuts and seeds. Consumption of these products is thought to have health benefits by lowering the dangerous **low-density lipoprotein (LDL)** levels.

Polyunsaturated

This fat structure contains the least number of hydrogen atoms. It is always liquid at room temperature and found in vegetable oils and oily fishes. It is also thought to reduce LDL and may have a positive effect on the beneficial **high-density lipoproteins (HDL)**.

There are other types of fat to be discussed briefly. These can be classified as:

- compound fats (including the low- and high-density lipoproteins)
- derived fats (incorporating cholesterol)

Compound fats

These are known as phospholipids, lipoproteins and glucolipids.

Phospholipids maintain the structure of cells and are essential in the blood clotting processes and in insulating nerve fibres.

Lipoproteins represent the main form of transport for fat in blood and are known to be of three different types:

- High-density lipoproteins (HDL) – known as the good cholesterol
- Low-density lipoproteins (LDL) – considered the bad cholesterol
- Very low-density lipoproteins (VLDL)

It is these components that are measured when cholesterol tests are completed.

Derived fats

The most common example from this group is **cholesterol**. Its structure contains no fatty acids but has the physical and chemical characteristics of fat. It is found in animal products only because it is produced from the liver of the animal. Sources include egg yolk, liver, kidney, shrimps, ice cream, cream cheese, butter.

Table 7.3 The major sources of fat

Saturated	Unsaturated	
	Mono-unsaturated	Polyunsaturated
Meat fat	Almond oil	Vegetable oils
Egg yolk	Olive oil	Fish oils
Dairy products	Rapeseed oil	Sardines
Palm oil	Avocado	Mackeral
Coconut oil	Seeds	

Role of fat

The roles of fat within the body are many and various:

- It represents the body's largest store of potential energy, with reserves sufficient to run for about 120 hours.
- It cushions vital organs.
- It insulates the body (male fat stores equal 15–18 per cent and females 20–27 per cent of total body weight).
- It is a major structural component of our cells.
- It provides us with essential fatty acids.

- It aids absorption of fat-soluble vitamins.
- It assists in the production of hormones responsible for blood clotting and the inflammatory response.
- It adds flavour to our diet.

Protein

Protein contains an additional component to both fats and carbohydrates. Its structure contains carbon, oxygen, hydrogen and **nitrogen**. Although energy production is not its primary use:

1 gram of protein contains 4 kcals of energy.

Proteins are built from **amino acids** (building blocks, of which there are 20 different types, both essential and non-essential). Eight of these cannot be manufactured from the body and therefore must be consumed in the diet. Sources include eggs, milk, meat, fish and poultry but these can also be high in fats and cholesterol, so low-fat options are healthier. Those from plant materials include nuts, seeds and whole-grain products.

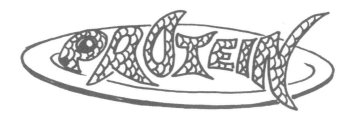

These sources can be classified as:

- complete: containing all essential amino acids (animal sources)
- incomplete: with one or more amino acids missing (plant sources)

Table 7.4 The major sources of protein

Complete (animals)	Incomplete (plants)
Eggs	
Milk	Seeds
Meat	Nuts
Poultry	Whole grains
Fish	

Role of protein

Protein is essential for:

- synthesis of cellular components (including DNA – the genetic material)
- the structure of hair, skin, nails, tendons and ligaments (structural proteins)
- enzyme production and hormone synthesis
- blood plasma (clotting agents – thrombin, fibrin, fibrinogen)
- production of haemoglobin (oxygen transport)
- the regulation of the acid-base balance of body fluids
- production of actin and myosin (muscle contraction)
- activating certain vitamin action
- energy production

If excess protein is consumed it cannot be stored; it is excreted by the kidneys. Excessive consumption over many years (as in the case of extreme body builders) can lead to kidney failure. Increased protein consumption may be necessary during adolescence (growth period), pregnancy, lactation and in the case of certain diseases.

Vitamins, minerals and water

Vitamins and minerals do not provide the body with energy. However, they are still essential, but are needed in much smaller amounts than the main nutrients.

Vitamins

Vitamins do not have a common chemical structure. They have to be consumed on a daily basis because the body can only synthesize one vitamin: Vitamin D. Vitamins can be found in both plant and animal sources:

- Plants: green leaves/roots of plants (manufactured during photosynthesis), seeds, grains and fruits
- Animals: meat, eggs, fish and dairy products

There are two classifications of vitamins:

- Fat-soluble
- Water-soluble

Table 7.5 Classification of vitamins

Fat-soluble	Water-soluble
Vitamin A	Vitamin B-1 (thiamin)
Vitamin D	Vitamin B-2 (riboflavin)
Vitamin E	Vitamin B-6 (pyridoxine)
Vitamin K	Vitamin B-12
	Niacin
	Folacin (folic acid)
	Biotin
	Pantothenic acid
	Vitamin C (ascorbic acid)

Role of vitamins

Vitamins themselves do not provide the body with energy. They serve as essential links to regulate metabolic reactions that facilitate the release of energy bound within food molecules and to control tissue synthesis. They are needed for growth and for the functioning of our immune, hormonal and nervous systems.

Vitamins cannot be stored but can be used repeatedly. Athletes need no additional supplements as all vitamins can be obtained from a balanced diet. However, the freshness of the food and the method of cooking can affect the amount of vitamins that can be absorbed by the body.

Minerals

These are a group of fifteen mostly metallic elements that enter our body through plants that absorb minerals from the soil and water. Minerals, like vitamins, contain no calories and are not an energy source but are essential to us in small amounts. They cannot be synthesized by the body, so must be obtained through our daily diet. How much of each mineral can then be absorbed from the food is dependent on many factors. It is known, for instance, that iron absorption is inhibited by caffeine.

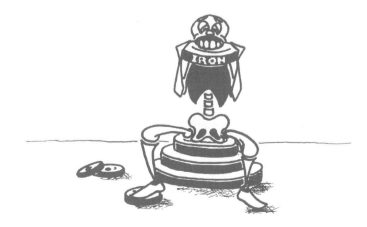

The minerals are classified as **trace** or **major** minerals. This does not, however, reflect their importance within the body.

Table 7.6 Classification of minerals

Trace	Major
Iron	Calcium
Zinc	Phosphorus
Iodine	Magnesium
Copper	Sulphur
Manganese	Sodium
Fluoride	Potassium
Chromium	
Selenium	
Molybdenum	

Role of minerals

Each of the minerals has a unique and essential role within the body. However this detail is beyond the scope of this chapter. Minerals in general are essential for the:

- formation of bones and teeth
- maintenance of normal heart rhythm, muscular contractility, neural conductivity and acid-base balance
- regulation of cellular metabolism

Water

This is essential to life; we cannot survive without it for more than a couple of days. It represents the body's transport and reactive medium and equates to about 60 per cent of our total body weight. Energy content of foods tends to be inversely related to their water content. The less water a food contains the more energy dense it is.

We all need to take in around 2–2.5 litres of water daily. This can be obtained from drinks, foods and from our metabolism as many of the by-products and end products of the reactions within our cells is water (refer back to the Chapter 6).

Water is lost from our bodies daily in a number of ways: through urine and faeces, evaporation from the skin, and from expired breath.

The role of water

Its main functions include:

- providing a medium for the diffusion of gases
- transporting nutrients, gases and waste products wherever necessary
- stabilizing heat fluctuations
- lubricating joints
- giving our body its form as water is non-compressible

Obesity

Obesity is an independent and powerful coronary heart disease risk factor that may be equal to that of smoking, elevated blood lipids and hypertension.

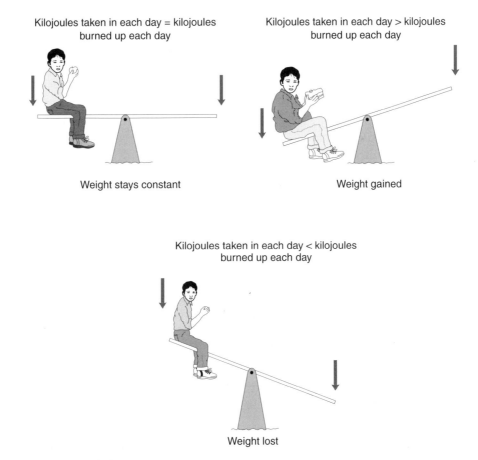

Figure 7.2 Energy balance

According to the **Health of the Nation Report (1994)** on obesity:

The prevalence of obesity in England has increased from 6% in men and 8% in women in 1980 to 13% in men and 16% in women in 1993. Based on current trends, the prevalence of obesity in the year 2005 would be around 18% of men and 24% of women. The health of the nation target is to reduce the prevalence of obesity to the levels seen in 1980.

Obesity often begins in childhood. An obese child is three times more likely to continue into adult obesity. Two critical factors in the development of obesity are food intake and energy expenditure.

Obesity could be due to overeating, possibly with a genetic background and certainly with environmental, social and racial elements. Other influencing factors that are being researched are eating patterns, biochemical differences in resting metabolic rate, basal body temperature differences, enzyme levels, brown adipose tissue deposits and levels of spontaneous activity ('fidgeting').

There are many obesity-linked disease risks, some of which are:

- impairment of cardiac function due to an increase in the heart's mechanical work
- hypertension and stroke
- pulmonary diseases and impaired pulmonary function due to the added effort needed to move the chest wall
- diabetes
- kidney disease
- gall bladder disease
- osteoarthritis, degenerative joint disease and gout
- several types of cancer

Regional fat distribution

It is not only overall fat content that is a danger, it is also where this fat is stored. The patterning of adipose tissue distribution, independent of body fat, alters the health risk of obesity. This is assessed by measuring the **waist-to-hip ratio**. Values over 0.9 are associated with increased risk of developing coronary heart disease.

Excess fat in this abdominal area (**central/android-type obesity**) is more active metabolically and more capable of entering into processes related to CHD than that located in the thighs (**peripheral/gynoid-type obesity**).

Common diets, dieting myths and theories

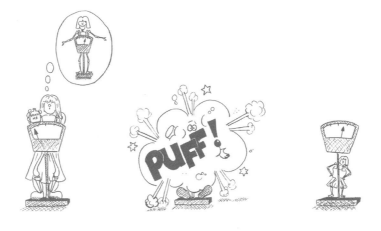

Common diets

1. Food combining diets

Examples: Hay diet and Kensington diet

Theory: That you do not mix carbohydrates and proteins in the same meal. It is based on the supposition that the enzymes used to break down each food group will work more efficiently if no other food group is present at the same time in the stomach.

Benefits: Makes people think about the foods they eat and possibly make healthier food choices as a result.

Drawbacks: Difficult to realistically continue over a long period of time. Makes it extremely difficult to eat out.

2. High-fibre diets

Example: F-Plan diet

Theory: The fibre expands and makes you feel full and therefore less able to eat high-fat foods.

Benefits: Speeds up the passage of food through the digestive system.

Drawbacks: Tastes poor and you need to drink plenty of water.

3. High-protein diets

Example: The Pennington diet

Theory: Low in carbohydrate and fat, high in protein. When in liquid form this 'protein elixir' contains artificial flavourings to make it palatable. It can also contain ground-up animal hooves and horns and pigskin mixed in a broth of enzymes and tenderizers to 'predigest it'. Protein diets suppress the appetite through the body's reliance on fat mobilization and excess production of ketone bodies.

Benefits: Reduction in fat intake.

Drawbacks: Potentially lethal. There is excessive strain on the liver and kidneys and risk of dehydration. If large amounts of lean tissue are lost, electrolyte imbalance can result that affects most metabolic processes.

4. Spot-reducing diets

Example: Hip and Thigh diet

Theory: That weight loss can specifically occur around this region if certain foods are eaten and an exercise plan is adhered to.

Benefits: It is essentially a healthy eating plan that is sustainable long enough to develop a lifestyle change.

Drawbacks: It perpetuates the myth that you can spot-reduce. This is not so.

5. Liquid diets

Examples: Slimfast (2 shakes and 1 meal per day), Cambridge diet and the Cabbage Soup diet

Theory: Based on severe calorie restrictions.

Benefits: Easy to prepare – this is one thing that makes it popular.

Drawbacks: Does not encourage a lifestyle change. You cannot stay on the diet for long; it does not encourage healthy eating choices, often tastes poor and becomes boring.

6. Low carbohydrate diets (ignoring overall calorific content of food)

Example: Drinking Man's diet and the Air Force diet

Theory: If minimal carbohydrate is available for energy, then body fat stores will be accessed more readily. Also high fat/protein diets generate excess ketone bodies (by-products of incomplete fat breakdown). These ketone bodies suppress appetite and cause urinary loss of these unused calories. This accounts for significant weight loss, despite a moderately high calorific intake. Dieters are told they can eat as much as they wish, so long as carbohydrate intake is restricted.

Benefits: Inclusion of rich foods may have psychological appeal and initial rapid loss of water may be an incentive.

Drawbacks: At most, the amount of calories lost in urine total 100–150 calories a day. This amounts to a small weight loss of 0.45 kg per month – not appealing when the fat content of the diet may be as high as 60–70 per cent. It has the potential for causing the body to lose muscle tissue as protein is used as a primary fuel to maintain blood glucose. It can raise serum uric acid levels and lower potassium levels that can facilitate cardiac arrhythmia, cause acidosis, aggravate kidney problems due to extra solute burden on the kidneys. It also causes blood lipid levels to rise, increasing CHD risk.

7. Metabolism increasing diets

Example: Herbal Chinese tea, grapefruit diet, pills (fat burners), amphetamines

Theory: Either stimulating Chinese herbs, acidic substances or drugs aim to increase the metabolism. This will have the effect of burning off more calories per day. If calories burned exceed those ingested, weight loss will result.

Benefits: Requires no thought or knowledge of healthy food options and food preparation. It is a quick fix.

Drawbacks: The herbs usually taste strange. Grapefruits become tedious and difficult to eat for long periods of time and there is no evidence to support the claims that it raises the metabolic rate. The pills and drugs have been known to have severe side effects on the cardiorespiratory system. In a small number of cases this has resulted in death.

8. One-food-centred diets

Examples: Grapefruit diet, Egg diet, Cabbage Soup diet

Theory: Low caloric intake favours a negative energy balance; certain foods are thought to burn off fat.

Benefits: Easy to follow. Has initial psychological appeal.

Drawbacks: Because it is too restrictive nutrients are generally lacking and the repetitive nature gives rise to boredom.

9. Slimming clubs

Examples: Weight Watchers (scales and points), Slimming World (sins), Hip and Thigh diet

Theory: That a specific menu plan developed by the company will guarantee effective weight loss.

Benefits: A group of like-minded people will provide support and encouragement. Specific meeting times encourage adherence to the programme.

Drawbacks: Tactics used are sometimes not psychologically beneficial, with guilt trips, sin foods and dependence on scales. Expensive to continue for a long period of time, so generally lifestyle changes are not adopted before individuals give up the programme.

10. Starvation diets

Example: Sub-1000-calorie diet, Slimfast, Bikini diet, fasting diets (detoxifying)

Theory: That severe calorie restriction will ensure a negative energy balance achieved quickly and maintained for as long as the diet is maintained. May be recommended in cases of severe obesity, with body fat totalling 40–50 per cent and above. Prescribed for up to three months, as a last resort before surgical intervention. The 'very-low-calorie-diet' approach assumes that abstinence from food may break established dietary habits, therefore helping long-term prospects of weight loss. Usually done under medical supervision.

Benefits: Large weight reductions in short timespan and reduction in exposure to temptation.

Drawbacks: Large loss of muscle tissue that may not return (leaving a greater percentage of fat than before). Lean tissue loss may occur disproportionately from critical organs like the heart. Poor success rate, ketogenic and often lacking in nutrients.

11. Yo-yo dieting

Although not a diet in itself this is important to mention here. The term denotes the cycle that is formed when an individual diets for short periods of time followed by periods of normal eating or bingeing. Usually the diet is a very low-calorie or starvation diet.

It is now known that this has a detrimental effect on the body's resting metabolic rate and fat stores. A well-documented change that occurs during weight loss through dieting is a dramatic and sustained reduction in the resting metabolic rate. This decrease can often be greater than the decrease attributable to body mass or lean body mass loss. Severe caloric restriction can reduce the resting metabolic rate by as much as 45 per cent. This reduction to the RMR is the body's way of conserving energy when calorie intake falls below the basic energy needs of the body. The depression of resting metabolism is enhanced with each subsequent attempt to reduce calorie intake. This considerably conserves energy and means that weight loss plateaus early. Dieters then consider the diet to be ineffective, become discouraged and return to pre-diet eating habits.

This 'yo-yo' effect is futile when attempting to permanently reduce body fat levels. Studies reveal that weight gain occurs more quickly with repeated cycles of body mass loss. Also, if the body is unable to regain its lean tissue at the rate at which it was lost through dieting, then it may be replaced by fat instead.

Further research has suggested that when obese people lose body mass, their fat cells increase levels of lipoprotein lipase (the enzyme that facilitates fat synthesis and storage). It makes it easier for these people to regain their fat. The fatter people are before the weight loss, the more of this enzyme they produce.

Current theories

The debate continues as to why the majority of diets are not successful long term. The reasons why some individuals become obese and others do not, despite calorific similarities, are also still under investigation. As an instructor you will hear individuals give their own opinion about why they feel they have been unsuccessful in losing or gaining weight. Some of these reasons will be touched upon below, but this is not a comprehensive list and further research will shed more light on the matter.

Set point theory

This advocates that our bodies have a natural set point – a specific weight that they will fight to maintain, regardless of our desires and activities. The body is thought to have an internal control mechanism, probably located deep within the brain, that drives the body to maintain a particular level of body fat. This level is thought to be as individual as an individual's resting metabolic rate. The only factors thought to alter this set point are amphetamines, nicotine and exercise. Dieting may have no effect on it.

This would mean that each time we manage to reduce the setting, the body will set in place mechanisms to ensure internal adjustments are made to replenish fat stores or resist the change. If this theory was proved this would give individuals an ideal excuse!

Fat cell genetics

Scientists are currently searching for the 'fat gene'. This will determine whether individuals are genetically programmed to become obese or overweight, despite their best efforts. It is still not clear whether we are all born with the same number of fat cells. If so, do overweight people grow more fat cells (hyperplasia) or simply store more fat in the cells that they have (hypertrophy)? Scientists are also investigating whether we can affect the number of fat cells we are born with. Studies have looked at the effects of nutritional practices of the mother during pregnancy, bottle-feeding and the early introduction of solid food. It is thought that the quantity and quality of food at this stage will affect the number of fat cells the child has.

Muscle fibre types

The ratio of slow- to fast-twitch muscle fibres an individual has affects their resting metabolic rate. The more lean muscle masses, the greater this value. Therefore, research has looked at issues related to muscle types and the associated genetics.

Slow metabolism claims

Larger individuals will often claim the reason they cannot lose weight is because they naturally have a slower metabolism. This has been proven not to be true – in fact, the opposite is true. Larger individuals will have higher metabolic rates, as it requires more energy to carry around more weight.

Enzyme activity (linked to fat metabolism)

Studies continue to delve into whether there is a difference in the activity and efficiency of the enzymes responsible for fat metabolism in individuals of normal weight and those who are obese. Research to date is inconclusive.

Appetite blurring

Investigations have been made into an obese person's ability to detect hunger pangs and signals that tell the body it is satiated (no longer hungry). Individuals of normal weight appear to detect earlier and more accurately when they are full.

Underestimating food intake

When food diaries are kept, the amount of food eaten daily is not accurately recorded. This is often because the higher-fat foods are blocked out from memory. These inaccurate assessments of ingested calories suggest that weight loss should be happening when it is not and leads people to conclude their bodies are incapable of losing weight or that whatever little food they ingest puts more pounds on them than other people!

Weekend overeating

This is when the individual sticks to a healthy eating plan from Monday to Friday and then binges on Saturdays and Sundays. This usually means that all the calorie sparing that has occurred during the week is cancelled and additional calories may be ingested above this. Weight loss is not likely to occur under this regime – indeed, weight gain may occur in many cases.

Time of day that you eat

It is often thought that the calories eaten at night are more likely to be laid down as fat, because of the inactivity and low energy requirements when asleep. However, what has been found is that food eaten late at night seems to be of a larger quantity and of higher fat content. This is particularly so if not much food has been eaten during the day and the bulk of the calories are eaten at this time. If this is the only time of day that you can eat, due to your lifestyle, then the body will utilize the food as it does at any other time of day. If the total calories ingested as food exceed daily energy expenditure, excess calories are stored as fat in adipose tissue.

It is the fat you eat that makes you fat

The composition of the diet influences the efficiency at which the body converts and stores excess calories as fat. About 3 per cent of the calories in ingested fat are required to convert these excess calories to stored body fat. About 25 per cent of the calories in carbohydrate are burned in the conversion process. It is easier to store excess calories as fat if they were ingested as fat, which is another reason to aim for higher carbohydrate-based meals (totalling 60–65 per cent of total calorie intake). It is worth remembering that fat contains twice the amount of calories than carbohydrates if eaten in the same quantity.

Table 7.7 Energy value of food sources

Food source (per gram)	Calories (in kilocalories)
Carbohydrate	4 kcal
Fat	9 kcal
Protein	4 kcal
Alcohol	7 kcal

Guidelines for effective weight management

It has always been understood that weight loss can only occur if the amount of calories ingested is less than those calories expended on a daily basis. There is no magic formula, potion or genetic discovery that can alter this. However, genetics and metabolism is thought to complicate this scenario. It is also now appreciated that the only real way to achieve and maintain weight loss is to combine exercise with healthy eating. This must become a lifestyle change and is best done through education and encouraging the individual to make the decision and direct these changes, which need to occur gradually and with support from family members, other individuals and possibly a counsellor, since it is often necessary to understand the psychological reasons we have for choosing certain foods over others.

Exercise for weight control

Evidence exists to show that excess weight gain throughout life often closely parallels reduced physical activity rather than increased caloric intake. Among the physically active, those who eat most often weigh the least and are the most fit. In the US and the UK caloric intake over the past 80 years have decreased, yet body mass and body fat levels have slowly increased. Americans now eat 10–20 per cent fewer calories than 20 years ago, yet they weigh 2.3 kg more. If dieting were effective, national body mass would be less, not more.

Some studies reveal that overweight/obese children may eat the same or less than normal weight individuals. However, obese children were shown to be less active than those of normal weight.

Arguments against using exercise as an effective and essential long-term component of weight management programmes include:

- Exercise would cause a concomitant increase in appetite and increased eating would offset any calorie deficit.
- The calorie-burning effects of exercise are small, and only make a small dent in fat reserves compared with starvation diets and other extreme measures.

The benefits of incorporating regular exercise into a weight management programme include:

- Increases in lean body mass raise basal metabolic rates, meaning that calorie expenditure will rise whether the individual is at rest or exercising.
- Exercise brings about enzymatic changes facilitating fat metabolism.
- Regular physical activity seems to contribute to the efficient functioning of the brain's feeding control centre. 'Creeping obesity' appears to be, in part, an inability to accurately determine the balance between energy expenditure and food intake. Active individuals are more likely to match their food intake with their energy expenditure.

TIPS FOR EFFECTIVE WEIGHT MANAGEMENT

Advise clients wanting to lose weight to:

1 Set realistic goals (amount of weight to be lost in what time frame).

2 Monitor body composition changes (choose the method most suited to the individual – clothes, belt, taped circumference measures, body fat, scales).

3 Lose only 1–2 pounds per week.

4 Keep a food diary.

5 Cut calories slowly.

6 Never consume fewer calories than needed to maintain the resting metabolic rate.

7 Consider food labels (fat content rather than calories).

8 Graze (eat 5–6 smaller meals throughout the day rather than 1–3 large meals)

9 Make gradual changes (to allow body and palate to adapt and promote adherence).

10 Complete a regular exercise programme (both cardiovascular and resistance exercises).

When advising clients you will need to consider psychological factors (why food choices are affected by certain moods, situations, people). Try to ensure there is support (friends, family, counsellor) and positive reinforcement is given regularly.

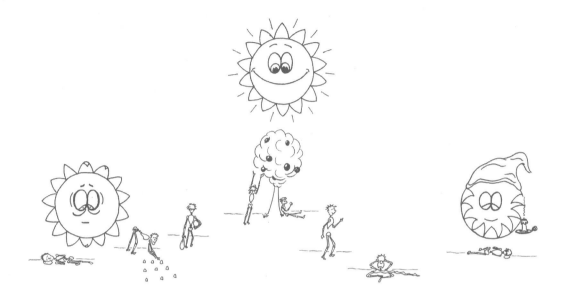

CHAPTER SUMMARY

- The basic six essential nutrients are: carbohydrates, fats, proteins, vitamins, minerals and water.

- Carbohydrates can be classified as simple or complex. Simple carbohydrates include glucose and natural sugars. Complex carbohydrates will encompass starches and fibre.

- Fats can be classified as simple, compound or derived. Simple fats include the saturated and unsaturated triglycerides. Compound fats incorporate HDL, LDL, VLDL. Derived fats include cholesterol.

- Sources of protein can be seen as complete (containing all essential amino acids) and incomplete (missing some amino acids).

- In our daily diet we should aim to consume 60–65 per cent of our calories from carbohydrates, 25–30 per cent from fat and 10–15 per cent from protein sources.

- Vitamins and minerals have to be eaten daily and are essential for various metabolic processes. Vitamins are classified as fat- or water-soluble, minerals as trace or major elements.

→

- Water is essential for life; the 2.5 litres needed daily are obtained from drink or food, or produced by the body. Water is lost through sweat, through breathing, and in the urine and faeces.

- Obesity is an ever-increasing problem and may be affected by: genetics, fat cell size and number, enzyme activity, exercise habits, environmental, social and racial elements.

- Diets are many and various and generally make large claims for quick weight loss. Theories are different but the result is generally that weight is regained after the diet is finished as no lifestyle change has taken place.

- The poor success rate of diets has led to theories including set points, fat cell genetics, metabolism defects, enzyme activity, appetite blurring, eating patterns, underestimating food intake, weekend binges.

- Exercise must be combined with a healthy eating programme for sustained weight management and reduction in the diseases associated with obesity.

- Effective weight management tips include: realistic goal setting; monitoring changes; slow weight loss; cutting calories slowly; never consuming fewer calories than needed to maintain the RMR; making changes gradually; keeping a diary; looking at food labels; grazing; considering psychological issues; providing support and reinforcement; and exercising.

Health screening

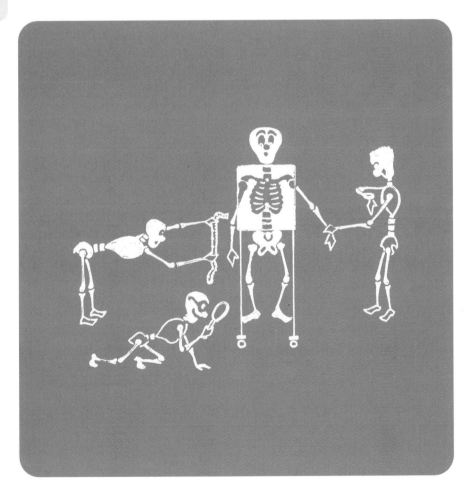

Topics to be covered in this chapter:

- The importance of health screening
- The PAR-Q
- Understanding coronary heart disease and risk stratification
- Blood pressure
- The medical clearance form
- The initial interview

Health screening can have different connotations for different centres and the instructors working within them. For both instructors and clients alike, it can be seen as a time-consuming procedure that could be an obstacle for people adopting a regular activity programme. If this is the opinion, then it suggests the instructor is not aware of the importance of screening procedures in terms of liability issues and individual programme prescription. The clients may be unaware of the fact that screening aims to ensure their safety and increase the suitability and effectiveness of any exercise they undertake.

The advice on screening procedures has changed over the past decade and it is important to be aware of current good practice. The ACSM (1998) recommends that a 'Physical Activity Readiness' questionnaire (PAR-Q) should be the *minimum* screening procedure undertaken by all participants. Any additional information provided by the participant or any medical referral information should be recorded clearly on a separate sheet of paper. This document should include the signatures of the participant and the instructor.

Health screening is not a one-off event, regardless of whether you are a gym instructor or a class teacher. You should continually check for any alteration in your participants' health status that may affect their ability to participate in your exercise programme or may increase the risk of a cardiovascular event occurring. In an ideal world, there also needs to be a two-way traffic of information happening between full-time instructors and the part-time or freelance instructors who may have contact with their clients.

The importance of health screening

The aim of a health screen is to ensure that every individual is suitable to partake in an exercise session and that you are aware of any conditions that may affect their exercise capability. This allows you to advise the participant on suitable adaptations or beneficial exercises, to monitor the problem or refer them to a medical authority if the condition is beyond your knowledge as an instructor.

The health screen is, therefore, recommended for the following multitude of reasons:

- It identifies individuals with diagnosed medical conditions.
- It identifies individuals at increased risk of disease.
- It provides you with a coronary heart disease risk profile of every individual.
- It provides you with an opportunity to take blood pressure (if resources allow).
- It alerts you to potential medical or range of motion problems.
- It may reduce the risk of a medical event or accident happening to the individual.
- It reduces the likelihood of legal proceedings being taken against you in the event of a medical event or accident.
- It reassures the individual that they have chosen the correct form of exercise to participate in – if they have chosen incorrectly, this can be an opportunity for you to suggest more relevant activities.
- It gives you valuable contact time with your member/class participant.
- It provides an opportunity to sell your other classes or club activities.
- It will make you look professional.
- It can improve relationships between you and your local doctors, physiotherapists, nutritionists and alternative therapists through referral procedures.

Health screening can be done in a variety of ways. Most class instructors will choose to do it verbally. If so, this is best done on an individual basis. This means that you need to make yourself available to your class before it begins, to welcome participants and ask the necessary questions (to be covered on the PAR-Q later in this chapter). It is fine to address the class as a whole, asking individuals to come forward with any concerns. This works best if you then give them the opportunity to approach you on their own as you are preparing the studio/tapes/equipment.

For gym instructors this process may be a routine appointment made by all new members. Usually the health screen takes the form of a written questionnaire, the **Physical Activity Readiness Questionnaire (PAR-Q)**. All information within this document should be treated as confidential. The participant should read and sign the document which is then safely stored under lock and key.

It is important to appreciate that, once this initial screening has been done, circumstances may not stay the same.

Members should be regularly re-screened and programmes adapted accordingly.

The class instructor should verbally screen even the most regular of participants as these may be most likely to train through recurring or new injuries or problems.

The Physical Activity Readiness Questionnaire (PAR-Q)

This is a questionnaire with a standard format that covers most of the major conditions that may be cause for concern when beginning an exercise session. It also allows you to build up a picture of an individual's **coronary heart disease (CHD)** risk factor profile. This is the identification of a number of factors that are known to be linked to a coronary event.

Any information collected on this form should be treated with the utmost confidentiality and subsequently stored in a lockable filing cabinet away from other members or class participants.

Under no circumstances should this information be left on a desk, filing cabinet or stereo unit in view of other people. Ideally, this information should not be displayed on programme cards, as much of the material will be of a sensitive nature. If you are working as part of a gym team, the information can be made available to other instructors who may need to refer to it if instructing the individual. However, beware of inputting this information onto a computer database. If this is done, you will need to be aware of the requirements of the **Data Protection Act** (1998).

It is not unusual during this screening process to find that individuals fail to disclose relevant or important details that may affect their exercise session. This may be because they do not realize their significance or they do not associate the problem with the question posed on the PAR-Q. It is therefore essential that you ask as many additional questions as you feel necessary to gain the information. Details of any condition or questions answered should be written down and once again kept confidential. If you give the individual any advice on receipt of this information, this should be noted alongside, signed and dated.

Although the individual will sign the PAR-Q (and maybe the additional note sheet), it is not a legally binding document. However, in the event of legal proceedings being taken against you, it will ensure that, from a legal standpoint, you have taken due care and attention to gain information, note details, and that this information has been verified and signed by the individual concerned.

Having gained the necessary information, it is essential that you understand the implications it may have for the exercise session and can identity when a doctor's referral is advisable.

Below is a copy of the PAR-Q followed by a breakdown of some possible concerns associated with answering 'yes' to any of the questions, with suggestions of possible follow-up questions that may be asked to elicit more detail.

Based on an individual's responses to the PAR-Q, the ACSM assign individuals to one of three categories according to the number of risk factors they have.

1 apparently healthy (none or 1 risk factors identified)
2 at risk (2 or more risk factors identified)
3 known disease (signs, symptoms and/or a diagnosis)

The ACSM suggest that medical clearance is required for individuals falling into the latter two categories.

It may not be easy to get the correct information from the PAR-Q if the individual is left to complete it on their own. There are helpful prompts that you can make that will assist them in giving you a fuller picture. There are always more questions to ask when a 'Yes' response is given to any question. Therefore, this chapter suggests some natural questions that may be asked, but never forget to write in detail the individual's response!

Physical Activity Readiness Questionnaire (PAR-Q)

If you are planning to take part in physical activity or an exercise class start by answering the questions below. If you are between the ages of 15 and 69 the questionnaire will tell you if you should check with your doctor before you start. If you are over 69 years of age and you are not used to being very active you should certainly check with your doctor. **Your instructor will treat all information confidentially.**

1 Has your doctor ever said you have a heart condition and that you should only do physical activity recommended by a doctor?   **Yes/No**

2 Do you ever feel pain in your chest when you do physical activity?   **Yes/No**

3 Have you ever had chest pain when you were not doing physical activity?   **Yes/No**

4 Do you ever feel faint or have spells of dizziness?   **Yes/No**

5 Do you have a joint problem that could be made worse by exercise?   **Yes/No**

6 Have you ever been told that you have high blood pressure?   **Yes/No**

7 Are you currently taking any medication of which the instructors should be made aware? If so, what? _____   **Yes/No**
_____
_____

8 Are you pregnant or have you had a baby in the last six months?   **Yes/No**

9 Is there any other reason why you should not participate in physical activity? If so, what? _____   **Yes/No**
_____
_____

→

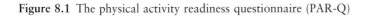

If you have answered yes to one or more questions

Talk to your doctor by phone or in person before becoming more physically active and before you have a fitness assessment. Tell your doctor about the questionnaire and which question(s) you have answered yes to. You may be able to do any activity you want – as long as you begin slowly and build up gradually – or you may need to restrict your activities to those which are safe for you. Talk with your doctor about the kind of activity you wish to participate in and follow his/her advice.

If you have answered no to all questions

You can be reasonably sure that you can start to become more physically active and take part in a suitable exercise programme. Remember – begin slowly and build up gradually.

Please note

If your health changes so that subsequently you answer yes to any of the above questions, inform your fitness or health professional immediately. Ask whether you should change your physical activity or exercise plan. Delay becoming more active if you feel unwell because of a temporary illness such as a cold or flu – wait until you are better.

I have read, understood and completed this questionnaire. All questions have been answered to the best of my knowledge.

Name	Signature ....
Address	Date ....
....	Phone No ....
....	
Emergency contact's name and phone number:	

Figure 8.1 The physical activity readiness questionnaire (PAR-Q)

Has your doctor ever said that you have a heart condition and that you should only do physical activity recommended by a doctor? YES

The umbrella term 'heart condition' includes huge numbers of medical conditions. The following represent the most common:

- Double/triple/multiple by-pass surgery – the coronary artery network is modified so that severely blocked arteries are by-passed and blood flow is diverted through blood vessels that are unaffected.
- Heart attack, technically termed myocardial infarction (MI) – the complete blockage of one of the coronary arteries results in insufficient blood supply available to the heart, causing the heart muscle to die. This is the end result if the above by-pass surgery is not performed.
- Angina pectoris or myocardial ischaemia – restricted blood flow to the heart, due to partially blocked coronary arteries, leads to pains in the chest. If left untreated, this can deteriorate and result in a heart attack.
- Cardiac arrhythmia – irregular heartbeats. In extreme cases this could result in ventricular fibrillation, where the heart muscle beats asynchronously, meaning that the blood flow is not delivered efficiently out of the heart and around the body. This can only be treated by shocking the heart (using a defibrillator); this causes the heart to stop and regain its natural rhythm.
- A hole in the heart – this could be between any of the four chambers within the heart and is often characterized by an additional 'whooshing' sound which can be detected when taking the blood pressure.

Questions that may need to be posed:

1 What is the exact nature of this heart trouble?

2 When did it occur?

3 Did it require medical attention?

4 Are you on any medication? Are there any side effects of this medication?

5 Do you have this medication with you? When do you take it?

6 Have you a family history of heart disease? At what age did family members suffer?

7 Have you sought your doctor's/specialist's permission to begin exercising?

Do you ever feel pains in your chest when you do physical activity? YES

Considerations:

- Angina pectoris or myocardial ischaemia – as described previously
- Shortened or damaged pectoral muscle – due to daily activities or muscle strain from unusual exercise
- Asthma – if the pain is linked to breathing difficulties

Questions:

Questions:

1 Does this pain occur every time you are active or only occasionally?

2 Does the pain increase with the intensity of the activity level?

3 Have you usually done a heavy weights session prior to the activity or done any upper body activity that you are not used to doing?

4 Do you have a stressful occupation or lifestyle? Does the pain coincide with periods of intense stress?

5 When you feel the pain in your chest, is it accompanied by difficulty in breathing? Do you suffer from asthma?

Have you ever had chest pain when you were not doing physical activity? YES

Considerations:

- Acute angina – an advanced form of angina that should be investigated
- Stress – this can include symptoms similar to a heart attack in some individuals

Questions:

1 Have you sought a doctor's advice on this?

2 Do you suffer from angina? Are you on medication?

3 Does this chest pain intensify if you become more active?

4 Do you have a stressful occupation or lifestyle? Does the pain coincide with periods of intense stress?

5 Was this pain experienced following an intense weight training session or blow to the chest?

Do you ever feel faint or have spells of dizziness? YES

Considerations:

- Hypotension (low blood pressure) – with values under 100/70 (although this will be dependent on the individual and what their normal resting blood pressure value is)
- Side effects of certain medications
- Hypoglycaemia – low blood sugar levels
- Pregnancy

Do you have a joint problem that could be made worse by exercise? YES

- Osteoarthritis – this is worn joints due to the degeneration of the articular cartilage covering the end of the bones, which causes excessive friction and pain within the joints.
- Rheumatoid arthritis – this is a chronic inflammatory condition affecting the joints. It is characterized by a swelling of the joint and pain during movement with reduced range of movement.
- Osteoporosis – 'porous bones': a reduction in bone density/strength. Bones become brittle and prone to fractures. Refer to Chapter 2 for more details.
- Ligament looseness/absence – unstable joints as ligaments have loosened through overstretching, an accident or the removal of a ligament that has snapped, again causing the joint to be less stable when under pressure.
- Muscular imbalance – one muscle in a pair is stronger. This can cause unnatural stress upon the joint.

Have you ever been told that you have high blood pressure? YES

This could indicate:

- Hypertension – blood pressure readings over 140/90 on more than two occasions
- Coronary heart disease
- Stress/anxiety – due to lifestyle, the screening appointment, first visit to the gym
- Side effects of medication
- Previous activity – if the individual has been active immediately before blood pressure is checked
- Ingestion of stimulants – nicotine, caffeine, drugs
- Infection/illness – if the individual is coming down with or recovering from an illness or infection
- Dehydration (through excessive alcohol intake or heat)
- Poor diet – high in saturated fats and cholesterol
- Pregnancy

Questions:

1 On how many previous occasions has it registered high?

2 Were there any explanations for this at the time?

3 Do you have a family history of high blood pressure?

4 Have you been ill recently?

5 Have you rushed here today or completed an exercise session already?

6 Do you have a stressful occupation or lifestyle? Does the pain coincide with periods of intense stress?

7 Do you smoke?

8 Have you recently drunk much caffeine or alcohol?

9 Do you eat a healthy diet?

Are you currently taking any medication of which the instructor should be made aware? YES

Questions:

1 What is the name of the medication?

2 What is this medication for?

3 How long have you been on it?

4 Do you suffer from any side effects?

5 When do you take this medication? When are you likely to exercise?

6 Do you need to carry the medication with you at all times?

Are you pregnant or have you had a baby in the last 6 months? YES

Considerations:

Pre-natal

- Balance, co-ordination and centre of gravity alterations
- Overheating (raising core body temperature) and dehydration
- Reduced blood flow to the foetus
- Pregnancy-induced hypertension – a precursor of eclampsia
- Effects of relaxin – ligaments loosen all over the body, making joints less stable/painful

Post-natal

- Relaxin – effects last for up to 6 months after the birth
- 8-week checkup completed – no complications
- 12-week checkup completed in the case of a Caesarean section

Questions:

1 Is this your first pregnancy?

2 What was your activity level pre-pregnancy?

3 Have you had a checkup (pre- or post-natal)?

4 How do you feel?

Is there any other reason why you should not participate in physical activity? YES

Question:

1 What is the reason?

This final question gives the individual time to reveal anything that has so far appeared irrelevant or has been forgotten about.

Understanding coronary heart disease and its risk factors

Coronary heart disease (CHD) is still the biggest killer in the Western world, responsible for four out of every ten deaths. If all CHD could be eradicated, our life expectancy would rise by about ten years. Physical inactivity has only recently been added to the list of factors that increase the risk of developing CHD.

The new emphasis within the fitness industry and the revised ACSM (1998) guidelines for health-related fitness are attempting to encourage the inactive 83 per cent of our population to become and remain active. The message being conveyed, that is backed up by substantial research, is that the level of activity required to impact the risk of developing CHD is low. Exercise intensity need only be around 50 per cent of an individual's MHR, the duration need only be around 30 minutes, cumulatively built up over the day, and this activity or exercise needs to be completed 5–7 days per week to maintain a regular habit.

> *Exercise is a stressful activity and places demands on a sedentary individual that are above normal levels. For this to be done safely, it is important to identify other factors that may suggest this could precipitate a cardiac event.*

CHD is a term that encompasses 20 different diseases. However, over 80 per cent of CHD cases are diagnosed as a condition called **atherosclerosis**.

Atherosclerosis is characterized by a narrowing and hardening of the arteries through deposits of cholesterol and calcium (known as **plaque**). This build-up of plaque on the inside of the arterial walls reduces the diameter of the blood vessels and makes it more difficult for the blood to flow through them.

Eventually, the plaque will completely block the blood vessel. If this is a vital blood vessel within the coronary network, a heart attack or death will result. Atherosclerosis is a normal part of the ageing process and occurs in all of us. However, the rate at which it occurs is dependent on a number of factors.

Risk factors increase the likelihood of the disease developing. If more than one risk factor is identified, the risk is greatly increased. Risk factors can be classified according to whether they are modifiable or not and whether they are actual risk factors or contributory factors.

The unmodifiable CHD risk factors

1 Family history (particularly significant in males under 55 years of age and in females under 65 years of age).
2 Gender – men are more susceptible.
3 Increasing age – CHD is far more prevalent in older people.

The modifiable CHD risk factors:

1 Cigarette smoking
2 Hypertension (>140/90mmHg)

3 High blood cholesterol (total serum cholesterol >200mg/dL or 5.2mmol/L)
4 Sedentary lifestyle (risk is twice as high for the sedentary)

Contributory CHD factors

1 Diabetes mellitus (fasting blood glucose levels >110mg/dL)
2 Obesity (Body Mass Index >30kg/m^2 or waist girth >100cm)
3 Stress
4 Type A characteristics (behaviours that include aggressiveness, ambition and anxiety).

Making reference to the above risk and contributory factors and the questions included within the PAR-Q, it is easy to see how you can develop a quick profile of an individual's CHD risk profile. This will give an indication of how likely they are to suffer from CHD, if they do not already. It also gives you sufficient information to suggest ways in which they can reduce their risk by modifying their lifestyle.

Blood pressure

Blood pressure readings are explained using two pressure readings – **systolic** and **diastolic** – expressed as systolic over diastolic.

> Systolic pressure represents the pressure within the arteries during the heart's contraction phase (systole means contraction).
> Diastolic pressure represents the pressure in the arteries as the heart relaxes (diastole means relaxation).

Consider the image of water flowing through a hose pipe. Individuals with low to normal blood pressure would be in possession of a large, wide diameter hose which allows the water to flow easily through the pipe. Individuals with hypertension would have a thin hose pipe with kinks in it that provides an intermittent high pressure water supply.

High blood pressure or **hypertension** effects many people especially in their later years. Although hypotension, low blood pressure, can be a problem as people faint or feel giddy it is rarely treated. From a health point of view high blood pressure is associated with increased risk of stroke, heart disease, kidney failure and peripheral vascular (blood vessel) disease.

In the majority of cases there are no obvious symptoms (**asymptomatic**) or single identifying cause of hypertension, but there has been a link with family genetics. Other factors that have been linked with blood pressure are dietary factors (such as sodium intake), obesity, cigarette smoking, inactivity and stress.

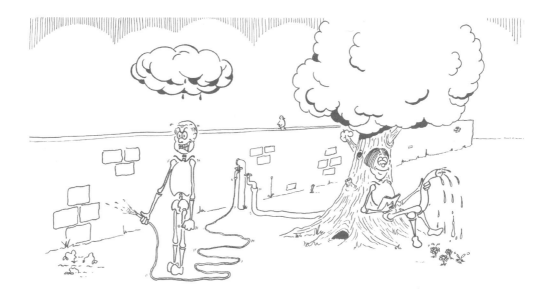

Exercise and blood pressure

Moderate exercise has been shown to reduce both systolic and diastolic blood pressure, especially in those individuals with moderate hypertension. Studies have shown that it is common for the blood pressure to decrease by about 10 mmHg through regular, moderate cardiovascular exercise. Resistance training is now also considered beneficial and has been shown to reduce blood pressures by about 3 mmHg. It is unclear if it is the exercise itself that makes the change in blood pressure, or other factors that have arisen as a consequence of exercising.

We do know that exercise reduces heart rate at rest, and during exercise it reduces the stress hormones that act on increasing heart rate and blood pressure. Exercise can also reduce body weight, which further reduces mild hypertension.

During exercise the systolic blood pressure will increase and the diastolic generally stays the same.

Taking resting blood pressure protocol

Blood pressure can be measured via a variety of blood pressure meters that vary in cost, accuracy and ease of operation.

- Mercury sphygmomanometer and stethoscope
- Air sphygmomanometer and stethoscope
- Automatic machine (no stethoscope required)

Before taking blood pressure using the mercury sphygmomanometer ensure the following guidelines are adhered to:

- Ensure that the individual has had sufficient rest and has not consumed alcohol and caffeine.
- The individual should sit upright with both feet flat on the floor.
- The left arm should rest on a table, palm up, with any clothing covering the arm removed or rolled up (as long as it does not cause discomfort or additional tension). The arm should be flexed slightly.
- Ensure that the mercury is released within the sphygmomanometer and that the pump bulb screw mechanism is tight.
- Remember to check the client's size of arm, as an extra large cuff may be required (14+ inch). If the cuff is too small, it will give an artificially high reading.
- Placement of the cuff is important. Wrap the cuff firmly around the upper arm at heart level, aligning the cuff pipe with the **brachial artery**, which runs along the inside of the arm. The cuff should be about 2–3 cm above the bend of the elbow.
- The stethoscope is placed in the **anticubital space** below the cuff.
- Pump the mercury column up to 160–200mmHg or 20mmHg above estimated systolic pressure.
- Once the blood has been cut off at the brachial artery then the pressure can be released from the bulb by slowly releasing the tightening screw. Aim to release the pressure at 2–3 mmHg per second.
- Listen for the first sound (the blood pressure coming back). This is known as the **first Karotkoff sound** and denotes the systolic blood pressure. Once the pressure is further released then the last sound heard, the complete disappearance of sound (the **fifth Karotkoff sound**) is the diastolic reading.

Many first-time exercisers will be apprehensive about having their blood pressure taken. This fact alone will increase their blood pressure. It is essential that you put them at ease and take time to explain how you will take the measurement and then what the reading means. Table 8.1 indicates the pressures that are within the 'normal' range and then categorises high blood pressure into various shapes.

Table 8.1 Resting blood pressure evaluation

Category	Systolic (mm Hg)	Diastolic (mm Hg)
Optimal	<120	<80
Normal	120–129	80–84
High normal	130–139	85–89
Hypertension		
Stage One	140–159	90–99
Stage Two	160–179	100–109
Stage Three	>180	>110

If your first reading is high, do not alarm the person. Wait for a while (ideally around 20 minutes) and repeat the procedure. The diagnosis of high blood pressure should never be made on the first reading. If the reading remains high after the second measurement, delay exercise and arrange for them to return 24–72 hours later for a third reading. If the reading is within normal limits on this final reading you can assume that external factors were artificially raising the reading on the first day. If it remains high on this final reading then refer them to their GP armed with a medical clearance form completed by you.

The medical clearance form

Medical Clearance Form

Name of fitness centre:

_____

Name & position of instructor: _____

Date: /   /

Reason for referral:

_____

_____

Dear Dr. _____

Your patient: _____

wishes to begin a regular exercise programme (programme attached) involving:

_____ (type, frequency, duration, intensity)

_____

_____

Please identify any recommendations or restrictions that are appropriate for your patient:

If your patient is taking medication that will affect his/her heart-rate response to exercise, please indicate the nature of the effect (raises, lowers, no effect):

Thank you,
Sincerely,

_____ has my approval to participate in the activity stated above with the recommendations or restrictions as detailed above.

Doctor's signature: _____

Figure 8.2 Medical clearance form

Following completion of the PAR-Q, if there is cause for concern then a medical clearance or referral form should be used. This should include as much information as possible for the GP, physiotherapist or other practitioner. Give as detailed information as possible about the exercise that you are planning to do with the client. Ensure you give a telephone number so the GP can contact you if they have any concerns or questions.

The initial interview

Initial Interview Sheet Instructor:	Date:
Medical details:	
Exercise history:	
Lifestyle considerations: **Likely barriers to exercise:**	
Goals (physical fitness/wellbeing) Short-term: Long-term:	
Signature:	

Figure 8.3 Initial interview sheet

Once an individual has completed the PAR-Q, assuming that they do not need referral to their GP, they can either participate in your class or embark on a gym session. For the latter to be most beneficial, you, as the instructor, will need to gather some further information.

In many centres the initial interview has replaced the standard and often compulsory fitness assessment. All the interview represents is a goal-setting session that considers the individual's:

- In depth medical details with your recommendations
- Past exercise history
- Time committed to exercise per session and per week
- Lifestyle considerations and barriers to exercise
- Exercise goals, whether fitness-orientated or wellness-based
- Short- and long-term goals

It is a good idea to use a template similar to that below to prompt investigation into the above areas.

Following this entire screening procedure, you should now be confident to instruct any individual through an exercise session. This may be a class with adaptations and modifications offered, or it might be a specifically designed gym programme that is achievable. The individual will have spent time getting to know you, will appreciate how professional you are and may have been advised on how to reduce the risk of developing CHD. Goals will have been set and will hopefully be reviewed regularly. More detail on this initial interview process and motivational techniques is to be found in Chapter 18, which considers how to promote regular physical activity.

CHAPTER SUMMARY

- Health screening will provide you with a CHD risk profile of the individual and alert you to medical problems that could affect their exercise suitability, effectiveness and enjoyment.

- PAR-Q stands for Physical Activity Readiness Questionnaire.

- On completion of the PAR-Q, the ACSM suggest that you assign individuals to one of three categories: apparently healthy, at risk and with known disease.

- 'Apparently healthy' individuals have none or one of the risk factors. 'At risk' individuals have two or more of the risk factors. Individuals in the 'known disease' category have received an official diagnosis and show symptoms.

- Medical clearance should be received on individuals falling into the 'at risk' and 'known disease' categories.

- Screening can reduce the likelihood of a medical event and your liability should this occur at your place of work. →

- CHD is an umbrella term encompassing 20 different diseases of the circulatory system.

- Atherosclerosis is the underlying factor in over 80 per cent of CHD cases. This is characterized by a build-up of plaque in the arteries surrounding the heart.

- There are modifiable and unmodifiable CHD risk factors, as well as contributory factors.

- Blood pressure represents the pressure of the blood flow against the artery wall. Systolic pressure is the contraction phase; diastolic the refilling phase of the cardiac cycle.

- A normal blood pressure value can be 120/80mmHg. Hypertension begins beyond 140/90mmHg.

- Individuals should be referred to their GP if the PAR-Q raises questions about their suitability to exercise. A medical clearance form should ideally be completed in as much detail as possible about the concerns and the suggested exercise session.

- The initial interview continues this information-gathering process before a personalized exercise plan can be designed.

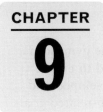

Workout structure

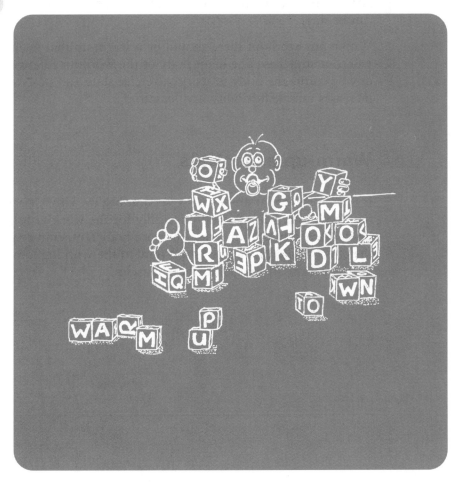

Topics to be covered in this chapter:

- ❏ Warm-up essentials
- ❏ Pre-workout stretching
- ❏ Cardiovascular training principles
- ❏ Resistance training guidelines and theories
- ❏ Cool-down components

When designing a workout, whether this is to be based in the gym or in the studio, there are basic principles that need to be observed to ensure an effective session. These principles can then be utilized, developed and adapted to suit any individual. In this way, fitness and health-related goals can be met.

Within any workout there should be a warm-up that includes some pre-workout stretches. The main body of the workout follows before the cool down returns the body to its pre-exercise state and post-workout stretches increases muscle flexibility and length.

Warm-up essentials

It is important that any exercise session begins with a warm-up. It prepares the body both mentally and physically for the work to follow. In any warm-up you are aiming to increase the core body temperature gradually. This has the effect of increasing the blood flow to the working muscles and allows a greater release of oxygen to these muscles.

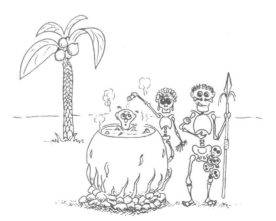

The physiological benefits in warming-up include:

1 Increasing core body and muscle temperature
2 Increased blood flow to muscles
3 Increased muscle elasticity
4 Higher metabolic rate and heart rate
5 Improved joint range of movement
6 The 'rehearsal effect'

Core body temperature, metabolic and heart rate

Exercise places additional stress on the body. As the muscles contract, circulation increases, heart rate rises and breathing rate increases as more oxygen is needed for the working muscles. Blood flow is diverted from vital organs to supply this demand.

More fuel is needed for the working muscles and the various metabolic processes that provide this additional energy. The by-product of these additional reactions is heat, which causes a rise of the core body and muscle temperature.

> *It is ideal if this exercise demand is increased gradually throughout a warm-up. The length of the warm-up will vary, depending on the activity to follow and the participants taking part.*

Muscle temperature, blood flow and elasticity

As muscles contract they demand more energy in the form of ATP and require additional oxygen delivery. Greater blood supply to these muscles is provided as a result of the increased heart rate, rising stroke volume and therefore, higher cardiac output. Once again, these factors contribute to the increase in muscle temperature. Muscles can contract faster and more efficiently when warmer and the blood supply can release oxygen at a faster rate.

> NB
>
> Warmer muscles are less likely to suffer injury. They can be compared to a piece of chewing gum. If a piece of chewing gum is stretched when cold and straight out of the wrapper, it snaps. If this same piece of gum is chewed for a few minutes first and then stretched, it can be stretched easily to several times its original length.

It would be incorrect to say that warming-up and pre-workout stretches *prevent* muscle injury, but evidence to date suggests that they may reduce the risk of injury. Whilst there is some controversy regarding the benefit of pre-workout stretches, they do no harm and hence it is best to follow this pattern.

Improved joint range of motion and the rehearsal effect

The warm-up phase of a workout stimulates production of synovial fluid within the joint capsule of freely movable (synovial) joints. This allows the joint to move fluidly through its full range of motion with reduced friction. The articular cartilage covering the ends of the bones within the joint absorbs some synovial fluid, which provides them with a greater ability to absorb shock as they become thicker. Refer to Chapter 2 for more detail on the structure of a joint.

> *Any warm-up must be specific to the activity that is to follow, which means that the range of motion required during the main body of the workout must be rehearsed. This ensures that the joint and surrounding muscles have gone through their full range of motion at a slow and controlled pace before this is done at greater speed and with greater force.*

The rehearsal effect practises movement patterns needed later, preparing the neuromuscular response patterns. Once the nerve-to-muscle pathways are activated, it is easier to repeat the movement and the reaction time becomes faster.

Psychological benefits to warming-up

The psychological benefits are also important. They allow the participants to prepare themselves mentally for the work to follow and to focus their minds on posture and technique. People bring a lot of mental baggage with them into the beginning of their workouts.

Components of a warm-up

> *The total duration of a warm-up will be 10–15 minutes. The length is dependent on many factors such as: the experience and fitness levels of the participants, the temperature of the environment, and the intensity of the work to follow. Within this 10–15 minutes all major joints should be mobilised, the pulse rate raised to just beneath the individual's training zone and the major muscles stretched in preparation for the workout.*

Every warm-up should contain a period of mobilization of the major joints, to increase the production of synovial fluid. This can be done simply and effectively in a number of ways.

The lower body can easily be mobilized through marching, side-stepping, walking on a treadmill, stationary cycling, or using other movements or cardiovascular machines suited to the workout to come.

Upper body mobilization can take place as the lower body is being mobilized and/or the pulse rate is rising, e.g. when cycling shoulder shrugs or rolls could be performed.

When considering the selection of mobilization moves, it is best to look at each joint, consider its potential range of movement, and combine moves in a way that fluidly works through the body.

The major joints that may need attention would be, from head to toe:

1 Shoulder/shoulder girdle
2 Elbows
3 Wrists (with certain sports/joint problems)
4 Spine (cervical, thoracic and lumbar)
5 Hip
6 Knee
7 Ankles

It is worth noting that the shoulders should always be mobilised before the neck.

It is important that most of the benefits of the warm-up are associated with the increase in core body temperature. Therefore, it is often advisable to incorporate some larger body movements with or between such isolation exercises.

The above mobilization moves should gradually raise the pulse rate, affecting the core body temperature and increasing circulation and blood supply to the working muscles. This initial component of the workout has the added effect of focusing the mind on the activity and away from daily stresses. Moves incorporated into this component should ideally prepare the mind and body for the activity that comprises the main body of the workout. This is best done by practising the moves in the warm-up that will be covered later during the session.

Pre-workout stretching

This section ensures that all the major muscles, now warmed, are further prepared for action in the aerobic phase by being taken through their full range of motion. This can be done in a controlled dynamic way, held statically at the end of their range of movement, or a combination of both. The choice of stretches is determined by the nature and content of the class or programme to follow and current thinking about stretching based on research data.

There continues to be a great deal of debate surrounding this section of the warm-up. Opinion is divided as to the benefits. The controversy is based around the fact that the stretches in this section are only held for about 6–10 seconds and some research has suggested that this is insufficient time to alter anything but connective tissue length.

In addition, it is often thought that holding a variety of static stretches for this time will cause the core body temperature to drop, and therefore negate the effects of the previous mobilization and pulse-raising, thereby perhaps even increasing risk of injury.

It is considered beneficial to include some range of motion stretching (not ballistic) with some static stretches. Even more beneficial if the participants have good co-ordination, is to combine stretches to reduce the time spent in this section and to add movement with or between each stretch to keep the pulse raised.

The choice of stretches is dependent on the nature and content of the workout.

The physiology of stretching

There are many different ways in which to stretch and much contradictory research on the subject. It is important for you to appreciate the different stretching techniques that can be used in a class or gym environment and to understand the mechanisms behind each. In this way, you can make your decision based on fact and the individuals in front of you.

Everyone differs in respect of their flexibility and it is important to make your participants aware of this and relaxed to stretch only within their own capabilities. This needs to be considered and alternatives should always be available for those who are very flexible, inflexible or have an injury-related range of movement restriction. Flexibility is specific to each joint.

Factors affecting flexibility

1 Genetics – some people are naturally more flexible than others.
2 Gender – possibly due to differences in muscle mass and connective tissue, but more likely connected to the types of activities undertaken by the different sexes in their formative years.
3 Age – flexibility declines with age at a rate of 1–2 per cent per year.
4 Practice – flexibility cannot be stored, it must be regularly practised.
5 Temperature – of the surrounding tissues and the atmosphere (time of day may make a difference, with 4–7 p.m. apparently being the most pliable time).
6 The flexibility, strength and bulk of surrounding muscles, tendons and ligaments.

Table 9.1 Soft tissue contribution to flexibility

Soft tissues	Percentage effect on flexibility
Joint capsule	47 (unchangeable)
Muscle and its fascia	41
Tendons and ligaments	10
Skin	2

Stretching can be split into two categories:

- Static stretching (active and passive)
- Dynamic stretching (range of movement or ballistic)

Static stretching

A slow, sustained stretching exercise that places a muscle in a lengthened position and holds that position for a few minutes. (Corbin 1980)

Static stretching can be further classified into **active** or **passive** stretches. There are many different ways to stretch the same muscle and it is important to build up a catalogue of stretches to offer individuals alternatives and adaptations based on range of movement problems, injury or postural issues.

An active stretch involves an unassisted movement requiring the strength and muscular effort of the agonist to hold the position.

For example, if stretching the quadriceps, the knee joint is flexed by the hamstrings and held in position with the heel close to the bottom. The

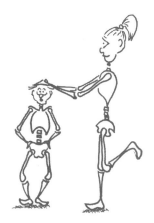

An active quadriceps stretch

hamstrings contract to maintain this position. As muscles work in pairs, this means that the quadriceps *must* be relaxed under these circumstances.

> *A passive stretch is accomplished through the use of an external force or prop such as a chair, wall or partner.*

For example, with the above quadriceps stretch, if the right quadriceps is being stretched, the right foot can be held in the right hand. This brings the heel closer to the bottom manually and allows the right hamstring to relax.

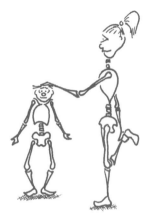

A passive quadriceps stretch

Dynamic stretching

> A type of stretching exercise involving bouncing or jerking to gain momentum in the body to enhance overstretching. (Corbin 1980)

This style of **ballistic** stretching has been synonymous with increased risk of injury for many years. The reason people continued stretching in this way was because gains in flexibility were supposedly greater than those available using static stretch techniques. Once again research and opinion are divided. Dynamic stretching does produce gains in flexibility but not significantly greater than that achieved through static work.

Dynamic ballistic stretching is applicable to those in specific sports that require their muscles to go through their full range of motion and beyond, at speed. If this is essential to the sport, then it is best to train the muscle to adapt to this, whether it is during football, karate or a dance routine. It does have its place, but must be done correctly, with the right people, and the benefits must always outweigh the risks.

Recently, **range of motion** stretching has gained popularity in the exercise to music world, and is a form of dynamic stretching. The muscle is taken through its full range of motion at a controlled pace, but not beyond. The whole movement may take 4–5 seconds to complete and is repeated 4–5 times.

It is important to understand that, despite the different types of pre-workout stretches available, they are all only **maintenance** stretches. Development of flexibility is only applicable at end of the workout. This is covered later in this chapter.

When completing any warm-up stretches always adhere to the following guidelines:

1 A minimum of 5 minutes of aerobic work should be completed beforehand.

2 Joint mobilization should always take place beforehand.

3 The atmospheric temperature should be monitored.

4 Stretches are combined with other body movements involving the large muscle groups to maintain core body temperature and pulse rate.

5 Hold these static stretches for an average of 8 seconds.

6 If doing range of motion stretches allow 4–5 seconds per movement and repeat an average of 4 times per muscle.

The warm-up is an essential part of any workout. Movements must be controlled and progressive in their range of movement. Until evidence conclusively proves otherwise, pre-workout stretching should be incorporated, probably as a combination of range of movement and static stretch techniques, while maintaining the core body temperature through rhythmic movements of the major muscle groups.

Cardiovascular training principles

Cardiovascular fitness is the ability of the heart and blood vessels to deliver an adequate supply of oxygen to the exercising muscles.

The aim of cardiovascular training is to develop the functional capacity of the central circulation, making the heart stronger, pumping more blood around the system, and to enhance the aerobic and anaerobic capacity of specific muscles involved in the activity.

If improvements to this ability are to be made, certain principles need to be adhered to. These principles are similar to those used to design resistance training programmes: **overload, progression, specificity** and **reversibility**.

Overload

> The cardiorespiratory demand placed on the body must be in excess of that which it is normally accustomed to handling.

Only in this way will the body find the need to adapt and change. Overload can be provided by extending the duration of the cardiovascular work over that which is normally completed or by increasing the intensity of the work.

Progression

Once overload has been provided, the body adapts by becoming more efficient at dealing with this increased workload. In order for further changes to be made, progression has to be enforced and a new overload applied.

Again the duration or intensity of the workload is increased. Once adaptations have taken place, the original overload has to be increased.

For example: An individual successfully completing a walk at 5.0 kph on 2 per cent gradient for 20 minutes may look to provide additional overload in one of three ways:

1 Maintain the speed and gradient but extend the time to 25 minutes.
2 Increase walking speed to 6.0 kph on this 2 per cent gradient and continue for 20 minutes.
3 Maintain the same 5.0 kph speed and time at 20 minutes but increase the gradient to 3 per cent.

Specificity

Adaptations to cardiovascular training are specific to the muscles used and energy systems called upon to provide the energy. These changes are not transferable across activities.

For example: adaptations are seen in the legs of endurance runners, but not in their upper body muscles. In long-distance swimmers, changes are seen across the whole body.

Reversibility

Fitness cannot be stored. Exercise must be performed regularly to gain and maintain noticeable benefits. If time is taken away from training or intensity is reduced, then previous adaptations will revert back to their original pre-trained state.

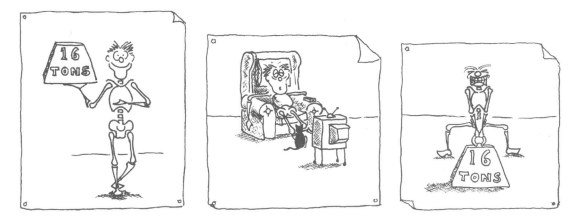

Changes within the exercised muscle tissue, resting heart rate reductions and stroke volume increases will all reverse.

This is an important concept to tell participants as they often return from a month's break or more and expect to return to exercise at their previous level of intensity and duration. This is not only demotivating for them but could potentially hold greater risk of injury.

The FITTA principle

Having considered the four basic principles of training, we can then apply the FITTA principle:

F   Frequency

I   Intensity

T   Time

T   Type

A   Adherence

To reiterate the ACSM (1990) guidelines for maintaining and increasing fitness:

Frequency   3–5 times per week

Intensity   60–90 per cent maximum heart rate (MHR)

Time   20–60 minutes

Type   maintained and rhythmical use of large muscle groups

Health-related fitness guidelines were then published by the ACSM (1998).

Frequency	5–7 times per week
Intensity	50–90 per cent MHR
Time	30 minutes (cumulative)
Type	maintained and rhythmical use of large muscle groups

The most noticeable difference between the two guidelines above is the level of intensity at which an individual is required to work. Represented as a percentage of their maximum heart rate, for maintaining and increasing fitness the lowest limit stands at 60 per cent. For health-related gains this has been reduced to as low as 50 per cent.

Firstly, it is necessary to know how to determine, accurately, a person's maximum heart rate (MHR) and secondly, it is essential to realize that every individual is different. This means that, for one person, working at 50 per cent of their maximum heart rate will be sufficient overload to produce change. For someone else, it will be necessary for them to work towards their 90 per cent MHR to produce overload.

Determining maximal heart rates

Before you can determine an individual's training zone, you need to have an idea of what that individual's maximum heart rate is and how it is calculated. This can be done in several ways, some more accurate and useful than others.

Completing a maximal heart rate test

This involves the individual completing an exercise until they can no longer do any more and their heart rate fails to rise any further. It is a hard and uncomfortable test, which can be done on various pieces of equipment, e.g. stationary cycle (Wingate test) or treadmill. This would be unrealistic and in many cases not advised for anyone but a trained athlete.

Using the maximal heart rate formula

This is the simplest and most often used formula. However, it is not the most accurate method, the actual MHR can vary from the figure calculated by 12–15 bpm, higher or lower.

The only information needed to calculate MHR is the individual's age. This is taken away from a standard figure of 220 bpm.

For example: for a woman of 30 years of age, her predicted MHR would be:

220 bpm − 30 years = **190 bpm**

To determine this woman's training zone for maintaining and improving cardiovascular fitness, using the ACSM's guidelines, we would then calculate 60–90 per cent of this MHR.

$190 \times 0.6 =$ **114 bpm** (60%)
$190 \times 0.9 =$ **171 bpm** (90%)

When exercising, this woman would then be advised to maintain her heart rate between these two values to overload her cardiovascular system. As the instructor, you would then specify the exact intensity of their workout.

Using the Karvonen formula

This is a progression on the above method, whereby the MHR can be calculated provided you know or can measure the individual's resting heart rate (RHR). This is a more accurate method as you are taking account of an individual variable. It is important to get as accurate an RHR as possible.

As above, we take the individual's age away from the standard maximum (220 bpm), then their resting heart rate is deducted, the percentages calculated and the RHR added back on afterwards.

For example: for a woman of 30 years of age with a resting heart rate of 72 bpm:

220 − 30 = **190 bpm**

Take the RHR away from this suggested MHR:

190 − 72 = **118 bpm**

It is this new figure that is then used in the calculations to locate the 60–90 per cent figures:

$118 \times 0.6 = 70.8$ bpm
$79.8 + 72 =$ **142.8 bpm** (60%)
$118 \times 0.9 = 106.2$ bpm
$106.2 + 72 =$ **178.2 bpm** (90%)

Monitoring exercise intensity

Having calculated the person's training zones, you need to know how to measure this intensity during a workout. Again there are a variety of ways to do this, some dependent on technology, others by simple observational methods. You have to adapt the technique to your resources, preference and the individual.

Heart rate monitors

A strap is worn around the chest and a watch on the wrist that records the individual's exact heartbeats per minute, based on readings taken every five seconds.

Manual pulse rate checks

These are easy to administer and are usually measured at one of two places – the radial (wrist) site or the carotid (neck) site.

Participants would locate their pulse at one of these sites using their first two fingers (not the thumb as this has its own pulse point). On your prompt they should count the pulse for 15 seconds and multiply the figure by 4 to determine the beats per minute. This figure should then fall between the two figures above that represent their 60–90 per cent training zone.

Rate of Perceived Exertion scale (RPE)

This is a subjective method and allows the individual to rate how hard they feel they are working against one of two recognized scales. The first scale was developed by Borg (1982) and participants rated their level of exertion from 6 to 20, 6 being no exertion and 20 being maximal exertion. This was later adapted by exercise practitioners, as 1 to 10 was an easier range for people to use.

This has been proved to be an accurate method, research revealing that it corresponds well with the actual heart rate values measured from individuals once they are used to this. As the instructor it is important that you introduce the concept at the beginning of the workout, giving participants imagery to express how they may feel as they progress through the scale and their workout.

An example of the scale is below:

The 15-point Borg scale

6   no exertion at all

7   very, very light

8

9   very light

10

11   fairly light

12

13   somewhat hard

14

15   hard

16

17   very hard

18

19   very, very hard

20   maximal exertion

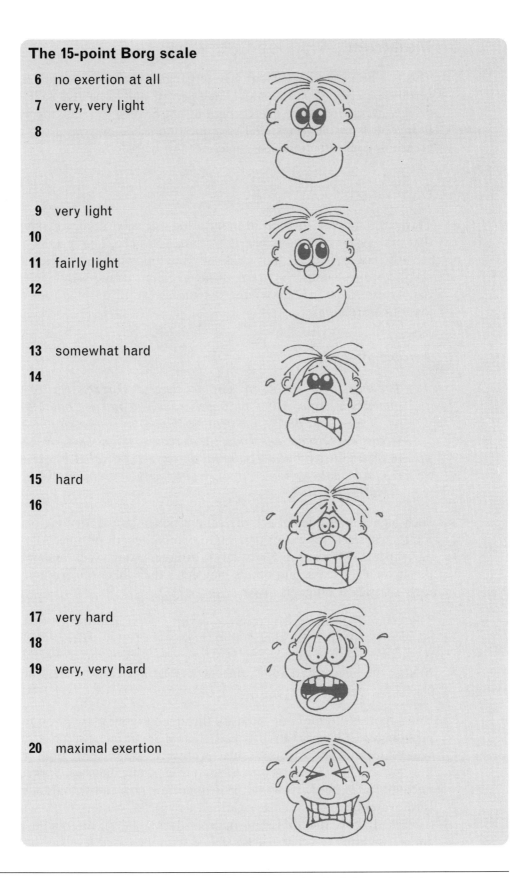

The talk test

This is a basic and convenient way of gauging exercise intensity and the aerobic capacity of participants. Each person should be able to hold a brief conversation while exercising, but not be able to relate their life story. If anyone is unable to respond to a question asked by you or too out of breath to count, then intensity may need to be reduced.

Observation

This is the simplest method of monitoring intensity. Look for symptoms that may suggest an individual is working too hard. This may be different for different individuals, but classically the following would indicate the need to reduce intensity: change of facial colour (some people will go very red, whilst others may go white), copious sweating, gasping for breath and loss of co-ordination.

Aerobic intensity

> *The meaning of the word 'aerobic' suggests that the level of intensity is sufficiently low to utilize oxygen and not build up an oxygen debt during the activity. This is in contrast to higher intensities, termed 'anaerobic', that require no oxygen for energy to be produced, but do build up an oxygen debt that has to be repaid by either a lowering of the intensity or stopping the activity altogether.*

Such higher intensities of activity cannot be continued for long periods: 3 minutes is generally considered a maximum length of time. All class participants will be at different levels of fitness, some will remain aerobic throughout the class, and others may enter their anaerobic training zone early on if their fitness is lower.

The main job of the instructor is to ensure, as far as possible, that every participant is working within their correct training zone; to have ways and means of monitoring this for every person and to be able to alter the intensity to adjust their workload if it is insufficient or excessive.

It is important to monitor intensity throughout your class or an individual's programme. If it rises too high participants are at increased risk of musculo-skeletal injuries and cardiovascular problems – quite apart from the fact that they are less likely to return to a class or workout that has worked them uncomfortably hard. However, it is important that individuals achieve cardiovascular and muscular **overload** during the session. Only when the body is worked above the level it normally is during daily living will it respond and adapt, initiating the changes associated with increased levels of fitness.

Resistance training

Resistance training is now more fashionable than ever, as clients are starting to realize the great advantages of performing these exercises in their training regime. This is linked to the introduction of studio-based resistance training classes that have recently gained in popularity.

This section aims to look at the concepts of resistance training in light of current research, together with the revised **ACSM (1998) guidelines** and to touch upon advanced training techniques.

We have already looked at the underlying physiological principles of muscle structure and function. It is now time to put this information into practice and appreciate the adaptations that occur as a result.

Basic resistance training guidelines

As with any issue of programme prescription, beware of looking for black and white answers, although there are some basic guidelines that need to be followed when structuring resistance sessions.

When deciding on what muscle groups to train and how many repetitions and sets to suggest, consider the following points:

- Level and experience of fitness of client
- Time available (total duration of session)
- Time of day that training will take place (peak time or day time)
- Client's goals
- Location of the machines (some resistance gyms are in separate rooms)
- Any joint problems

Exercise selection order

Ideally, any programme of resistance training should involve all the major muscle groups. There are a number of basic rules when designing any programme.

- Ensure that you train larger muscle groups first, as they are more fatiguing, and then follow them by medium and progressively smaller muscle groups.
- Consider the agonists (prime movers) and synergist muscle groups used in each and every exercise within the programme. You would not want to pre-fatigue muscles that are to be used later in the workout. An example of this would be doing the triceps pushdown before the chest press or doing biceps curls before the lat. pull down. Refer to Chapter 3 for revision of the roles a muscle can play and Chapter 4 for exercise analysis methods.

- The abdominals and erector spinae muscle groups are the supporting postural muscles; therefore you want to work them at the end of the session when they are no longer needed.
- Think about balance. Always ensure that the agonist and antagonist muscle(s) get sufficient work. Imbalance can lead to injury. Be aware of the number of sets that you are doing for each muscle group. For example you do not want to work six sets biceps and then two triceps!

Table 9.2 General order of a resistance training programme

Exercise	Major muscle groups
Leg extension/leg press	Quadriceps muscle group
Seated leg curl/prone leg curl	Hamstring muscle group
Hip adductors	Adductor muscle group
Hip abductors	Abductor muscle group
Bench press/fly	Pectorals major
Chin/lat. pull down/row	Latissimus dorsi
Shoulder press/lateral raise	Deltoids
Biceps curl	Biceps brachii
Triceps push down/triceps extension/dips	Triceps brachii
Dorsal raise	Erector spinae
Ab. trainer/abdominal curl	Rectus abdominus

Frequency

During training the muscle tissue undergoes a degree of micro trauma which needs a repairing and rebuilding period to be able to adapt and cope with the next stress.

DID YOU KNOW?

These physiological changes usually take approximately 48–72 hours and each new workout should take place when this activity has been completed. For this reason it is counterproductive to train the same muscle groups in successive days.

Each individual has a different time frame and ability to recover so frequency will be a question of trial and error. If you are still achieving strength gains, no matter how small, each workout, then it can be said that your training frequency is appropriate. A training diary can be useful unless you have an excellent memory. In his research, **Westcott (1996)** found that two or three strength training sessions weekly using a whole body approach produced excellent results for most people. He noted that two strength sessions a week were 75 per cent as effective as three in muscle strength and lean tissue improvements.

Repetitions (reps)

Repetitions can be defined as:

> The number of times you lift and lower the training resistance without resting (Westcott 1996)

An example would be in the biceps curl, where one repetition would represent one movement bringing the bar towards the upper body and then slowly returning it to the start position.

Westcott (1996) found from his research that our ability to perform a given number of reps can be dependent on our predominance of fast- or slow-twitch fibres. People who had a fast-twitch predominance had the least endurance and vice versa. On the basis of his findings he concluded that those with low-endurance muscles (fast-twitch predominance) generally gained better results by training with 5–8 repetitions (taking 6 seconds for each set). Those with a higher level of endurance-based fibres (slow-twitch predominance), gained better results in the 12–15 rep range.

Different clients will have different strength goals when it comes to resistance training. What they mean by the term 'strength' often differs dramatically. You will need to distinguish when 'strength' means strength and when it means endurance or muscle tone. There are three commonly used terms used to define the different types of strength goals. The number of repetitions in any set vary, depending on the goal.

Table 9.3 The recommended level of repetitions

Training goal	Number of repetitions
Muscular strength	6–8 reps
Muscular hypertrophy	8–12 reps
Muscular endurance/toning	12–15+ reps

Westcott (1996) summarized his research on repetitions:

- You need to make every repetition count by using the correct technique.
- Slow repetitions require more muscle tension than fast repetitions.
- Slow repetitions are highly effective for strength development.
- Training with 8–12 reps is highly effective for increasing muscle strength and mass.

Sets

The definition of a set is:

> the number of times you perform repetitions of a given exercise (Westcott 1996)

For example, if you perform ten leg extensions, rest one minute and then complete another ten reps you have completed two 'sets' of exercise.

Current thinking dictates that one-set training may have advantages over multi-set training. Westcott (1995) and **Starkey** et al. (**1994**), found that one-, two- and three-set training were equally effective for increasing muscle strength. Such research has profound implications for those who lack time to complete their workout because it suggests that we do not have to complete multiple sets. However, for advanced clients one set may not be a realistic or effective method.

Activity order and interaction

The decision on whether to place resistance work before or after the cardiovascular work in a programme is sometimes a difficult and disputed one. Much research has looked at the potential gains to be had in resistance training before cardiovascular work and the results have been inconclusive. The effects do not appear to be significant. Therefore, it is usually best to place the activity first that represents the client's highest priority.

Exercise resistance, progression and overload

Overload, as we have investigated previously, is a key issue within strength training. Overload suggests some notion of progression using the FITTA principles so that the muscles adapt. But what are the best ways of doing this?

Adaptation, which is what most people want from their exercise programme, has been shown to increase when participants have gone to fatigue, or momentary muscular fatigue. A number of issues are brought to mind.

It appears that each person has a different threshold as to what they consider to be fatigue. Clearly previous experience may play a part in this, and certainly the person's level of motivation. Designing a resistance training programme is a difficult balance between potentially increasing the risk of injury whilst creating enough fatigue to create an adaptation.

We can be quite scientific by using a percentage of one-repetition maximums and also looking at different ways of creating adaptation. Later we will look at more advanced methods but quite simply we can provide overload by regularly increasing the load, repetitions, number of sets or by using a training partner or spotter.

Speed

Westcott (1996), from his research, rated speed in three ways.

- **Fast**, where you cannot stop the resistance and momentum is emphasized. This reduces the muscular effort involved and increases the risk of injury. Each repetition may last only 2 seconds.
- **Moderate**, where there is a reduced emphasis on momentum. This increases muscular effort and reduces the risk of injury, with speeds of 2–4 seconds for each repetition.
- **Slow**, which is characterized by complete control, minimizing momentum and maximizing muscular force. Each lifting repetition taking 4 or more seconds to complete.

Westcott found that there was a slight improvement overall in strength in the slow speeds. Moderate and slow repetitions were found to be more effective than fast. He noted that there was a higher level of muscle force generated and a longer period of muscle tension when using slow to moderate speeds.

> Westcott (1996) recommended 6-second repetitions: 2 seconds lifting and 4 seconds lowering.

Range of movement

Muscular adaptation is specific to the movement in which it has been trained. It is suggested that we use the full range of movement to develop full range gains. An example of this would be training chest to gain strength in this area by undertaking the chest press. If we only train in the upper region of the movement then that is where we would gain strength; not in the whole range of movement.

 As an instructor, you need to consider that each of us has a different range of movement. The full range of movement that one person has may be totally different from that of another. One positive note is that the position for the full range of movement to occur has been shown to increase a person's joint flexibility as well as increase strength.

Always balance full range of movement with potential for injury. Just because an individual can move a joint through a large range of movement does not mean they should do that during an exercise.

Breathing

The best piece of advice for participants here is to breathe! Breathing can be difficult for the beginner to think about, especially when they are trying to remember all the other instructions you will have given them.

Opinion is divided on the best way to breathe during exercise. Some recommend breathing *out* on the exertion; and others recommend breathing in on the exertion. At present it seems preferable to breathe out on the exertion, both because it seems natural for the majority of people and because it decreases internal pressure as the external musculature pressure increases.

Some people may find this alien to them and they should find the way that suits them, but be aware that clients must never hold their breath as this will increase internal pressure, which, coupled with the external pressure of muscular contraction, can limit blood flow to the heart and brain (**valsalva manoeuvre**). Always control your breathing while focusing on postural stability.

Adaptation

There are many factors that impact upon development and maintenance of muscle mass and many studies have investigated the underlying causes of adaptation. Currently the main areas thought to impact the rate and extent of adaptation are:

- genetics
- environmental factors
- neuromuscular factors
- nutritional status of the individual
- current physical activity and exercise levels

One of the fundamental adaptations to resistance training is an increase in muscle mass. The enlargement of muscle fibres, or specifically the increased cross sectional area, is known as **hypertrophy**. This adaptation in turn gives the muscle fibres an increased ability to develop force.

What actually happens in hypertrophy is:

- The cells' myofibrils have thickened and increased in number.
- Additional sarcomeres are formed, by increased protein synthesis and a reduction in protein breakdown.

It does appear that these adaptations are affected in differing degrees by the following factors:

- Gender
- Intensity rather than duration of exercise
- Whether or not your client is an advanced trainer
- The specificity of the exercises

Overtraining symptoms

As discussed briefly in Chapter 1, when a body does not recuperate between workouts, there is a drop in performance. It is then easy to get into a 'more is better' approach, with disastrous consequences.

Below are some signs of overtraining:

- Extreme soreness or stiffness the day after training
- Unwanted decreases in total body weight
- Lack of motivation
- Loss of appetite
- Swelling of the lymph nodes in the neck/armpit
- Constipation or diarrhoea
- Drop in physical performance
- Lowered resistance to exercise
- Inability to complete a training session

Factors to help reduce overtraining:

- Sufficient rest
- Eating sufficient for needs
- Periodization of training
- Gradual increments in training
- Listening and responding to the body
- Looking for early warning signs
- Keeping a training log

Summary of ACSM Statement on Muscular Fitness (1998)

The combination of frequency, intensity and duration of regular exercise has been found to be effective for producing a training effect. The interaction of these factors provides the overload stimulus. In general, the lower the stimulus the less the training effect.

These recommendations should be used in the context of the participant's needs, goals and initial abilities. In designing a programme for an individual you need to provide the proper amount of physical activity to attain the maximal benefit and the lowest risk. Emphasis should be placed on factors that result in permanent lifestyle change and encourage a lifetime of physical activity.

- Resistance training should be an integral part of an adult fitness programme and of sufficient intensity to enhance strength, muscular endurance and maintain fat-free mass.
- Resistance training should be progressive in nature, individualized and provide a stimulus to all the major muscle groups.

- The effect of resistance training is specific to the area of the body being trained.
- Muscular strength and endurance are developed by the progressive overload principle. Any magnitude of overload will result in strength development, but heavier resistance loads requiring maximal and near-maximal effort, will elicit a significantly greater training effect. Muscular endurance is best developed using lighter weights with a greater number of repetitions.
- Intensity and volume of the resistance training programme can be manipulated by varying: the weight (load), repetitions, rest intervals between sets and the number of sets completed. Caution is advised for eccentric training as the potential for skeletal muscle soreness and injury is increased; especially in untrained individuals.
- To some extent both muscular strength and endurance are developed under each condition but each loading scheme favours a more specific type of neuromuscular development. To elicit improvements in both muscular strength and endurance, most experts recommend 8–12 reps per set – however, a lower rep range of 6–8 reps, with a heavier weight, may optimize strength and power.
- Repetition maximum refers to the maximal number of times a load can be lifted using good form and technique before fatigue.
- Muscular strength and endurance can be developed by means of static (isometric) or dynamic (isotonic) exercises. Dynamic exercise is often recommended, as it best mimics everyday activities.
- Resistance training for the average participant should be rhythmical, performed at a moderate to slow, controlled speed through the full range of movement and with a normal breathing pattern during the lifting movement. Heavy resistance exercise can cause a dramatic acute increase in both systolic and diastolic blood pressure, especially when the valsalva manoeuvre is evoked.
- Improvement in strength from resistance training can be difficult to assess because increases in strength are affected by the participant's initial level of strength revealing their potential for improvement. The average improvement in strength for sedentary young to middle-aged men and women, for up to 6 months of training, is 25–30 per cent.
- Consider the time it takes to complete a well-rounded programme. Programmes lasting longer than an hour have been shown to be associated with greater drop-out rates. Multiple set regimens may provide greater benefits if time allows but the difference in improvement is usually small.
- For the more serious weightlifter a regimen of 6–12 reps of 1–3 sets using periodization techniques usually provides greater benefits. It is also worth mentioning that the regimen of using heavy weights and few repetitions and multiple sets may not be suitable for adults with different goals from the athlete. The risk of orthopaedic injury and precipitation of a cardiac event in middle-aged and older participants is also a concern here.
- Programme variation may also be a factor in resistance training outcomes.

- Resistance training equipment may provide better feedback as to the loads used but calisthenics and other resistance activities can still be effective in improving and maintaining muscular strength and endurance.
- In the light of current research the following is recommended for the average healthy adult: one set of 8–10 exercises that condition the major muscle groups (arms, shoulders, chest, abdomen, back, hips and legs), 2–3 days per week. Most people should complete 8–12 repetitions of each exercise, however for older and more frail people (approximately 50–60 years of age or above) 10–15 repetitions may be more appropriate.
- Research supports this minimal standard for the adult fitness and health model for resistance training. It appears that resistance training 1–2 days a week elicits optimal gains in strength for the spine and 3 days per week for the appendicular regions of the body.

The cool-down

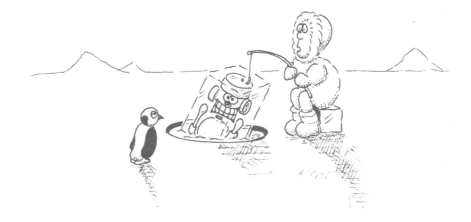

This is a vital section of any class and should last about 5–10 minutes. The aim is to increase flexibility, empty the mind, relax the body and leave the participants refreshed and alert on leaving the studio or gym.

As with the preceding three sections of the class, the cool-down can be sub-divided into three different components:

- Flexibility
- Relaxation
- Revitalizer

It is important that all participants are brought back to near-resting levels in terms of their core body temperature, heart rate and mental state at the end of their workout. Their metabolic rate, however, may remain elevated following the exercise session for an hour or more, depending on the nature and intensity of the activity.

The main reasons that it is important to cool down are to:

- reduce delayed-onset muscle soreness (DOMS)
- improve flexibility
- release stress
- aid relaxation

Flexibility

Muscles are best stretched when they are warm and pliable. At this stage of the workout the muscle temperature should still be raised. The muscles worked during the resistance section may still be tense and shortened and in need of lengthening before they cool down.

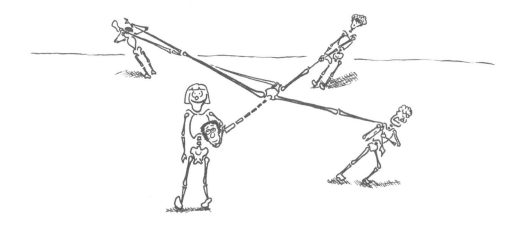

Care should be taken during this section to structure it so that each stretch follows smoothly on from the other, without great changes to body positioning. During the stretching section, the relaxation process will hopefully have begun.

The content of the component may vary considerably between classes and programmes. One reason for this lies in the muscle groups that have been chosen to be stretched. This will be dependent on:

- the choreography within the aerobic section or selection of gym machines chosen
- what muscles, if any, were stretched post-aerobically
- what exercises were completed during the resistance section
- the participants' needs

Once the muscle groups to be stretched have been chosen, the instructor has to decide which will undergo **maintenance** stretches and which need more advanced **developmental** work.

Maintenance stretches

These are held for 6–10 seconds, as all stretches were during the warm-up section of the class. The muscle is taken to the point at which tension is felt in the belly of the muscle. This position is then statically held for 6–10 seconds and released.

Muscles that are stretched in this way will not require additional length and flexibility, either because it is difficult to adopt the position that allows increases in flexibility to occur, or simply because these muscles are of no benefit to us in a lengthened state.

The muscles that are usually given only maintenance stretches are listed below. This list precludes an injury or range of movement issue that may mean one of these muscles needs additional focus.

- sternocleidomastoid
- deltoid
- biceps
- triceps
- rhomboids
- trapezius
- latissimus dorsi

- rectus abdominus
- obliques
- quadriceps
- gluteal group
- abductor group
- anterior tibialis
- soleus

Developmental stretches

These are held for longer, for 15–60 seconds and beyond. Current research suggests that the optimal time is 30 seconds considering the time restrictions that your average client will be facing.

Muscles are taken to their point of tension, as with maintenance stretches. The position is held until the feeling of tension subsides, once this has happened the stretch is increased by taking the limb into a position that allows the muscle to be lengthened further.

The stretch should never be forced. If the limb begins to shake, release the position slightly. Important points to remember are that the muscle being stretched should remain as relaxed as possible and that breathing should be deep and regular.

Muscles needing to be stretched developmentally include those that are shortened regularly during daily activities. For example, if your daily job involves much seated computer work, then the pectorals, hip flexors and hamstrings will shorten and can cause postural problems.

Muscles that may need to be stretched in this way include the following:

- pectorals
- erector spinae
- hip flexors

- hamstrings
- adductors
- gastrocnemius

Both types of stretches are static in nature. There are no bouncing or ballistic-style stretches. There are other, more advanced static stretching methods that can sometimes be seen within classes:

- Proprioceptive neuromuscular facilitation (PNF)
- Contract–relax–agonist–contract (CRAC)

Both techniques should be done with experienced participants only and can be more effectively done on a one-to-one basis, rather than in a group situation.

Before either of these two methods can be understood, it is essential to introduce the two protective muscle reflexes that lie within the muscle and tendon complex:

- The stretch reflex (myotatic reflex)
- The inverse stretch reflex (golgi tendon organ reflex)

Greater flexibility gains can be made by appreciating how these operate, so that they can be utilized. If they are ignored and worked against, few, if any, flexibility gains are made and injury risk could be greater.

The stretch reflex

The muscle must have a way of relaying information to the brain and spinal cord. This is needed to inform the brain what state the muscles are in, whether they are relaxed, contracted (under tension) or being stretched. This sensory organ is located within the belly of the muscle, running parallel to the muscle fibres and is called the **muscle spindle**. The role of the muscle spindle is to protect the muscle from being overstretched.

> *When a muscle is stretched impulses are sent via the sensory nerve to the spinal cord. If the tension within the muscle is such that it is at risk of being overstretched, impulses are sent to the muscle via the motor neuron. This causes a reflex contraction of the muscle, causing it to shorten.*

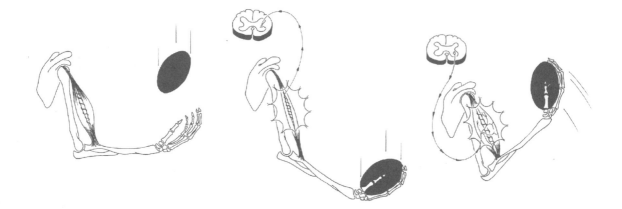

This reflex response is variable and dependent on two factors:

- The amount of tension within the muscle
- The rate at which the muscle is stretched or lengthened

The faster the stretch is performed the greater the magnitude of the reflex response. This is why it is thought that ballistic stretching may increase the risk of muscle injury. Bouncing at the end of a muscle's range of movement and beyond, evokes a violent stretch reflex and can increase the risk of muscle tearing.

Stretches like PNF and CRAC are advanced forms of assisted stretching, using a partner or an external resistance of some kind. They both aim to bypass this stretch reflex reaction so that the muscle can be taken to a longer length without a reflex shortening response that would otherwise work against this. To do this, these stretching techniques utilize the other reflex: the inverse stretch reflex.

The inverse stretch reflex

This is another protective mechanism. The sensory receptors this time are located within the tendon of the muscle. These are the **golgi tendon organs**. They respond to tension within the muscle and the degree to which the reflex is evoked is related to the force of the stretch, but not the rate of lengthening.

> *If the muscle is placed under great tension, the golgi tendon organs relay this to the brain and spinal cord and cause the muscle to relax. It does this because to contract the muscle when under such great tension would cause more damage to the muscle. If you evoke this reaction when stretching, the relaxation of the muscle can allow the stretch to be taken further.*

If we compare the connections within the spinal cord between the stretch reflex and the inverse stretch reflex, you can appreciate how the latter operates.

The sensory neurons (from the golgi tendon organs) do not link directly to the motor neurons, as in the stretch reflex. Here within the spinal cord there is an additional neuron that links the two: the **inhibitory neuron**. As the name suggests, this neuron receives information from the sensory neuron and connects to the motor neuron telling it to relax the muscle, not to shorten it. It inhibits the contraction of the muscle.

For the inverse stretch reflex to be evoked, there needs to be a high level of tension within the muscle. Normal static stretching procedures do not excite this reflex response. However, both PNF and CRAC involve contraction of muscles during the stretching process. Contraction builds sufficient tension in the muscle for the inverse stretch reflex to come into play.

Relaxation

Hopefully, your participants will have begun relaxing during the stretching component of this cool-down section, providing there have been smooth transitions between stretch positions and the music has been of a suitably slow or instrumental nature. This component gives participants a further 3 minutes to unwind, empty their minds and release any tension remaining within the worked muscles. The format of this particular section can differ widely between class instructors and is not generally seen within a gym programme.

There are probably three main variations seen:

1. Music appreciation

On playing one track of music of your choice, you instruct participants to adopt a comfortable position of their choosing. They are to close their eyes, breathe evenly and deeply and relax their entire body. They are to empty their mind of any thoughts but the music and you allow them to drift off into their own worlds for the duration of the track. On completion of the track, bring people slowly back to reality; take a minute to bring them safely to their feet.

2. Visualization

Once again with music playing in the background, you allow participants to relax and empty their minds. You then take them on a journey in their mind, e.g. they are to picture themselves on a sandy beach that expands for miles. The sky is blue, there is not a cloud in sight. The sea laps gently at their feet . . . However, be careful with this one as you can take participants into too deep a relaxed state, to the point of hypnotism. When you have completed this, people need time to come back to the present and focus on where they are before coming safely to their feet.

3. Progressive relaxation

This is a technique involving a contraction of a muscle group or body part, followed by its relaxation. For instance, with participants lying on their backs, eyes closed, breathing deeply and regularly, you instruct them to contract (tighten) all the muscles in their arms, hold for 3–5 seconds, then relax. Repeat three times per body part/muscle group, concentrating on the relaxation phase, and the weight of the limb relaxing into the floor. You work down the entire body, finishing with an entire body clench and relax.

Consider your choice of music carefully for this section. Often instrumental tracks are best. Lyrics can often be distracting from the relaxation process, or remind a participant of a problem at home, with a partner, etc. This can be upsetting if you hit on someone's 'our tune' and they have just split up.

You might wish to reconsider using relaxation tapes containing water sounds or waterfalls. However, any pregnant women in the class may feel uncomfortable as this could lead to an association with needing the toilet or their waters breaking.

Revitalizer

> *This small and final component only lasts about 1 minute. Its role is to ensure that participants are awake and alert before they leave the studio, following the relaxation phase.*

It can be dangerous to allow individuals to leave the studio too relaxed – they may walk into someone, fall down the stairs, or walk in front of a bus! This component, therefore, uses upbeat music, perhaps similar in tempo to the warm-up. You get them on their feet, moving around, checking their co-ordination. This is an excellent chance to make an impression on your class. Stylize this component to make the class remember you and leave the class on a high. Make it fun!

The cool-down section of any class is an important section and yet is one that is often hurried or cut out completely if time runs away with the rest of the class. Stress-related illnesses are affecting more of our population each year. These final 5–10 minutes of the class can leave people feeling more relaxed and refreshed and allow them the opportunity to do nothing, for which they might not otherwise make time. This could significantly reduce stress levels in many people. Make time for it!

CHAPTER SUMMARY

- The warm-up is the preparation phase of any exercise session that raises muscle and body temperature, heart rate, co-ordination levels and aims to reduce the risk of injury as a result.

- The warm-up can be divided into three sections: the mobilizer, pulse-raiser and stretches.

- The mobilizer aims to take the major joints in the body through their full range of motion, slowly and in a controlled manner.

- The pulse-raiser is faster, involving more movements off the spot, aimed at increasing heart rate and introducing movement sequences.

- The stretches are maintenance stretches only, held for 6–10 seconds. These can be a combination of static and dynamic stretches. It is important to keep the pulse rate raised during this section.

- Stretching is affected by genetics, age, gender, temperature of the room and muscles and practice. Care should be taken and instructions should be clear.

- The four cardiovascular training principles are: overload, progression, specificity and reversibility.

- These principles are then applied to the frequency, intensity, time and type (FITT) principle. →

- The maximal heart rate or Karvonen formula are the easiest ways of calculating training zones.

- Exercise intensity can be monitored via observation, talk test, RPE scale and heart rate monitoring methods.

- When designing resistance training programmes consider exercise selection order, reps and sets, frequency, speed, range of movement, breathing, adaptations and recovery.

- Overtraining symptoms are recognizable as extreme soreness, loss of appetite and a decrease in physical performance.

- The cool-down consists of three sections: the flexibility section, relaxation and the revitalizer.

- It is an essential section to allow the body to return to its pre-exercise state with regard to heart rate and core temperature.

- The benefits of this section include increased flexibility of certain muscle groups, reduced muscle soreness (DOMS), and stress release.

- The flexibility section contains examples of both maintenance and developmental stretching.

- More advanced static stretching techniques include PNF and CRAC.

- These above methods use the stretch reflex and inverse stretch reflex to increase flexibility safely and effectively.

- Relaxation can mean a 3-minute music appreciation period, visualization or a progressive relaxation session.

- The revitalizer ensures that everyone is alert and co-ordinated and ready to leave the studio.

Gym instruction

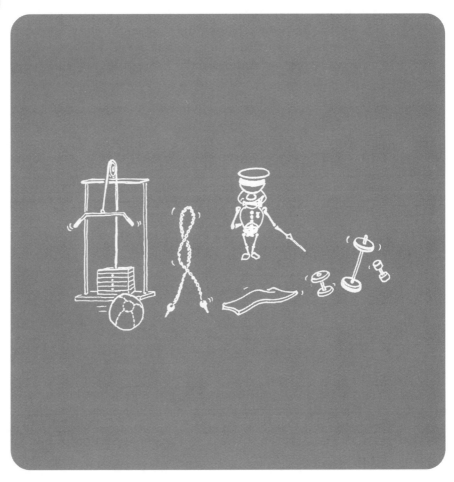

Topics to be covered in this chapter:

- The changing role of the gym instructor
- Cardiovascular machine instruction
- Free weight spotting techniques
- Exercise prescription issues
- Case studies for programme design

Gym instruction used to be seen as an easy and predominantly social job in which your time was spent in a pleasant environment, talking to people with whom you had lots in common. Even five years ago there was no nationally recognized gym instruction qualification. Consequently, the fitness industry is filled with instructors with a huge variation in knowledge, experience and communication skills. Gradually, the people working within the gym environment are being regulated and standards are rising. It is no longer uncommon to find instructors with degrees and/or a range of industry-specific qualifications.

It is now accepted by both employers and participants that gym instructors should hold a nationally recognized qualification to enter the industry and, as they gain experience, that they should maintain professional development through attendance at other specialist courses or conferences.

This chapter will consider some of the basic skills now required for you to cultivate in your role as an instructor. The two previous chapters have covered the essentials of the screening procedures and the structure of the workout. Since resistance training was discussed in some depth in this latter chapter it will not be considered again here except for free weight spotting techniques. This chapter also focuses on the variety of cardiovascular machines at your disposal and touches on exercise prescription.

The changing role of the gym instructor

In addition to the changing face of fitness instruction qualifications available today, the actual tasks a gym instructor is asked to carry out have also altered dramatically. Today's gym instructor needs to be multifaceted. Ideally, instructors need to have class teaching skills in addition to the original gym floor knowledge. As more centres also become more holistic in their activities, many instructors become involved in massage and relaxation along with pool and spa maintenance.

The potential jobs that may be included in an average day as a gym instructor are:

- Equipment maintenance and cleaning
- Health screening appointments
- Gym inductions
- Fitness assessments
- Programme writing
- Instructing spin cycling classes
- Instructing gym circuits and studio circuits classes
- Instructing body pump classes
- Instructing Concept II rowing classes
- Pool and spa testing
- Taking personal training sessions

The most fundamental skill a gym instructor must have is the ability to correctly demonstrate exercise technique on all the cardiovascular, resistance machines and free weights. This necessitates an in-depth understanding of how to operate each one and how to present this to clients in a simple, memorable and effective way. In a sense, the gym instructor's job is to do him or herself out of a job. Your aim should be to ensure that, on their next visit, the client is clear and confident to operate the machines without the help of an instructor. This then frees instructors to focus on other aspects of their training such as education.

When instructing a client on any machine it is useful to include the following information:

- Name of the machine
- Function of the machine (cardiovascular or resistance)
- Muscle groups worked
- The movable and adjustable parts of the machine
- How to programme the machine and increase the intensity progressively
- The correct posture and technique
- The sensations likely to be felt while exercising on the machine
- How this machine will assist the client to reach their goals

Cardiovascular machine instruction

With an ever-expanding fitness industry comes an ever-expanding list of gym equipment. Whilst it may seem confusing, there are underlying principles that can be applied in the set-up and use of any machine.

The following section gives some general guidelines for common cardiovascular machines. It is not an exhaustive list by any means, and obviously does not take into account individual makes and models. The aim here is not to give guidance on individual programme settings but to give some pointers as to the techniques, teaching points, and the machine's basic use.

For each machine you are given background information, main teaching points, advantages and disadvantages and lastly common errors specific to each machine. These are correction opportunities, used by the instructor, on the gym floor when a client is not using correct form.

The stationary cycle

Background

In most gyms there is a selection of cycles to choose from:

- Upright cycle
- Semi-recumbant cycle
- Cycles with movable arms
- Spinning cycles

It is usually individual preference that dictates which model is used, as there is little difference in which muscles are recruited. The upright cycles appeal as they are most familiar; the semi-recumbent models offer a seat with back support and the pedals are situated so that the client is pedalling from a 45° angle as opposed to a 90° angle. This may offer a little more support for those worried about their posture on the bike and some feel it is more comfortable. In the last few years spinning cycles have become popular in gyms. Set-up procedures on these can mean many different adjustments, depending on the make and model. The main safety factor that makes this cycle different from others is that it has a **fixed direct wheel**. This means that for every revolution you do, so does the wheel. Unlike a normal bike, if you stop pedalling it does *not* free-wheel, as the pedals always spin with the wheel. Therefore, if you have built up momentum and suddenly attempt to stop using your leg strength, it can cause damage to ankle and knee.

The set-up on most bikes is similar but we are not concerned here with what buttons to press, merely to ensure that the client is adjusted correctly and maintains a comfortable position throughout.

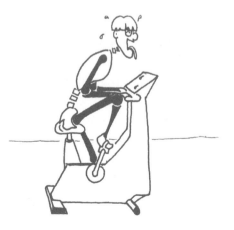

Correct technique and posture

Ensure that the seat height is appropriate to the client.

One way to do this is to get the client to stand next to the bike and measure up the hip joint against the seat height. When the client is standing with feet shoulder-width apart in an upright posture, the hip joint should be level with the top of the saddle.

Another way is to get the client to sit on the bike. When the client's feet are flat within the foot strap, and the client starts pedalling, there should be a *slight* bend in the knee. This ensures that the client does not lock-out the knees as this causes stress on the knee joint.

If the seat is *too* high the hips rock from side to side, and this can put undue strain on the back. If the knee is *too* bent, this not only makes pedalling harder, due to the force angle, but can also put undue strain on the knee.

It is a good idea to mark the number or hole position of the correct seat adjustment onto the client's card.

Ensure that the foot strap is a comfortably tight fit.

Not many people adjust the foot straps because it is time-consuming and sometimes hard to adjust correctly, but it is worth doing. The strap not only ensures that the foot won't slip, but also ensures that the rider is cycling efficiently. By having the foot in the strap correctly, force can be applied on the up stroke as well as the down stroke. If needed, more power can be added throughout the whole pedal revolution.

Ensure posture is correct when pedalling.

Clients should have an upright position with retracted scapula, chest lifted, and abdominals tight. More serious cyclists may maintain a 'racing' position (forward flexion) with their elbows rested on the handlebars. If clients insist on holding this position focus on a neutral spine position making sure they are not slumped over the handlebars.

Ensure that the client pedals at the correct speed.

For the majority of gym users a rate of 70–90 revolutions per minute (RPM) is appropriate. It is worth pointing out to the client that if they pedal too slowly they will generally feel additional tension against the pedals, too fast and tension can be reduced, making the exercise easier. Some models of cycle will prompt a specific speed and may even cut power if the speed is insufficient.

Advantages of the cycle

- Good choice for beginners as they feel 'safe' due to its ease of use and familiarity.

- Quick learning curve.
- Intensity can be lower compared to other machines.
- It supports body weight, so can be less fatiguing for the heavier client.

Disadvantages of the cycle

- Sometimes it can be hard for the client to get a balance of the correct RPM.
- If the seat height is incorrect the experience can be unpleasant or painful.

Common errors while cycling

- Bike seat not set up correctly so that the knee is too bent or locked out.
- Foot straps not set correctly and therefore do not allow correct foot position and transfer of power from the legs.
- RPM is too high or too low.
- Poor posture, slouching or adopting a forward flexed position.

The rower

Background

The rower is an excellent piece of equipment that incorporates both lower and upper body exercise. It is weight-bearing, as the body weight is supported on a sliding seat. The rowing action, if broken down, can actually be quite technical, and in consequence some people are actually discouraged from using it. The rower has had some bad press claiming that it is too hard and intensive to use and that it should not be used by those suffering from a bad back.

The first criticism arises from the fact that most people do not understand the correct stroke action. They either see a hard-core gym fanatic going hell-for-leather and sweating buckets, or have tried rowing and become exhausted quickly, due to inefficient technique. The second criticism is a fallacy because as long as you are teaching the correct rowing technique then the client should have little difficulty, dependent on the exact nature and severity of their back problem.

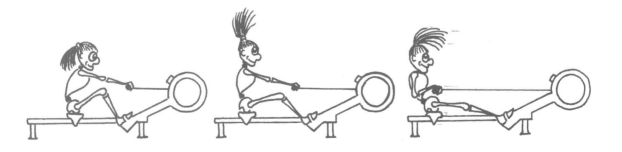

There are now a variety of rowers on the market:

- Most common are the Concept II rowers that utilize air resistance to increase loading.
- Machines with built-in screens allow you to visualize rowing down the river and use electromagnetic resistance.
- Water rowers actually contain water that provides the resistance to the rower's stroke and supposedly simulates competitive rowing most effectively.

Whatever the machine type, the following will give some guidance as to set-up procedures and main teaching points.

Let the client know that the seat moves and ensure that the client's T-shirt is tucked in

Clients have been known to fall off seats due to their T-shirts getting trapped in the seat mechanism.

Show the basic adjustments for resistance, stroke rate and time

In the example of the Concept II rower there is a small screen with which the client must be familiar. As with most machines there is a quick-start programme. This means that the client can start straightaway without putting in their time or distance and stop when the allotted distance/time comes up.

Get the *client* to enter in the variables. Show them how to adjust the resistance against the handle and what stroke rate they should aim for. A higher stroke rate is not always necessary. A slower more efficient stroke is more efficient. The tension adjuster should not always be put up to the maximum as the upper body can tire quickly causing local muscular fatigue and technique can suffer as a consequence.

Ensure the handle is in the clip for ease of use once the foot straps have been done up

Quite often a client has limited flexibility to be able to reach the handle if it is not in the correct holder. They would then have to undo the foot straps.

Show the foot strap position and how to adjust for foot size

The footplate should be adjusted so that the strapping goes across the widest part of the foot. This is generally about level with the lowest lace of the shoe. Ensure the client adjusts their own position so that they are sure of how to adjust it on their next visit.

Explain the start, mid and final positions

The client begins with the bar in hand, sitting upright with elbows slightly bent. Movement is initiated by the legs as pressure is applied through the feet and the legs straighten. Once the bar has passed the knees the arms come into play. The bar is pulled into the body at the level of the mid-abdominals. The return phase begins with the arms straightening past the knees. The legs then bend to return the body to the start position, still maintaining an upright posture.

Make note of the following teaching points:

- Keep shoulders in line with hips throughout the movement.
- Explain that the majority of the power should come from the legs, not the arms.
- Keep knees in line with the feet.
- Ensure that the legs extend but don't lock.
- If the arms are always quite bent then it can be more fatiguing on the upper body.
- Keep wrists in a straight position as the bar approaches the body.

Advantages

- It works both the upper and lower body.
- It supports body weight.
- It can promote good core stability (as it is essential to focus on good form).

Disadvantages

- Some clients might find it hard to master the technique.
- Some clients are put off using it if they have any back weakness, in the belief that rowing is bad for the back. This is a fallacy as, if technique and form are optimal, rowing can promote back strength.

Common errors

- T-shirt hangs out
- Incorrect foot plate positioning
- Locking of legs in the extended position
- Rolling of the wrists as the bar is brought into the chest
- Poor postural control throughout movement
- Letting bar come too high or low
- Using a shortened range of movement. This increases strokes per minute but decreases stroke efficiency
- Leaning backwards excessively from the hip
- Misalignment of ankle, knees and hip

Treadmill

The treadmill has to be the most popular piece of cardiovascular equipment in the gym and most gyms would be wise to include a number of these. They are effective for both walking and running although you do not *have* to run. The treadmill is comparatively easy to use once the client has built up confidence about their walking/running style. Some people feel as though they are having to learn to walk again. Although the moving belt actually stays in one place, it does make co-ordination suffer, which can put some people off using it. Make sure that extra time is allowed for clients to get used to the machine and that demonstrations are clear and offer lots of teaching points.

Explain the set-up and how to reduce speed and stop the machine making reference to any safety cut-out clips that can be attached to the client.

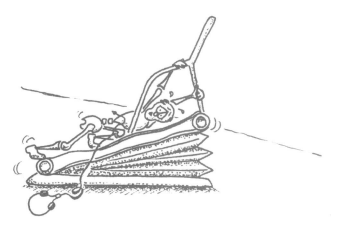

Stand with a foot either side of the belt

This not only puts less strain on the motor but means that the machine does not start with a jolt – which can be unnerving for first-timers.

Test the belt with one foot first

This gives the client a feel for the belt speed and can be reassuring because the belt can appear to be moving a lot faster than it really is.

Strike the belt with heel then toe

This helps with balance. If the toe strikes first, this usually makes the client lean forward. It also disperses the forces through the feet more efficiently, thus reducing impact stresses. Always ensure that appropriate footwear is worn; no bare feet.

Keep central to the belt

If the client stays central to the belt they are less likely to fall off.

Look straight ahead, not down at your feet

It does not help balance when the client is not looking where they are going.

Initially hold rail for balance

The client can hold onto the rails, but it does reduce the exercise intensity and could, if continued, cause lumbar region problems. When the upper body is fixating and the lower body is moving it causes too much rotation in the lower spine.

Make note of the following teaching points:

- The client should keep close to the front of the machine – this will reduce the tendency to creep back which can cause them to fall off.
- The client should keep an upright position and use the arms for balance. If they let the arms swing normally, it can help them get into a rhythm to aid co-ordination.
- As soon as the client is confident, try to coax them to take the speed to the correct intensity.
- Let your client know that it is perfectly normal to get off the machine and feel as though they have just come off a ship!

Advantages

- It is weight-bearing so can be useful for calorie expenditure and preventing osteoporosis.
- It can offer a safe, low-impact workout for more sedentary clients and an effective impact workout for those clients wishing to run.
- Clients can use it effectively and easily and often feel comfortable to work for longer periods of time.

Disadvantages

- The technique feels different from normal walking and can feel strange to clients who have never used a treadmill before as it has a different proprioception. This can be discouraging.
- Clients are often frightened of the machine, especially of falling off.
- Clients tend to hog the machine and stay on it for much longer periods than other machines.

Common errors

- Not letting go of the front bar once balance has been accomplished.
- Pushing hard with the feet whilst leaning forward.
- Running action at walking speed.
- Moving off the centre of the belt and losing balance.
- Looking down at the belt.

- Having the gradient up too high and 'hanging off' the front bar!
- Not staying close to the front of the machine/wandering close to the back of the treadmill.
- Staying on the toes when walking.

Stairs and steps

Background

There is often a lot of confusion between stairs and steps and their use. The main difference between the two is that stairs have an independent action, in that when you press one of the pedals down it will not affect the other pedal. The steps are dependent in that when you press one of the large footplates down, the action causes the other pedal to move. They work in unison.

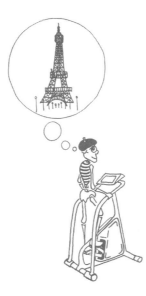

Stair climbing action

There seems to be a great deal of controversy over the various stepping styles. When demonstrating the stairs the action should not be short steps with a small range of motion, but deeper steps, without hitting the top or bottom bump stops. Everyone has their individual differences in style but this will hold true for most people. Feet should be kept flat against the stair platforms. Teach the client to focus on bringing the knees up, as opposed to pushing down hard on the foot platforms, as this can make it harder. Some clients are put off by the stair action as it takes a little getting used to. It is probably best to set the resistance a little higher than anticipated initially, as this reduces the client's feeling that the stairs are falling away underneath them.

Stepper climbing action

Using the stepper requires a slightly different action because you want a full range of motion, full extension of the legs, without locking the knees out. Beware of using momentum to rebound off the bump stops, this will add to the impact and can make it easier. Keep the feet flat on the step platform, allowing for individual differences in ankle flexibility.

General teaching points that can be applied to both the stepper and the stairs are as follows:

Keep an upright position on the machine, look straight ahead with chest up

Clients' posture tends to suffer as they get fatigued, so check and correct posture.

Don't lock out the arms on the rails

Clients have a tendency to lock out their arms to take some weight off their legs to make it easier to complete the stepping. This can put extreme pressure on the elbows. You can hold onto the rails at the front lightly as long as you are not hanging on for dear life!

Advantages

- They offer a challenging workout.
- They are weight-bearing.
- They are excellent at expending calories.
- They work well at targeting lower extremities as well as providing a cardiovascular workout.

Disadvantages

- Clients find ways of cheating. Correct form must be used at all times to get the maximum benefit from both stairs and steps.
- Both machines can be taxing for the more sedentary person, so care must be taken in setting the right levels and evaluating whether the client is suited to the machine.

Common errors

- Wrong depth of step
- Clients allowing the step to bounce off the bump stops and propelling themselves skyward!
- Clients have the incorrect tension settings – either too much resistance, which causes them to stay at the top of the movement and feel they are stepping through treacle, or too little resistance, where they find themselves sinking towards the floor.
- Clients supporting their bodyweight by hanging on to the supports or locking out their arms to take some weight off the legs.
- Leaning over and forwards from the waist.

Cross-trainers

The trend at present is to develop cardiovascular machines that incorporate both upper and lower body. Common cross-trainers are:

Nordic Ski

A simulated cross-country skier, which incorporates the skiing action of the arms, moving backwards and forwards, and the sliding action of the legs. These particular machines tend to be used more at home.

Versa climber

An upright machine where the feet are secured in foot straps and the arms hold onto adjustable bars. The arms and legs work in unison. Various options include additional resistance and a seated version. The trick to using the versa climber is to have smooth movements and not to overextend the arms and legs when moving. Some people tend to use quick short movements but ideally the movements should encourage full range of movement without this extending into a full stretch. A common problem is that people set off too quickly – it is best to pace yourself! It can be quite a hard machine, so would probably suit a fitter client.

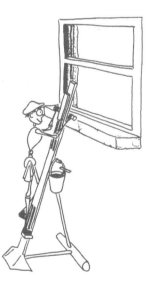

Reebok Skywalker

Similar to the action of the Nordic Ski but you are suspended off the floor into giant footplates. The arms are involved by pushing and pulling on the handles and the legs swing backwards and forwards. It could be quite intimidating for the beginner, due to the sheer size of the machine!

Elliptical trainer

This requires a combination movement of a treadmill and cross-country ski action where the legs move in a figure of eight. Resistance can be varied by moving the ramp at the front of the machine either up or down. The action can be reversed so that the legs are travelling backwards. This is a low-impact machine that is gaining popularity.

Advantages

- They offer variation from the normal workout and challenge the body in a way it may be unaccustomed to.
- They can offer a time-efficient workout for the client as most work upper and lower body.
- Most are weight-bearing improving bone density.
- They offer a high-intensity, low-impact exercise option.
- The resistance adjustments work well to increase muscle tone.
- Due to the different joint actions involved in some of these machines, they can replicate sporting activities and help to provide sport specific adaptations within the working muscles.

Disadvantages

- Techniques can be tricky to master.
- Heart rate can increase easily due to the use of upper and lower body muscle mass and weight-bearing effect, therefore clients can go beyond pre-set heart rate parameters.
- Some of the cross-trainers may be more suited to the fitter clientele only.

Common errors

- Feet sliding or moving from foot plates.
- Postural changes from the upright position.
- Locking of limbs, either knees or arms.
- Wrong resistance settings causing unnatural movement patterns.
- Not allowing the heel to rise in its natural movement.

This covers the main types of cardiovascular machines found within gyms, although new products are being developed all of the time. Our attention will now turn to resistance exercises. As most resistance machines have clear instructions available, for the user and the instructor, on their sides, the focus of this chapter turns to instruction tips relating to free weights exercises.

Free weights instruction

The following tables summarize the most common free weights exercises for the major muscle groups. They cover:

- muscles used
- correct set-up procedures
- essential teaching points

Dumbell front raise

Muscles used
Deltoid.

Set up
Feet hip width apart facing forward, knees soft, abdominals tight, upright posture, shoulders back (hips, knees, feet in alignment).

Teaching points
Start with palms facing you, elbows slightly bent. Raise dumb-bell out in front of body to shoulder level. Keep elbows bent throughout the movement and wrists in line with forearms.

Additional information
It can be easier on the shoulder and more 'functional' to do it in a 'thumbs up' position.

Single arm row

Muscles used
Latissimus dorsi, biceps brachii, posterior deltoid.

Set up
Lent on bench with body parallel to floor. One knee on the bench, with same side arm resting on the bench with elbow bent. Head in line with spine. Other leg is extended back with knee bent. Exercising arm elbow slightly bent.

Teaching points
Arm extended slightly forwards from shoulder. Dumb-bell moves in either a diagonal or arc towards the hip, letting the elbow extend beyond the body. The torso stays stationary and the abdominals tight.

Additional information
More upper back can be targeted if the elbow is taken directly out to the side and up.

Dumbell bent arm pullover

Muscles used
Latissimus dorsi, pectoralis major.

Set up
Lying on bench, with one dumb-bell held in both hands at lower sternum level. Neutral spine. Keeping elbows slightly bent. Palms up with dumb-bell discs up to ceiling.

Teaching points
Let the dumbbell go back to shoulder level, keeping elbows fixed in bent position. Watch wrists are not extended. Return to top position.

Additional information
Ensure that the elbows stay fixed and do not straighten throughout the movement.

Behind the neck press (barbell)

Muscles used
Deltoids, triceps brachii.

Set up
Once barbell is behind neck, ensure upper arm is parallel to floor, elbows at 90°, wrists in line with forearms. Knuckles up hand position. Neutral spine. Head up. Do not lock out in top position.

Teaching points
Feet hip/shoulder width apart, knees soft, abdominals tight, head up, shoulders back. Wrists in line with forearm, knuckles up.

Additional information
People have different ranges of movement for this that may limit their movement capabilities. This can be quite damaging for the shoulder joint.

Shoulder press (dumb-bell)

Muscles used
Deltoids, triceps brachii

Set up
Feet hip/shoulder width apart, knees soft, abdominals tight, shoulders back, arms out to side with elbows at 90°, wrists in line with forearms, knuckles up.

Teaching points
Move the dumb-bell upwards and inwards in an arc so that at the top of the movement dumb-bells are overhead close to each other. Do not lock elbows, keep wrists in line with forearm.

Additional information
It may be easier on the shoulder joint if arms are brought slightly forward. Hands do not have to be facing front (palm forward), they can be slightly angled.

Lateral raise

Muscles used
Deltoid

Set up
Feet shoulder/hip width apart, knees soft, abdominals tight, shoulders back, looking ahead. Elbows slightly bent.

Teaching points
Taking the arms away from the body to shoulder level. Elbows stay slightly higher than hands. Palms stay parallel to floor throughout. Elbows are maintained slightly bent.

Additional information
Leaning slightly forward from the hip brings the medial deltoid on top of the shoulder and is said to create a greater contraction to the target area.

Barbell upright row

Muscles used
Deltoids, trapezius, biceps brachii

Set up
Feet shoulder/hip width apart, knees soft, abdominals tight, shoulders back, upright position. Holding bar at about shoulder width, knuckles facing the floor.

Teaching points
Leading with the elbows, palms stay facing the body, the bar stays close to the body. The elbows are raised until the upper arm is level with the deltoids. Keep the body erect.

Additional information
Be aware that traditionally this is done by a close grip, but this may limit ROM. Ensure the body maintains upright with neutral spine.

Bench press (barbell)

Muscles used
Pectoralis major, triceps brachii, deltoids

Set up
Lying on the bench, neutral spine, abdominals tight. Once bar is in hands, keep wrists in line with forearms, knuckles up, elbows slightly bent, bar kept at lower sternum level.

Teaching points
Bar hand width position can be ascertained by taking the bar down so upper arms are parallel to floor and elbows are then 90°. Arms are taken to a straight but not locked position.

Additional information
Depending on the height of the bench, it may be necessary to raise the feet up. The bar need not come to the chest, the length of the bar travel is dependent on the upper arm being parallel to the floor.

Chest press (dumb-bell)

Muscles used
Pectoralis major, triceps brachii, deltoid.

Set up
Lying supine on the bench, neutral spine, abdominals tight. Dumb-bells held with wrists in line with forearm, knuckles up, palms facing forward, elbows slightly soft. Dumb-bells held at lower sternum level.

Teaching points
Dumb-bells taken back in arc, so that upper arm goes parallel to the floor and elbows are at 90°. On the upward phase, dumb-bells return in an arc so that in the top position the dumb-bells are close together. Do not lock arms.

Additional information
Weights are controlled and not 'banged' together at the top!

Dumb-bell flyes

Muscles used
Pectoralis major, deltoids.

Set up
Lying supine on the bench, neutral spine, abdominals tight. Dumb-bells held with wrists in line with forearm, knuckles up, palms facing each other, elbows slightly soft, with arms extended. Start with dumb-bells close.

Teaching points
Dumb-bells are taken straight out, whilst elbows are maintained soft, until the upper arm is parallel to the floor, and then returned. Ensure arms are not straightened on the downward phase.

Additional information
A variation offers the arms to go out in an arc whilst palms face forward instead of together.

Dumb-bell prone fly

Muscles used
Posterior deltoid, rhomboids, trapezius.

Set up
Lying prone on the bench, neutral spine, abdominals tight. Arms are taken out so that there is a 90° angle at the armpits and the body, and arms are in a 'T' shape. Dumb-bells are held with palms down, knuckles up, elbows slightly bent.

Teaching points
Arms are brought up and back, whilst maintaining elbows bent. Arms are taken behind the body to whatever ROM is. All the movement comes from the shoulder.

Additional information
A variation of this is where arms are kept at 90° at armpit, but elbows are bent at 90° and palms face towards the feet, knuckles down.

Supine triceps press (barbell)

Muscles used
Triceps brachii.

Set up
Lying supine on bench, neutral spine, elbows pointing to ceiling, with elbows bent and palms facing the ceiling. Elbows kept at shoulder width.

Teaching points
The arms are extended at the elbow whilst keeping the elbows fixated. Wrists are kept in line with spine. Be careful to straighten, but not lock the elbows.

Additional information
To make it slightly harder, keep the elbows slightly facing back towards your face (45°).

Single arm triceps press (Dumb-bell)

Muscles used
Triceps brachii.

Set up
Sat in an upright position, neutral spine, abdominals tight, shoulders back, feet flat on floor, knees at 90°. The exercising arm is raised up so that the elbow is pointing to the ceiling, hand behind. The other hand supports the exercising arm.

Teaching points
Maintaining an upright position, extend the arm so that the arm straightens but not locks.

Additional information
This can be done lying in a supine position with either one or two arms.

Barbell curl

Muscles used
Biceps brachii, wrist flexors.

Set up
Feet shoulder/hip width apart, knees soft, abdominals tight, shoulders back, upright position. Barbell is at a comfortable distance (usually slightly wider than shoulder width), elbows slightly bent. Wrists in line with forearm.

Teaching points
Barbell is raised whilst maintaining elbows fixed into side, wrists stay in line with forearm throughout. Careful not to take arms away from the body and lean back.

Additional information
Take into consideration the 'carrying angle' of each individual.

Seated dumb-bell curls

Muscles used
Biceps brachii, wrist flexors.

Set up
Sat down in an upright position, neutral spine, abdominals tight, shoulders back, feet flat on floor, knees 90°. Elbows into side of body, palms up with wrists in line with forearm, elbows slightly bent.

Teaching points
Dumb-bell is raised with elbows fixed into side of body until full ROM achieved. Upper body is kept upright. Wrists kept in line with forearm.

Additional information
It may be helpful to use an adjustable bench to support the back.

Barbell squat

Muscles used
Quadriceps, gluteus maximus, hamstrings.

Set up
Bar is placed on top of back (trapezius) via squat rack or clean and heave movement. Feet hip/shoulder width apart, knees soft, abdominals tight, shoulders back, upright position. Slight forward flexion looking ahead, neutral spine.

Teaching points
On the downward movement, head looks ahead maintaining neutral spine, sit back and allow the body to move downward taking the lower body no lower than 90°. Pause momentarily, keeping neutral spine bar staying central to the body, forcing up until knees come to slightly soft position.

Additional information
Those with longer limbs need not necessarily go down to 90°. Aim to keep heels to the floor. It may be a good idea to practice without weight first as it is quite a technical exercise.

Modified Clean and Heave Exercise (broken down)

Exercise One – Dead Lift

Muscles used
Erector spinae, quadriceps, gluteus maximus, hamstrings.

Set up
Bar is kept slightly over the feet, feet shoulder width or slightly wider, knees soft, abdominals tight, neutral spine, chest up, shoulders back, looking ahead, grip bar at about shoulder width using an overhand grip, keeping elbows very slightly bent.

Teaching points
From the pick up position, spine is kept neutral, abdominals tight, chest up, looking ahead. Raising up with feet flat on the floor, the upper body pulls the bar, keeping the chest lifted, into a standing position with knees/elbows slightly bent. The body is now erect ready for phase 2.

Additional information
The next movement brings the bar travelling upwards close to the body using momentum to get it to an upright row.

Exercise Two – Upright Row (Catch)

Muscles used
Deltoids, trapezius, wrist flexors.

Set up
Knees stay soft, abdominals tight, upright position. The bar stays close to the body. Elbows lead until upper arm is parallel to floor.

Teaching points
Leading with the elbows, palms facing the body, keeping the bar close. Looking ahead, abdominals maintained tight.

Additional information
Once the bar is up by the upper chest, the wrists are rotated and the arms dropped underneath. The body drops underneath allowing the bar to be caught whilst the knees are softened to take the force of the bar.

Exercise Three – Shoulder Press (Heave)

Muscles used
Deltoids, triceps brachii.

Set up
Bar is resting close to body by upper chest, wrists stay in line with forearm, keeping an upright body position, knuckles up.

Teaching points
From this position, the body position is dropped and a little momentum from the body gets the bar travelling upwards, the arms extend and straighten, keeping wrists in line with forearm. The knees bend a little to take the force of the weight.

Additional information
On the return the bar is brought to the upper chest, wrists rotated, bar is kept close to body to the upper thighs and then returned to the floor always maintaining neutral spine.

Free weight spotting techniques

Gym safety is imperative, and part of that safety, from an instructor's point of view, is spotting.

> Baechle (1994) defines spotting as 'actions taken by the spotter to protect the lifter from injury', and the spotter as 'someone who assists the lifter in the execution of the exercise'.

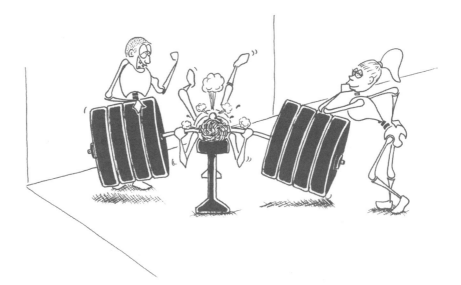

The spotter has three main functions. In order of importance they are:

1 To protect the lifter from injury (and to avoid injury to themselves).
2 To recommend technique changes to improve the quality of execution and therefore benefit the lifter.
3 Motivating the litter to achieve greater overload and intensity.

Before spotting

- Not everyone will ask you to spot, so be aware that some people may object to being touched. Ask beforehand, to make sure that they are aware of what you intend to do.
- Ensure all extraneous equipment is cleared from the area where you are spotting, so that the client and the spotter come to no harm.
- Other users must be informed to stay clear, if attempting a lift such as a barbell overhead lift, so that there is no interference, and therefore no accidents.

- Ensure that you are able to safely control the weight that your client is lifting. Consider whether it is necessary to have a **second spotter**. If in doubt – get another spotter! Never take on a spot if you feel it is beyond your capabilities alone.
- Ensure that there is good communication between you and your client. Ensure that the client knows the correct technique for the chosen exercise.
- If the client is advanced they may have a preference as to where they would like you to spot them. Make sure that this is communicated prior to the lift. However, you must do what is safest for the client and yourself!
- As a spotter, ensure that you are in the optimum position to spot from.
- Before the lift ensure that the weight is evenly loaded and that the barbell/dumb-bell is safe for use. Especially ensure that collars are secure.
- Ensure that you both know the exact number of repetitions required, prior to the lift.
- Allow the client time to focus on the lift as, if it is a heavy weight, it may need a lot of concentration.
- If the client is using dumb-bells then generally it is preferable for them to lift the weight from the rack or from the floor. If the spotter tries to pass the weight it could be dropped. This principle can be applied to barbell exercises apart from ones where there is a rack. Here the spotter may assist the client to the start of the exercise.

During the lift

- Pay attention at all times. Focus entirely on the client. You need to be aware of any problems and be ready to offer assistance in an instant.
- Make sure that you have an optimum grip on the barbell dumb-bell so that if the client suddenly becomes fatigued you will be able to take the weight. Generally, it is best to use an over grip, with fingers and thumb wrapped around the bar.
- Just as before the lift, ensure that any communication is clear and direct.
- Get in position ready to spot. With your hands and the client's hands in position ensure that both parties are ready. Ask the client if they are ready, and then you can assist in lifting the weight to the start position. Don't let go until the client has said that they are okay. Some spotters say 'Your bar' to which the client says 'My bar'. This ensures that there is no confusion over the handing over process.
- Don't over spot. There is nothing more infuriating than a spotter who lifts too much of the weight or lifts too early on in the lift. Not only are you robbing the lifter of the required overload, but also you diminish the sense of achievement.
- The client should indicate whether they need you to spot, but always look for non-verbal cues and signs that they may want assistance. Obvious cues would be poor technique, uneven weight distribution and grimacing facial expression.

- Offer words of encouragement, but at the right time. A few words from the spotter can give an extra kick of motivation to do 'just one more rep!' Just ensure that the client knows his/her limits.
- Don't distract the client at any time during the lift. Idle chatter does not go down very well.
- Ensure that the weight is safely on the floor or put back in the rack holder before you consider the lift accomplished.

After the lift

- Review the exercise by discussing: use of correct assistance, correct intensity, exercise form and overall effectiveness.
- Ensure that the weights used are returned to the correct area and that it is left safe for other users.

Spotting guidance

Table 10.1 serves as a guide to assist in free weight exercises. It may be necessary to do some techniques slightly differently, so you just need to use common sense. In general it is best to spot near the weight. As with many skills, spotting techniques improve with experience. Each client will demand different things from you. In turn you will learn how to deal with each client, to maximize their effectiveness and safety.

Table 10.1 Spotting positions

Exercise name	Position of spotter(s)	Hold position on client or equipment
Barbell squat	Preferably one either side, standing at each bar end. Single spotter stands behind client.	A spotter stands holding each bar end, as opposed to the client. Single spotter holds client's upper torso just under armpits. Can also support close to waist.
Static dumb-bell lunge	Just behind client.	Hold on waist.
Barbell bench press	One spotter stands at each end of the bar. Single spotter stands behind client's head.	One spotter holds each bar end. Single spotter holds on to bar with palms facing self, close to the client and bar.
Dumb-bell fly	Behind client. A kneeling position can be more comfortable.	Clasp on wrists
Dumb-bell bench press	Behind client.	Clasp on wrists.
Seated barbell shoulder press	Standing behind and above client, preferably on raised platform.	Holding onto bar.

Table 10.1 (*cont'd*)

Exercise name	Position of spotter(s)	Hold position on client or equipment
Standing lateral raise	In front of client.	Holding on to or just supporting the wrists.
Prone reverse fly	Kneeling in front, just beside client's head.	Holding on to or just supporting wrists.
Barbell upright row	Standing in front of client.	Holding on to or just supporting bar.
Triceps kickback	Standing beside the client's exercising arm.	Holds on to or supports the exercising arm.
Barbell prone triceps extension	Kneeling or standing behind client.	Holding on to or just supporting barbell.
Dumb-bell prone triceps extension	Kneeling or standing behind client.	Clasping wrists.
Seated single overhead dumb-bell extension	Standing beside or behind the client on the exercising arm.	Clasping wrist.
Barbell curl	Standing in front of client.	Supporting the bar.
Standing dumb-bell curl	Standing in front of client.	Holding wrists preferably, otherwise just supporting them.
Dumb-bell calf raise	Standing behind client.	Holding on to waist.

Exercise prescription issues

For any gym programme to be safe and effective and to allow individuals to achieve their fitness goals a number of different factors have to be considered. Having obtained in-depth information regarding the individual's goals, current activity levels, medical or injury issues and their likes and dislikes within the gym environment you are ready to design their programme card.

Programme prescription is a controversial and creative area that is continually developing in the light of new research and training methods. However, in general, cards need to be tailored to the individual as specifically as possible, reviewed regularly and adapted to continually progress the individual towards their goals. Writing a standard programme for every individual will not enable their goals to be met as effectively or within the desired time frame. It also leads your client to become demotivated and to stop attending the gym.

It is best to begin with a blank programme card and an open mind containing many questions. Think of every piece of equipment available, constantly return to your individual's goals and desires and balance the two to create a programme that can be adapted and redesigned as and when necessary to ensure progressive overload occurs along with enjoyment of the routine.

Table 10.2 Gym programme overview

Component	Content	Duration
Introduction	Self Health and safety Programme card	5–10 mins
Warm-up	Mobilization Pulse-raiser Preparatory stretches	5–15 mins
Main body of programme	Cardiovascular session Resistance session	10–60 mins
Pulse-lowerer	Cardiovascular cool-down	3–5 mins
Floorwork	Abs and back training	5–15 mins
Cool-down	Flexibility Relaxation Revitalizer	5–15 mins
End session	Ask for feedback, any questions Inform of procedure on next visit and where to go for assistance if necessary Thank them, praise them, say goodbye	2–3 mins

Nothing is necessarily right or wrong. Just be prepared to justify every decision and make it relevant to your client's goals and all the initial interview information.

The questions you need to ask

When designing a programme of activity for clients it is important to consider all the variables. Once you have completed a programme use the following template to analyse its effectiveness and see whether it is safe and effective.

- Have you considered all the components of fitness?
- What were your client's specific goals?
- Are the goals prioritized?
- Have you written the programme taking into consideration all lifestyle and time constraints?
- Have you applied the specific adaptation to imposed demand (SAID) principle?
- Do you feel that the programme is suitable to cause adaptation?
- Is there any information regarding progression?
- Is your warm-up sufficient and relevant?
- Do you need to apply any specific mobilization prior to increasing intensity?
- Are the stretches chosen for the preparatory section suitable? →

→

- Is the intensity chosen for the cardiovascular section adequate?
- Are the cardiovascular machines set out appropriately to allow for a maintenance of heart rate?
- Within the resistance section, have you considered the following factors: reps and sets for goals, choice of machines or free weights, balance of agonist and antagonistic muscles, larger muscle groups first, erector spinae and rectus abdominus last, secondary muscles not brought in prior to primary fatigue, i.e. triceps before chest press, type of contraction, speed of movement, rest periods, etc.
- Can you periodize or split the programme in any way?
- Is the programme realistic for them to achieve?
- Have you considered using any other club facilities in the programme?
- Have you chosen specific developmental stretch areas?
- Is the cool-down effective?
- Have you included sufficient information for them to follow the programme and understand it without you present?

Case studies for evaluation of programme design

SCENARIO 1

Mrs Jones is a 56-year-old administrator. She has had a deskbound job all her life and decides to take up more regular physical activity.

She is concerned about the onset of osteoporosis and wants to increase her bone density and get generally fit.

She would like to do some CV work and some resistance work but has never used any equipment before and is a bit apprehensive about using the gym. She can come in three times per week.

She has no coronary heart disease risk factors other than being over 50, and has no injuries.

SCENARIO 2

Mr Roberts is a 60-year-old retired business executive. He has always had a sedentary job and drove a lot. The only activity he previously undertook was squash, and he played this on a fairly regular basis (twice weekly).

He would like to get generally fit by doing some CV work and some resistance work, feels that his flexibility is limited, and wants to lose some weight. He can come in up to three times a week.

He has a weak lower back with no specific disc problem, is slightly overweight, and also smokes over 20 cigarettes a day.

SCENARIO 3

Sarah Thomas is a 24-year-old nurse, who would like a programme written to improve her hockey. She is currently a club player for the 2nd team and wants to improve her performance to get in the 1st team as she feels that it is her fitness that is letting her down, not her skill.

She wants a gym programme that will improve her stamina, strength and flexibility that relates to her centre half position.

She has no injuries but gets the occasional twinge from her knee. This has never stopped her training at all. She can come in four times per week.

The aim here is to write a programme that can be used in the gym and incorporates their wishes. Analyse the data given, showing why you have designed each aspect of the programme that way.

CHAPTER SUMMARY

- Ensure that you demonstrate each piece of equipment before the client and allow the client to programme the machine in order to gain confidence.

- When demonstrating any piece of equipment inform the client of the name and function of the machine, what muscles it works, what posture and technique to adopt and how this relates to their goals.

- The spotter's responsibility is to ensure the safety of the lifter and to ensure correct technique of the lift with maximal weight.

- Different information needs to be given to the spotter before, during and after the lift.

- Programme prescription can only be done after many questions have been asked. All programmes should be balanced, goal-orientated and prioritized. Specific overload needs to be applied, progressive and realistic. Recovery should be planned.

Circuit training

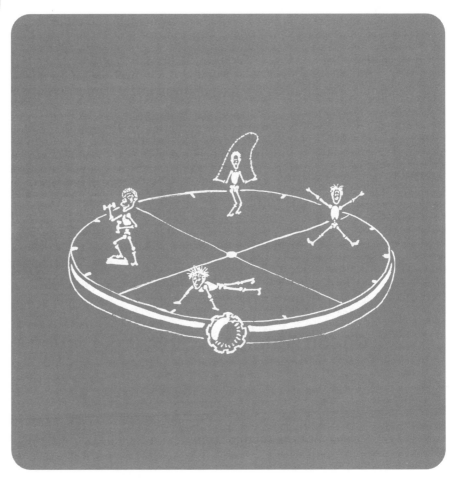

Topics to be covered in this chapter:

- Technical definition
- The benefits of circuit training
- Class design principles
- Different class formats
- Class layouts
- Teaching skills and motivational methods
- Sport-specific circuit programmes

Circuit training as a structured exercise session was introduced into England in the 1950s. Originally it revolved around free weights with machines being introduced at a later date. It remains a popular class format as it appeals to a variety of individuals, whether male or female, trained or untrained, as any class can be adapted to suit any ability or fitness level.

Generally, less co-ordination is required to complete a circuits class and this format may, therefore, encourage a crossover between the gym and the studio especially if the class itself is not run within the gym environment. Depending on the selection and sequences of exercises, a circuits class can be tailored to be specific to a particular sport or to target a specific energy system.

Circuit training is an instructor-led multi-activity workout, allowing for a more personal touch than within the gym, and perhaps encouraging individuals to train harder or more efficiently than they would on their own. It encourages cross-training, adds variety to a gym routine and encourages social interaction between participants who are often paired.

Circuit training technical definition

The planned execution of a series of exercises, in a predetermined sequence, for an allocated time or number of repetitions.

The benefits of circuit training

Regular attendance at a well-structured circuits class will provide the same benefits as any other mixed cardiovascular and resistance exercise session.

Many claims have been made to suggest that circuits can provide greater benefits than other forms of exercise, through increased metabolism before and after the session and increased body fat-lowering potential. However, research has been inconclusive due to the lack of a standard in the experimental design.

In general, the benefits can be seen as:

- providing a full body workout
- training all five components of fitness
- offering a multi-level challenging workout for anyone
- being space and time-efficient
- requiring little co-ordination
- being sport-specific and aiding cross-training goals

The location can also be varied depending on the facilities and the equipment available.

Studio circuits

This is the most common environment. Any amount of the normal studio equipment used in aerobics and step classes can be utilized. This will be a familiar style of class for anyone from the armed forces and represents the standard image of a circuits class, with stations placed in a circle around the perimeter of the studio.

Gym circuits

This is a slightly newer format and can involve any number of the cardiovascular and resistance machines usually found in the gym. However, some gyms have gone a step further and introduced specialized equipment for these activities. This generally means there is a set area for the classes and the equipment is easy to operate and quick to adapt to different fitness levels and body shapes. Air pressure machines are ideal in this situation, as the machines resistance can be altered at the touch of a button. These machines are also time-efficient in that they allow for resistance to be applied in both directions.

For example, on a knee extension machine the quadriceps extend the knee on the initial phase and the hamstrings then flex the knee to return the machine to the start position. This is an example of **dual concentric**

contraction action and is similar to the way muscles work in water as discussed in Chapter 14.

Spin circuits

With the introduction of studio or gym-based cycling classes, there have been many classes alternating between resistance stations and these specialized cycles.

Outdoor circuits

These can also be labelled 'cross-training sessions' and are very popular in the summer months as they add fun and variety to your normal class format. Consider whether any additional insurance cover is required for outdoor sessions at your centre. If you have a flat grassy area then equipment may be utilized. More commonly, the emphasis is on body weight, partner resistance and the creative use of various obstacles and structures like park benches en route.

Some leisure centres have what they call 'trim trails' around the perimeter of their property. Along this running trail are a number of stations with set exercises suggested at each. Just be careful with uneven ground, unsafe structures and the likelihood that some class members may suffer from hayfever or have an allergy to bee stings! Consider an additional and specific PAR-Q related to outdoor training.

Aqua circuits

Water provides additional resistance and support for any cardiovascular and resistance exercise and is, therefore, an ideal environment for circuits. Intensity can be raised without the sweating responses and feelings of discomfort experienced on land. Higher-impact activities can be added to the class without an increase in the risk of musculo-skeletal stress or impact injuries. It can be an invaluable aspect to a rehabilitation programme. The exact content and equipment used in these classes are discussed more fully in Chapter 14.

Class design principles

The basic class structure is similar to that for either a gym programme or exercise to music class. The one additional element within a circuits class is what is called the second pulse-raiser that occurs after the pre-workout stretches. This is aimed at raising the intensity of the class to that suitable for participants to enter the circuit.

Circuit training class overview

- Introduction to yourself, the venue and class structure
- Circuit station demonstration
- Warm-up (mobilization, first pulse-raiser and pre-workout stretches)
- Second pulse-raiser
- Main body of circuit
- Pulse lowered
- Floorwork
- Cool-down (flexibility, relaxation and revitalizer)
- Feedback from class

Screening

As with any class or activity, you should determine if the participants are suited to the class format and content and if there are any contraindications, medical problems or injuries that may affect their ability to complete the circuit.

This can be done in two ways:

- Written screening (via PAR-Q form)
- Verbal screening

At the very least, the latter should always take place at the start of every class, giving individuals the opportunity to come to you privately with any questions or revelations they may have. This is best done while you are rewinding music tapes or laying out the circuit cards.

This procedure is particularly important for any new participants. Whenever possible, these individuals should be talked to and introduced to the circuit before the start of the class. A careful eye should be kept on them during the class for the first week.

The warm-up

The reasons to warm up are the same as with any other class or workout. All moves should be relevant to mobilizing each major joint and to the content of the class. The intensity should be progressive and the impact should be low within this initial warm-up phase. There is plenty of opportunity within the second pulse-raiser to increase intensity and to add impact in preparation for the circuit. Within this initial section the joints are less able to deal effectively with the stress associated with high-impact moves. In addition to this, the intensity has a tendency to drop a little during the pre-workout stretch session, so from this perspective there is little point in increasing the intensity before these have been completed.

The content of your warm-up will depend on a number of factors:

- The location of the class (gym, studio or outdoors)
- The space available
- The equipment available
- The content of your main circuit
- The co-ordination level of the class
- The preferences of your class
- Your confidence, as an instructor, with aerobic moves

The particular style of your warm-up could fall within any of three categories:

- Aerobic-style
- Running
- Participants are pre-warmed

Aerobic-style warm-up

Typically, your regular circuit training attendees will not voluntarily attend an aerobics class, and therefore, do not feel too comfortable with co-ordinated moves to music. However, to achieve the benefits of a warm-up, the major joints of the body need to be taken through their full range of movement. The heart rate needs to be raised and the way to achieve this is to involve movements of these major muscle groups; perhaps rhythmically.

If an aerobic-style warm-up is chosen, make it simple, with early cueing, and amend the format if there is negative feedback after a couple of weeks. Remember that anything new is generally resisted for the first couple of weeks until people feel more comfortable and confident.

Running

If the studio is sufficiently large, more of a running-style warm-up can be completed. The content of this style of warm-up, as the name suggests, is predominantly running around the perimeter or length of the studio. The speed of the circuits or shuttles will progressively increase throughout the warm-up until they end on a sprint. Although this is a simple and familiar format for many circuit attendees, it can alienate newcomers or the less fit. It is not uncommon for the participants to be working maximally after only ten minutes of activity!

The structure of this warm-up style needs redefining. 'Gradual' and 'progressive' are the key terms to apply. Initially, the class should be instructed to walk, as the level of impact, as well as intensity, needs to be gradually applied to the body. Low-impact options should be given throughout to ensure you are catering for all ability levels. The warm-up is performed with or without music. If music is played, it is for background purposes only, with no emphasis on working to a beat.

Whatever the chosen style of the warm-up, the moves need to replicate the moves to be done during the circuit.

Pre-warmed

In the case of a gym class or a spin circuits class situated in the gym, you may find that participants turn up already warmed, or do so under your instruction on the nearby cardiovascular machines. However, you can lose a little control over your participants. You rely on them arriving early enough to warm themselves sufficiently and there may be no specific rehearsal of moves to be completed in the circuit.

Main body of circuit

Circuit classes contain a variety of exercises, each exercise being labelled a **'station'** on the circuit. This station could involve a cardiovascular or a resistance exercise for a certain duration (number of seconds) or number of repetitions.

Between stations there is a rest, recovery or transfer time, that allows the individual to regain their breath, rest their muscle fibres and set up correctly for the next exercise. One of the ways in which circuits are recognized as time-efficient is because this rest period can be active rest. In other words, while one body part is worked another rests, so there is activity almost continuously throughout the duration of the class.

Depending on the nature of the circuit, any fitness component can be emphasised. This would lead to a variety of class names:

- aerobic circuit
- strength circuit
- endurance circuit
- plyometric circuit
- power circuits
- step circuit
- aqua circuits

The same factors need to be taken into consideration when designing any of the above classes.

Factors under review include:

- choice of exercises
- sequence of exercises
- intensity
- the work/rest ratio
- the overall volume of work (affected by the above)

Usually most formats revolve around a mixture of cardiovascular and resistance stations, sometimes alternately, depending on the fitness component to be emphasized and the ability level of the class. In addition to the different components of fitness, both the anaerobic and aerobic energy systems will be utilized.

Choice of exercises

The beauty of circuit training lies in the fact that such a variety of exercises can be included in any circuit of any style. This enables participants to work each muscle in different ways to maximize fibre recruitment on resistance stations. With the cardiovascular stations the inclusion of some simple equipment means that you can make the station fun while asking the individual to work at a higher intensity than they normally would without the equipment. An example of how this works can be seen on skipping stations.

The exact stations you decide to put into your circuit will depend on many factors:

- the available space
- available equipment
- transfer time necessary
- the training objective
- consideration of muscle balance
- fitness and skill levels of the class

Sequence of exercises

This needs to ensure even distribution of mechanical stress on the joints and physiological stress on the cardiovascular and energy systems. Care needs to be taken not to overload any particular muscle group. This is a common problem for the deltoid as it is active in all upper body exercises except for those where the deltoid is the antagonist. This needs clever sequencing of your upper body stations to ensure the deltoid can recover before being asked to work again.

Common pre-fatigue issues are seen when the triceps dips station precedes the press-up station. Unless you are working with an advanced group and it is your intention to pre-fatigue the triceps, avoid this amount of overload for your average participants.

The format of your class will alter your sequence of muscle groups. Never forget that, if you have designed a circular circuit, the first station follows the last station. It is easy to pre-fatigue or excessively overload a joint or muscle group in this situation.

It is now generally agreed that, unless you are working with advanced groups, your main circuit stations should not contain any abdominal or lower back stations. As these are the postural muscles that are actively working throughout the circuit to maintain good posture, they should not be unduly fatigued during the circuit. If they are included, you are likely to see a reduction in form and exercise technique that could lead to injury.

On a more positive note, it is essential that your participants reach their desired target heart rate zones and the sequence of stations should enable this to happen.

Intensity

One of the significant benefits of circuit training is that individuals can monitor and alter their own exercise intensity at any stage throughout the class. This is provided that you explain to them that they are responsible for monitoring this and that there are clear options for them to take to increase or decrease intensity.

The methods for altering intensity on cardiovascular and resistance stations will differ and need to be made very clear to your participants.

Methods of increasing cardiovascular station intensity include:

- increasing the speed of the exercise
- increasing the size of the move
- adding arm patterns
- adding travel to the move
- adding impact

Methods of increasing resistance station intensity:

- ensure full range of motion
- increase the resistance
- reduce the speed of the exercise
- place the emphasis on the eccentric phase of the exercise

The aim of the resistance station is to reach momentary failure of the muscle group through local fatigue. It is your responsibility to ensure that each participant is working within their capacity and reaching this point. With cardiovascular stations participants should reach their target heart rates. This suggests the need for you to monitor their intensity to ensure that this is happening. There are five commonly used methods. Each method should not be viewed as a separate entity; it is wise to combine methods to ensure accuracy.

- Heart rate monitoring
- Manual pulse checks
- Rating of Perceived Exertion Scale (RPE)
- Talk test
- Observation

Work/rest ratio

Having made your selection of exercises for your circuits class, you need to decide for how long you wish your participants to be working on each of these stations and how much recovery you will allow them between stations. These timings can dramatically alter the amount of work completed in a circuits class. Your decision will be based on a number of factors:

- The duration of your class – usually 45 or 60 minutes.
- Total number of stations within your circuit.
- The emphasis of the circuit – whether endurance- or strength-based.
- The equipment available to you.
- The ability level of your class.

Some examples of work–rest ratios commonly used in classes are given below.

Table 11.1 Work–rest ratios

Work time	Rest time	Ratio	Class emphasis
60 seconds	No recovery	1:0	Aerobic endurance (advanced)
60 seconds	30 seconds	2:1	Aerobic and muscular endurance (beginners)
60 seconds	120 seconds	1:2	Muscular strength
45 seconds	15 seconds	3:1	Aerobic and muscular endurance (intermediate)
30 seconds	30 seconds	1:1	Aerobic and muscular endurance (beginners)

Active recovery

Recovery time allows muscles to rest before they are required to work again or allows time for the heart rate to fall between cardiovascular stations. However, for intermediate to advanced groups recovery can be **active**. This means that not all activity is stopped between stations. While the lower body muscles may be recovering, the upper body muscles can be worked. This makes the best use of time within the circuit while still ensuring that the work being done is effective.

Other class design considerations

Circuit cards

These should clearly identify each station, having written and visual descriptions of the exercise, although they should not be relied upon for execution of correct technique.

Information should include:

- The number of the station
- The name of the exercise
- Whether it is a cardiovascular or resistance station
- The muscle group worked
- A diagram of the start and finish positions
- An easier and a harder alternative
- Three specific teaching points

This information must be backed up by the instructor. These cards can be individually designed and laminated by you or bought from various organizations.

Music

The music structure will be covered in more depth in Chapter 12. The advantages and disadvantages of music need to be touched upon here. Typically many circuit-training instructors will be used to teaching without the use of music. This is useful as the centre may not have a suitable stereo and there is then no pressure for you and your participants to work to the beat of the music.

Advantages of using music

- Adds motivation and fun to the class.
- Creates an atmosphere.
- Can increase the effort that participants put into the exercises by working to a fast beat (on cardiovascular stations).
- Can get the class working together.
- Can be used to cue the station changes.

Disadvantages of using music

- Can make participants feel unco-ordinated if they cannot work to the beat.
- Can encourage exercises to be done too quickly (both cardiovascular and resistance).
- Can reduce the effectiveness of your verbal cues (due to competition).
- May necessitate the use of a microphone (cost implications).
- Choice of music may not appeal to your class.
- The need to use PPL licensed or PPL-free tapes (cost implications).

Current licensing laws mean that a PPL licence should accompany all tapes (unless PPL-free). If an ordinary CD or tape is to be played, the centre itself should still have a licence to play music to an audience.

There are many companies on the market now that provide class tapes. Some companies using original recording artists ask you to pay a monthly subscription for which you will receive a set number of tapes per year.

Circuit equipment

The list of equipment suitable for circuit training is long and varied. Obviously, the limitation will be cost, in terms of what you are willing to buy or what is available at your centre. You will need to be clear on how to use each piece of equipment safely and effectively and know suitable alternatives for use by individuals of different ability levels.

Whether you are bringing your own equipment into classes or using the centre's own kit, it is essential that every piece should be checked to ensure it is in good working order. This means you, as the instructor, getting to the venue early to check the equipment. Before the start of the class, it is advisable to get the participants to double-check all equipment. This will put your mind at rest and alerts the class to the potential dangers of each piece of equipment so that if any should become dangerous during the class they will be able to identify this to prevent an injury from occurring.

Due to the nature of a circuits class there is ample potential for an accident due to:

- The high intensity of some of the exercises
- Quick changes from station to station
- The way equipment can be thrown to the floor
- The fact that equipment can be tripped over

Encourage your class to place equipment on the floor, safely at the edge of the room, using correct lifting technique. This will ensure that your equipment and the participants' lower backs will last a little longer.

Typical equipment found in circuit training classes

- Rubber bands and resistance tubing
- Body bars and barbells
- Dumb-bells
- Medicine balls
- Stability balls
- Steps
- Slides
- Rebounders
- Skipping ropes
- Cones
- Spacehoppers!

Instructor equipment

To appear professional and prepared there are a number of items that you, as the instructor, should consider bringing to your circuits class:

- Circuit cards
- Stopwatch
- Whistle

- Stereo
- Microphone
- Water
- Towel

Different class formats

Combination cardiovascular and resistance circuit

The heart rate remains elevated, particularly if there are only short rest periods and quick transfer between the stations. Usually CV and R stations alternate.

Work period: 30–45 seconds
Rest period: 10–15 seconds

Strength circuit

The work periods are reduced, with longer rest periods, involving equipment or machines to achieve overload. Can involve partner work or small groups to provide a spotter.

Work period: 6–10 reps or 30–60 seconds
Rest period: 1–3 minutes

Utilizes advanced training techniques:

- Super sets – working the same muscle groups in succession in different exercises.
- Matrix training – using partial repetitions at the bottom and top of the ranges of motions in addition to full range of movement exercises.

Pure aerobic circuit

Can build upon endurance or work specifically to increase anaerobic thresholds.

Work period: 30 seconds–5 minutes
Rest period: none–2 minutes

Class layouts

Your circuit stations can be organized in a variety of ways, limited by the shape of the room, presence of pillars, other obstructions and equipment to be utilized. Some of the different layouts are described below, but this is not an exhaustive list. Use your imagination and your venue creatively.

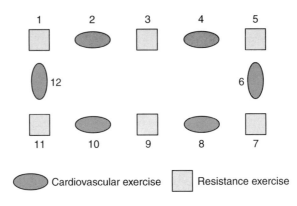

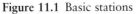

Figure 11.1 Basic stations

Figure 11.2 Double circle

Outer circle: the aerobic circuit

Inner circle: the strength circuit

Options

- Concentrate on one circuit then the other.
- Alternate the stations between the two circles.
- Work in pairs and swap with partner.

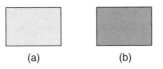

Figure 11.3 Double squares

Circuit a: upper body exercises

Circuit b: lower body exercises

Options

- Class in two groups completing one circuit before transferring.
- Class in pairs and swapping after each station.

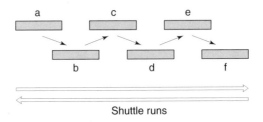

Figure 11.4 Zigzag

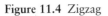

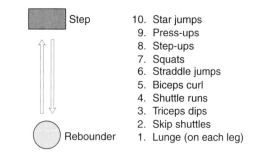

Figure 11.5 Ton-up circuit

Lucky dip

This can apply to any design of circuit. On approach to the station an individual picks a card from those face down by the station. Either this station alone or the whole class completes the exercise chosen. This can apply to the whole circuit or can be used as an activity to bring the class together and concentrate on a particular aspect of fitness.

There are a multitude of other layouts that can work well, keeping your clients interested, motivated and returning to your classes.

Teaching skills and motivational methods

As with any class, your personality will be a factor in who attends it and its nature and emphasis. Whether your class is based in the gym or studio, there are a number of essential skills you will need to demonstrate to ensure it is safe, effective and motivating. These skills are considered in depth in Chapter 15. Some essential points are mentioned here, specific to circuits instruction.

- Organization
- Clear and correct exercise demonstration
- Observation of all participants at all times
- Clear corrective techniques
- Plentiful teaching points
- Early, continuous and various cueing techniques
- Knowledge of suitable adaptations
- Understanding of training principles and exercise selection
- Motivating while controlling competition within the group

Continual observation of the class is difficult in this environment because of the number of people doing a number of different exercises. It is imperative that you, as the instructor, keep your body open to the class and not to turn your back on any individual. When you see incorrect technique, you need to correct it quickly, being careful not to block out the remainder of the class as you turn your attention to one individual.

Methods of correction

These methods are the same, whether the class is exercise to music, step or circuit training-based. Your observation methods need to be more developed in a circuit training environment because, in general, each individual will be doing a different exercise and there are as many different teaching points as there are participants. You will need to develop eyes in the back of your head and rapid, efficient methods of correction.

- Give general teaching points to the class.
- Re-iterate and rephrase teaching points.
- Give specific teaching points.
- Use positive teaching points (rather than negative).
- Make the corrections quickly – recorrect if necessary.
- Ask before using hands-on correction.
- If wearing a microphone, remove it before talking to an individual.

Motivational methods

As ever, motivational methods will depend on the style, goals and participants within your class. There will usually be different methods of motivation used at different stages of the class. For instance, early on the class praise technique, controlled speed and full range of motion on each station. This will ensure correct posture and technique for the later, possibly faster, sections of the class. Towards the peak, focus on positive feedback to individuals on their effort and good form. Voice volume may be elevated and mimicking exercises may play a key role.

All styles and classes will differ. Find the style that suits you and your class, whilst attempting to vary your methods to keep participants working to the best of their ability.

The most common technique is raising the voice and 'bullying' individuals to raise cardiovascular intensity or complete another set of resistance work. Alongside this there are sometimes forfeits for not increasing the intensity as instructed. Although this is one method that can work with advanced groups, you must be aware of the fact that this style is not appreciated by the majority and you must never overlook the fact that an individual may not complete your instructions because they physically cannot do so. You must tailor your methods to the variety of individuals within the class and not adopt a blanket approach.

Forfeits can be used effectively. If you are asking the group to perform a specific exercise with good form and they fail to follow your instructions, then you add an additional exercise into the floorwork section that aims to improve this weakness. Beware of using forfeits carelessly. There is no point in asking a group to complete another high-intensity station because they did not seem to put sufficient effort into the previous high-intensity cardiovascular station. They may simply be trying to tell you they are too tired. Adding a forfeit station will then demotivate them. Forfeits must remain motivational and maintain the balance of your circuit in line with your goals.

Motivational methods could contain all or some of the following:

- Energy and enthusiasm – through your voice, posture and facial expression.
- Encouragement – making eye contact with and giving verbal feedback to every individual.
- Group praise.
- Individual praise.
- Mimicking the action of exercises alongside individuals.
- A variety of exercises specific to the needs of the group.
- A variety of motivational styles to suit the group.
- Use of relevant and good choice of music.
- Effective use of forfeits.

Spotting techniques

You, as the instructor, will effectively be spotting for all your class participants, ensuring good technique, correcting if necessary and giving assistance when required. Alternatively, you can partner up participants to spot for each other on certain circuits. They can also encourage each other and inspire each other to work harder than they would on their own. This is usually done with more advanced groups, as understanding of correct form is needed first.

True spotting techniques are generally associated with free weight strength training sessions where absolute fatigue of the muscle group is achieved and the participant is at risk of injury if they fail to complete the final lift. This could mean that they drop the weight or trap themselves under it. This is unlikely to be the scenario in your circuit but you should keep alert to this possibility.

In large classes of over 30 participants, it is wise to employ an additional person to walk around the class to assist you in correcting technique and ensuring good posture. These individuals are often referred to as spotters.

Circuit demonstration

This can be done at one of two stages of the class:

- Before the warm-up
- After the warm-up

If all class participants are on time and attentive then demonstrating before the warm-up can be an easy option. You can then repeat instructions during the warm-up. Circuit cards at each station will then back up these verbal directives.

If you choose to demonstrate the circuit following the warm-up, you will then have to keep your participants warm as you take them round the circuit, ideally by getting them to replicate the movement to be performed at each station. It is easy to negate the effects of the warm-up by allowing the pulse rate to drop and muscles to cool as they concentrate on what you are demonstrating.

Sport-specific circuit programmes

Although the details of sport-specific training are beyond the scope of this chapter, it is worth taking a brief glance at the considerations necessary to plan for a sport-specific circuit. This will, hopefully, start you thinking about further skills and formats that can be incorporated into these classes.

The main considerations when planning any sports circuit include:

- Establishing which muscle groups are involved with the sport.
- How are these muscle groups used? (What type(s) of contraction predominate?)
- Looking at the muscle groups not so involved and aiming to keep a balance to prevent injury.
- What are the specific joint actions involved?
- What speed of movement around this joint is necessary?
- What energy systems are most relied upon?
- Are there specific flexibility needs?
- Appreciating the idea of periodization – the seasons and cycles within any sport.
- Being aware of the psychology – working alone, pairs or in a small group.

The most important aspect of this circuit is that it has to mimic, as closely as possible, the movements needed in the sport.

Circuit training classes have the potential for enormous variety and can be some of the most interesting and varied classes that your participants attend. Class formats, layouts, and individual stations can be differed regularly and easily. Fitness goals can be achieved in a time-efficient manner while in a safe and motivating environment. Differing ability levels can be catered for with ease and sport-specific aspects can be tailored to suit certain individuals. Essential observation, motivation and correction skills need to be at the forefront of any instruction, making the whole experience positive, safe and effective.

CHAPTER SUMMARY

- Circuit training represents the planned execution of a series of exercises, in a predetermined sequence for an allocated time or number of repetitions.

- Circuit training is considered a time- and space-efficient, challenging and balanced workout that requires little co-ordination but plenty of variety.

- Circuits can take place in the gym, studio, pool and outdoors.

- Resistance can take the form of gym equipment, portable equipment, body weight, partner resistance and water.

- Portable circuits equipment includes rubber bands, barbells, dumb-bells, medicine and stability balls, steps, slides, rebounders, skipping ropes and cones.

- Class structure is the same as that of any other class bar the addition of a second pulse-raiser between the warm-up and main body of the circuit.

- Warm-up (and first pulse-raiser) moves should be low-impact and replicate the moves to be performed at the stations and can be in the style of an aerobic class or walking.

- Each station should have two alternatives, one always offering a low-impact move, to accommodate for mixed-ability participants.

- When designing a class, consider carefully the choice, sequence and balance of the exercises, the work–rest ratio and the intensity of each station.

- Each circuit card must contain clear information on the number of the station, the nature and name of the exercise, muscles worked, start and finish position, and teaching points and should give an easier and a harder alternative.

- The instructor must come prepared with a stopwatch, whistle, pre-prepared circuit cards, water, towel and stereo and microphone (if applicable).

- Class layouts can differ to add variety but must be clear to avoid confusion.

- Teaching skills need to include quick correction techniques and strong motivational methods tailored to the individual needs of the participants.

- To assist the observation and correction procedures a spotter may be utilized.

- Sport-specific circuits require an in-depth analysis of the sport in question and should reflect this by targeting the relevant energy systems and muscles used, joint range of movement and flexibility needs as a minimum.

Exercise to music

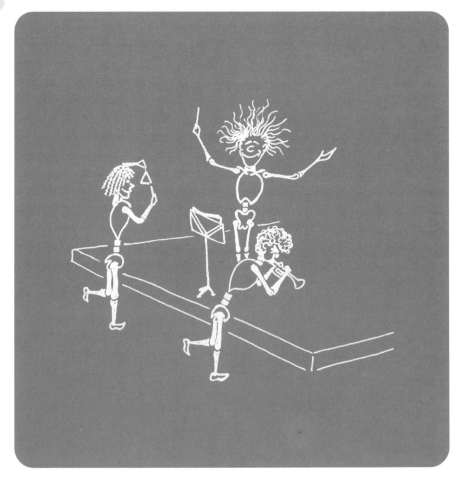

Topics to be included in this chapter:

- Benefits of exercise to music
- Class design principles
- Different class formats
- Music theory and appreciation
- Exercise to music choreography

Exercise to Music came to Britain from the United States. It became popular in the early 1980s. This class format originated at the Coopers Institute in Texas in the 1970s and was known as 'aerobics'. People such as Jane Fonda and the 'Green Goddess' spread this concept far and wide, along with the image of lycra, leotards and leg warmers. The class style was energetic and high-impact. The goals of the class included 'going for the burn', sweating profusely and completing the class on all fours – sometimes literally with the Rover's Return-style floorwork exercises!

This introduction to exercise to music certainly encouraged a large proportion of the female population to become interested in group exercise. As it developed and matured throughout the decade, exercise to music became the first nationally recognized qualification within the fitness industry. The certificate first appeared in 1986 and has become increasingly popular. Although class exercise has diversified greatly since the first aerobics classes, exercise to music has set the defining standard for the other teaching disciplines certificates.

Benefits of exercise to music

To use the term 'aerobics' to describe exercise to music classes is technically incorrect. As detailed in Chapter 6, we know that for an activity to be classified as strictly aerobic it must be of sufficiently low intensity for oxygen to be utilized throughout. However, many exercise to music classes involve participants working anaerobically for certain sections of the class. This may be programmed into the choreography or may mean that the individual is simply less fit and has a low anaerobic threshold.

Exercise to music classes can provide a multitude of benefits to participants. Many of these benefits will be identical to those suggested for circuit training in the previous chapter. Others will more closely reflect benefits of step aerobics and aqua aerobics that are the focus of Chapters 13 and 14 respectively.

Most obvious benefits to an exercise to music class include:

- Improvements in the five components of fitness.
- Improved posture.
- Increased music appreciation and co-ordination.
- Assists in weight maintenance.
- Social interaction.
- Increased adherence levels to a regular exercise programme.

Class design principles

Many of the basic class design principles covered in Chapter 11 relating to circuit training will be identical to those considered for exercise to music. For instance, the need to warm up progressively remains the same and the components within this section are identical. The main section of the class is where the differences are seen. This is called the aerobic curve and will be considered in some depth later in this chapter. The nature of this section is more progressive than that found in the main body of a circuits class and is segmented into three specific components.

The floorwork is called the muscular strength and endurance section. Like circuits, it needs to contain abdominal and lower back work to improve the core stabilization muscles. However, it may include work on many other areas of the body too, provided that the overall section provides a balance of the muscle groups and you have ways to effectively provide overload for each participant.

The final cool-down section will be similar to other class structures although the emphasis may alter, depending on the goals and needs of the group.

Exercise to music class overview

- Introduction to yourself, the venue, and class structure
- Warm-up (mobilization, first pulse-raiser and pre-aerobic stretches)
- Aerobic curve (build-up, peak and build-down)
- Post-aerobic stretches
- Muscular strength and endurance (MSE)
- Cool-down (flexibility, relaxation and revitalizer)
- Feedback from class

Warm-up

Mobilizer

As detailed in Chapter 9, the warm-up aims to raise the pulse progressively, ensuring all the joints and muscles pass through their functional range of movement. Generally in your average exercise to music class the mobilizer and pulse-raiser sections are combined. As most pulse-raiser moves mobilize the joints of the lower body there is little need to statically mobilize these. It is fairly easy to mobilize most joints in the upper body by performing a variety of arm patterns. Remember that range of movement should be increased gradually and limited use of high or overhead arm patterns will be included at this early stage as these raise the heart rate quite dramatically.

Usually the only joint mobilization move that is seen isolated within a warm-up is that for the spine. Always ensure that the core body temperature and the temperature of the muscles surrounding the spine are sufficiently high before performing these movements. It is quite common for these moves to be performed in the later stages of the warm-up after the pulse-raiser or maybe between the pre-aerobic stretches.

Pulse-raiser

The pulse-raiser should aim to increase the co-ordination of the class gradually by progressively building small routines, similar in style to those to come within the aerobic section. Some of the low-impact versions of the moves needed in this later section should be introduced to the class at this stage. All moves within this section of the class should remain low-impact.

Pre-aerobic stretches

Opinion is still divided as to what type of stretches, if any, are relevant or effective at this stage in the class. Most instructors currently tend to favour dynamic range of movement stretches in preference to static stretches. Range of movement stretches maintain the elevated pulse rate and replicate the way the muscle is going to be used during the class. Many instructors combine both types of stretches by performing dynamic stretches and then holding the static position for the usual 6–10 seconds. The decision is yours and should be based on what your group feels comfortable with and can perform effectively.

Make any range of movement stretches slow and controlled insisting on correct posture and correct technique.

Essential considerations when designing the pre-aerobic stretch component include:

- Which muscles need stretches?
- Keep the number of stretches to a minimum required for the aerobic section.
- Decide on whether the stretches will be dynamic or static.
- Demonstrate the correct posture and alignment.
- Use profile positions for some of the demonstrations.
- Maintain the pulse rate between stretches.
- Make transitions between stretches smooth.
- Inform your participants which muscle they are stretching, where they will feel the tension and how this should feel.
- Walk amongst your participants to observe and correct positions.

It is ideal to introduce the method of monitoring intensity that you intend to use throughout the class within this section, particularly if using the rating of perceived exertion scale. The class will need the warm-up as their reference point.

The warm-up is an essential and memorable part of the class. You should start the class as you mean to go on and begin positively and full of energy. It is your opportunity to make an impact on the class and show them how professional you are. If you are covering for a regular instructor do not make the mistake of apologizing to the class for the fact that you are there instead! This may make some of the class believe that you are not as good. Let them make their own minds up at the end of the class instead. Many of your participants may be in the class half-heartedly or their minds may still be at work. Wake them up and make them glad they attended.

- Smile and tell the class they are in for a great time!
- Demonstrate good posture and strong movement quality.
- Mobilize all joints.
- Progressively raise the pulse rate.
- Introduce moves to be used later in the class.
- Introduce cueing methods to be used later in the class.
- Introduce your methods of monitoring intensity.
- Take all muscles to be used through their full range of movement.
- Stretch the muscles to be used in the class.
- Show control of the class if changing direction.
- Develop a rapport with the class.
- Assess ability and fitness level of the class.

The aerobic curve

This is the all-important component for many of your class participants. They will be there to burn calories, learn new routines and have some fun. It is in this section that you can put your creativity to work. However, this can be the most frustrating section when you first begin to teach. The music speed will be faster, the movements quicker and usually more complex. There will be less time and opportunity to provide teaching points and early cues for your class. This does get easier with practice, but only once you have learnt your routine inside out. If your brain is occupied with remembering what is coming next, you will dramatically reduce both your teaching skills and the enjoyment to be had by the participants in your class.

The **aerobic curve** is generally visualized as following the shape shown in Figure 12.1. A common mistake made within this section of the class is to raise the intensity too quickly in the build-up without sufficiently breaking down the moves.

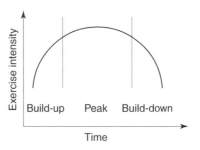

Figure 12.1 The aerobic curve

The build-up

The build-up phase gradually raises the pulse into the participant's training zone. The level of impact will be generally low with a concentration on the other methods of raising intensity such as increasing the travelling and adding arm patterns.

The peak

The peak is reached through a gradual layering of the moves. They become more high-energy, with a selection of higher-impact options. Intensity should be checked during this component and alternatives offered verbally and visually demonstrated to ensure that you allow for all ability levels. Be aware of the symptoms of overexertion and attempt to get verbal feedback from the class regularly throughout this whole section.

The build-down

The build-down reduces the intensity of the class and is usually performed to music of similar speed to the build-up. This will be slower than that within the peak. The moves within the build-down can replicate the moves performed in the build-up, but must be in reverse order. Alternatively, you could include some moves that may be introduced into the peak of the class in the following weeks. The end result should be that the pulse rate returns to about the level it was at the end of the warm-up. Now post-aerobic stretches can be performed effectively as the muscles are very warm.

Post-aerobic stretches are performed on muscles for two reasons:

● Muscles that have been used within the aerobic section of the class and will not be used during the MSE section are better being stretched from a standing position.
● Muscles have not been used or pre-aerobically stretched but will be used in the MSE section.

Muscular strength and endurance (MSE)

Following the build-down you must double-check that all muscles to be targeted in this component have been stretched before they are worked.

Essential considerations necessary when designing this section

- All muscle groups must be balanced, e.g. if the biceps are targeted, the triceps need attention too.
- All equipment necessary to provide an overload is available to the class.
- The whole class is facing the same way so that you can demonstrate and observe easily.
- Transitions between exercises must be smooth.
- Your demonstrations are clear, strong and in the correct teaching position for your class to observe safely.
- Your cueing skills are effective and relevant to the position the participants will be in to perform the exercise.
- The music is of the correct speed to make the exercise controlled and the full range of movement is possible at the joint.
- You should walk around the class to correct participants and motivate individuals.

Cool-down

This section differs little in content and structure from gym programmes, circuits, and step classes. Once again Chapter 9 details the reason and basic content of this section. This section is very beneficial for your participants and as much thought and planning should go into it as goes into the main part of the class.

There are now a greater number of classes that specialize in these components alone. The increased demand is due to the rise in the number of stress-related illnesses and the more holistic approach to exercise and the emphasis on wellness and relaxation.

Flexibility

As with any class, the flexibility component needs to reflect the content of the class and any additional needs of the class. All muscles worked in the MSE section need stretching. Any remaining muscles used in the main aerobic section that were not stretched post-aerobically need to be included.

Your most difficult decision concerns which muscles are to be developmentally stretched and in what position, with what options. Remember that muscles are chosen to be developmentally stretched for a number of reasons:

- They should have the capacity to be lengthened.
- Their opposing muscle does not need to be developmentally stretched.

- They are regularly shortened during everyday activity, which has caused a postural problem.
- They require additional length to perform everyday activities.
- There is a specific limitation to their current range of motion.

As with earlier stretch components, consider the smooth transition between positions and clear teaching points that enable the participants to adopt the correct position effectively and to know they are feeling the right sensation in the correct muscle.

Relaxation

Different methods of relaxation were touched upon in Chapter 9. Consider which method suits your class, your voice, the time remaining to you and the time of day when the class is taking place. You will tend to find that with early morning classes there is less of a need to focus on relaxation, as they are with you in order to kick-start their day, not to return to bed on leaving you. However, evening classes often enjoy a longer relaxation component.

Try different methods with your class and get their feedback, remembering that it may take a participant a couple of sessions to feel comfortable with the different methods. Some individuals, no matter how hard you try, will find it difficult to empty their minds and relax in an environment that is not familiar to them. As with all other sections of the class, you need to cater to the majority so beware of becoming overly influenced by the opinions of one or to participants.

Revitalizer

This is, probably, the most underutilized component of any class. Once again, consider your group and your own style of teaching to ensure that this final section does not appear out of sync with the rest of the class. Never forget that this will be what your class remember as they leave the studio. Their decision to return to you may be based on the feelings they have as they walk out of the door. Therefore, it makes sense that you leave them smiling and feeling good.

Different class formats

Due to the massive explosion of group exercise classes over the past decade, numerous different formats and class styles have developed. Although there are many workshops that provide certificates of attendance for these different class formats, there remains one basic exercise to music certificate recognized at the national level.

Many different classes have grown out of a demand by participants and desire by instructors to alleviate the boredom of just one format. Classes reflect the trends within the industry. Initially, the popular high-impact classes turned low-impact due to the increased incidence of repetitive loading injuries. This transition was aided by the research that identified that a higher percentage of fat was burned when performing low-intensity exercise.

The following is not an exhaustive list but represents some of the most common formats found in clubs today:

- High-energy (impact aerobics)
- Low-impact aerobics
- Fat-burning aerobics
- Hi/low aerobics
- Body conditioning
- Power aerobics
- Stretch and relaxation classes
- Funky aerobics
- Salsa aerobics
- Pre and post-natal aerobics
- Seniors aerobics
- Aero skip

Some focus on a couple of class components only; others introduce influences from the dance arena; yet others are tailored for a specialist population; while the rest include equipment to add variety and focus.

Regardless of the name or focus of the class, they all utilize music to add enjoyment, create an atmosphere and direct the speed of the moves. An understanding of the structure of music is necessary to be able to use it to full effect.

Music theory and appreciation

Music is central to the planning of any exercise to music class. Choice of music is not easy, as there are many factors that need to be considered:

- speed of music
- music phrasing
- suitability for class participants (not just the instructor!)
- music susceptibility

Speed of music

Music speed is measured in **beats per minute** (bpm). If you march in time to the music each foot strike is one beat. The speed of the music that you use for a class will depend on the participants and the section of the class for which it is intended.

Recommended speeds:

Warm-up	128–136 bpm
CV section	130–160 bpm
MSE	Depends on exercise
Cool-down	Any – generally much slower (except revitalizer!)

These speeds will give you an idea of what to look for – especially if you are purchasing pre-mixed tapes. In a beginners' class you would look for slower speeds, whilst in an advanced class you will tend to use higher speeds. Beware when the speed goes above 155 as often this means that, due to the fast speed of the music, a full movement cannot be performed and thus the intensity of the exercise decreases.

Whilst the number of beats per minute provides a guideline, the best way to evaluate a piece of music is by listening to it and performing an exercise to it to see if it is suitable (is it marching speed, jogging speed? etc.).

Music phrasing

Music phrasing is all about the structure of a piece of music.

A story is structured in chapters, paragraphs, sentences and words. A poem is structured in lines and verses.

Music is also structured. Its smallest unit is a beat. Most beats are then structured in groups of 8, then 16 and then 32. When choosing music for an exercise to music class, it is useful to have all music structured into groups of 32 beats and use this to plan routines. In some music, you will find odd beats. When these are present in music it can make it more difficult to plan the exercise, especially when there are lots of then. These groups of odd beats are known as **bridges**.

Songs are also structured into verse, chorus and instrumental parts. These too can be used in planning routines.

Music order		*Phrase*
Introduction		Intro
Verse		A
Chorus	B	
Verse		A
Chorus	B	
Instrumental		C
Chorus	B	
Verse		A
Chorus	B	

Once you know the structure of the music you need to work out how many beats there are in each section. Listen to the introduction and count the number of beats. An easy way of keeping count is to use a tally, with one line (I) to represent each group of eight beats. If there were 32 beats in the introduction this would be written:

Phrase   Beats

Intro   IIII   or   (4 × 8)

Often the verse and chorus of a song are the same length, so the music breakdown may look like:

Phrase   Beats

Intro	IIII	or	(4 × 8)
A	IIII IIII	or	(8 × 8)
B	IIII	or	(4 × 8)
A	IIII IIII	or	(8 × 8)
B	IIII	or	(4 × 8)
C	IIII	or	(4 × 8)
B	IIII	or	(4 × 8)
A	IIII IIII	or	(8 × 8)
B	IIII	or	(4 × 8)

By understanding how the music is structured you can plan how you are going to use each of the beats of music and what exercise you are going to do for each part.

Example 1

Phrase beats   Exercise

Intro	(4 × 8)	2 × 8 Marching – feet together
		2 × 8 Marching – feet wide
A	(8 × 8)	2 × 8 Shift weight
		2 × 8 Shift weight and lift alternate shoulders
		2 × 8 Shift weight and roll alternate shoulders
		2 × 8 Shift weight and half circle alternate arms
B	(4 × 8)	2 × 8 Step together
		2 × 8 Double step
A	(8 × 8)	2 × 8 Single step with bicep curl
		2 × 8 Double step – arms forward
		2 × 8 Single step with bicep curl
		2 × 8 Double step – arms forward

Suitability of music

When choosing music, you need to find music that your class participants are going to enjoy. The music you choose is likely to depend on the age of the participants; however, there are some great 50s, 60s and 70s compilations that all ages like. Whilst the music should be aimed at the participants, it also needs to motivate you and, most importantly provide a clear beat that you can hear. Music will vary depending on the section of the class.

In the warm-up you will want to find something with a strong beat that is going to get everyone's attention – remember the first few minutes are when your class form their first impressions.

The cardiovascular section should sound energetic. Try not to use monotonous music – again music with a strong beat is very helpful here. There is a greater choice of music for the MSE section. This doesn't need to be as energetic as the warm-up and CV sections and can vary widely in speed.

There is also a good deal of choice for the cool-down section of the class, however, there are a few points worth noting. Sad songs can upset people, as can love songs, especially if someone on the class has just split up from their partner. For the relaxation part, it's nice to use music without any words.

Music licensing

In order to play music to an audience you need a PPL licence. It is the responsibility of the instructor to ensure that this licence is in place before they start playing music, not the responsibility of the centre.

The licence you require is different from that required by centres to play background music, so you need to check the details. Most health and fitness centres will hold this licence but some places still require instructors to get their own. If you are setting up your own classes in a village or school hall, you will need to get your own licence. You are not allowed to play music that you have recorded from the originals onto a blank tape. This is illegal. People who have been caught playing music they have recorded have been fined several thousand pounds! Alternatively, you can use licence-free music (known as PPL-free).

The music you play and the way in which you interpret the beat will determine the moves you plan into your class. The moves need to be thoroughly planned and progressively built into routines. The next section will provide some ideas of what moves are commonly included in classes and how they are strung together.

Exercise to music choreography

Once instructors have mastered the essential teaching skills their attention will turn to issues of choreography. Many people feel concerned that they have only a few moves to draw on and that their classes may become boring. Others will have the ideas but fail to teach these sufficiently or link them smoothly and have enormous difficulty remembering it all. There are many different ways to structure a class and variety can be added without using your entire repertoire of moves in one class. The way you can remember routines will depend on practice, the choreography structure you adopt and the music you use.

What is choreography?

The word 'choreography' often makes people apprehensive when considering the content of their classes and there are many misconceptions about it. All this term refers to is the moves you link together within your class to produce a training effect and to provide interest and enjoyment.

Here are some basic rules to consider:

- All choreography is essentially built from about six basic moves.
- There are no new moves, just different combinations.
- Choreography does not have to be complex to be interesting.
- Simple choreography can be very high-intensity.
- Complex choreography can lose intensity and, therefore, have a reduced training effect.

How to build up a catalogue of moves

As stated above, one way of thinking of choreography is that, when considering the lower body patterns, all moves are derived from six very basic steps. Therefore, when building up a catalogue of moves, it makes sense to take each one of these basic moves and attempt to progress it in as many ways as possible to develop more moves.

The six basic moves to work from could be:

- March
- Side step
- Box step
- Half jack
- Knee lift
- Hamstring curl

If you observe any aerobics class it should become apparent which one of these basic moves is the base of each combination.

Once you have chosen a basic move, consider the different ways it can progress. Considering the lower body movements only for now, most moves can:

- Be low-impact
- Be high-impact
- Have a power option

Taking any of the above three options, the move can be further varied by:

- Timing (half time, double time)
- Travel (forwards, backwards, sideways, in a circle)
- Repeater options (double, triple)
- Rhythm (syncopations, pauses, down-beat emphasis)
- Arm patterns

The variety of alterations we can make to any move makes it unlikely that any two instructors will teach the same moves in the same style.

For example, a march:

Low-impact	Basic march (right, left)
High-impact	Basic jog
Power option	Run 1,2,3, with power knee hold
Timing	Sprint (double speed)
Travel	Forwards and backwards
Repeaters	Double hops on each foot
Rhythm	Ponies
Arm patterns	Double punches overhead and to the floor

This process can be done for every one of the above moves. Complete the table below.

Table 12.1 Choreography progressions chart

Move	*Low-impact*	*High-impact*	*Direction/travel*	*Power option*
March				
Side step				
Box steps				
Half jacks				
Hamstring curls				
Knee lifts				

Understanding linking, progression and class structure

Having completed the above process for all six moves, you should have enough choreography to fuel half-a-dozen classes. Your next challenge will be to link these moves smoothly together, grouping moves into routines and then remembering the entire sequence! Although this seems a daunting process, there are methods that will ease the brainpower required.

Linking moves

Unfortunately, not every move is easily compatible with every other. You usually discover this mid-way through your class, as you realise that what worked in your living room has not transferred to the studio so smoothly! This is why it is always advisable to plan and practise every class before trying it on a group of unsuspecting class participants who have paid to work out.

> **EXAMPLE 1**
>
> Try linking the following moves together and appreciate why one flows together better than the other does.
>
> 1 A single grapevine travelling right and then back to the left followed by 4 single side steps travelling to the left first.
>
> 2 As the above but the 4 single side steps travel to the right first.

The issue of what moves link together best is generally an issue of weight transference. It is extremely difficult to move to the left if you have ended the previous move with your weight on your left foot. It is easy to move in the direction of the leg that is lifted or has the least weight through it.

If your previous move ends with equal weight through both legs you could choose to move in either direction, leading with either foot. In this case, make sure that you clearly cue which direction you wish the class to move in. If left to their own devices you will find that half the class will instinctively move to the right, the rest to the left. This could end in collisions!

> **EXAMPLE 2**
>
> Try linking another two moves together – 4 box steps on the right leg, followed by 4 knee lifts.
>
> Do this in a group and you will find that not everyone will move together. Where does the problem lie and how can you minimize the risk of this happening in your classes?

There are some even very simple moves that can be completed in different ways. This can cause confusion during routines. You can either choose to stay clear of these problem areas or ensure your cueing is early and precise.

Progressing moves

Obviously, when completing the choreography sheet you have effectively progressed the basic moves in a variety of ways. This can be via:

- Larger range of movement
- Travelling
- Adding repeaters
- Adding impact
- Adding arm patterns

Progressions should be included gradually with you always demonstrating and giving your class the option of maintaining the low-intensity or impact option at all times. This should be reinforced verbally to allow all levels of ability to participate comfortably in your class.

When designing your routines remember your aerobic curve. This should progress throughout the aerobic section smoothly. Whatever method of structuring your class you choose you must ensure that intensity is maintained even when introducing a new move or routine. This can be accomplished by keeping your class doing a basic but intense move (e.g. jogging with double punches overhead). Arm patterns are key at this stage. Once the arms drop, the intensity drops very quickly.

Each routine working towards the peak section of your class should include larger, more intense moves (possibly more complex depending on the class description). Consider the following routines and determine which will maintain heart rate best and how the other could be modified to do the same.

EXAMPLE 3

Routine 1:

4 single side steps starting right, 4 scoops forward and 4 knee lifts back. 2 single grapevines travelling right, 1 double grapevine, 4 jumping jacks repeat grapevines travelling to the left.

Routine 2:

2 single grapevines travelling right, 1 double grapevine, 4 jumping jacks repeat left. 4 scoops forward, 4 heel digs backward, 4 half jacks on the spot.

Class structure

There are a number of equally effective options in structuring the aerobic section of your class. These differences can add variety to your class and help you remember routines.

- Verse and chorus
- Add-on choreography
- Combination add-on choreography

Verse and chorus

This is one of the most straightforward methods of choreographing and perhaps one of the easiest for both you and your class to remember. It was used a great deal when people made their own tapes for their classes (before music licensing was enforced) and when popular music contained obvious verses and choruses, as in the days of Kylie Minogue and Rick Astley. Now with continuous music tapes it is harder to do.

In this option you simply assign a set routine to the chorus and a different routine to the verses of a particular track. This means that your participants continually come back to a familiar routine when the chorus returns. It also means you have to know your music to cue them on time. Each verse may then build in intensity and complexity.

EXAMPLE 4

- **Verse 1:** 4 marches forward and backward and 4 single side steps to the right; repeat × 4
- **Chorus:** single grapevine right and left and 2 box steps leading right, single grapevine left and right and 2 box steps leading left
- **Verse 2:** 4 marches forward and backward and 4 single side steps; turning 90° repeat around the room.
- **Chorus:** as above.

Add-on choreography

This style simply means that you continuously add moves in a linear fashion. It is a very popular method of structuring the aerobic section, but can be difficult for you and your class to remember. You also need to be aware of how many times you repeat the initial moves within the routine.

EXAMPLE 5

- 4 single side steps
- 4 single side steps + 4 scoops forward and backward
- 4 single side steps + 4 scoops forward and backward + 2 double side steps
- 4 single side steps + 4 scoops forward and backward + 2 double side steps + 4 single grapevines
- 4 single side steps + 4 scoops forward and backward + 2 double side steps + 4 single grapevines + 8 jogs forward and backward →

→

- 4 single side steps + 4 scoops forward and backward + 2 double side steps + 4 single grapevines + 8 jogs forwards and backwards + 4 double grapevines

- 4 single side steps + 4 scoops forward and backward + 2 double side steps + 4 single grapevines + 8 jogs forwards and backwards + 4 double grapevines + 8 full jacks on spot etc. . . .

Combination add-on choreography

Now instead of simply adding on one move at a time, you add on separate sequences or routines. This can be easier to remember and less repetitive than the above method, as you will not repeat the first routine as many times as the first move above. You may also decide to assign each routine a name, a style or to characterize it by a particular move.

EXAMPLE 6

Routine A   8 single side steps
4 scoops forward and backward
2 Double side steps right and left

Routine B   2 marches forward and backward in four counts
4 half jacks
4 spotty dogs

Add routine A + B

Routine C   Single grapevine right and left
2 box steps right leg
Repeat starting grapevine travelling left first

Add routine A + B + C etc . . .

How to vary basic moves

This can be done using a variety of methods:

- Changing the speed of the move (half time or double time)
- Adding rhythm changes (syncopated – jazz; pauses and down beats – hip-hop)
- Music style (salsa, jungle, classical, hip-hop, live band, country and Western, themed – Christmas, films)

Each one of these methods will give a different flavour to even the most basic of moves.

The following table suggests some ways to add variety to some familiar and less familiar moves. However, by far the best approach is to find yourself an empty studio and play some music and see what moves come naturally to you.

Table 12.2 Choreography suggestions

Move	Low-impact	High-impact	Progression		Direction
Angels		Angel	Farmer Giles		Sideways
Box step/ easy walk/ v-step	Box step	Jump back × 2	180° on jumps	Funky jack	On the spot
Grapevine	Grapevine	Add jump on end	Double	Add 180° during double	Sideways, diagonal
Hamstring curl	Hamstring curl	Hopscotch – add jump and travel	Repeaters × 3 or × 5	Single, single-double with 180°	On the spot, forward and backward
Heel digs	Heel digs	Add jump	Double speed	Syncopated – 1,2,3-hold	On the spot, forward and backward
Highland fling	Knee lift tapping toe across	Add jump	360°	—	—
Jack	Half jack	Jumping jack	Cross feet and turn 180°	Power jack	On the spot, forward and backward, circle
Knee lift	Alternate knee lift	Add jump	Doubles	Add 360°	On the spot, forward and backward, circle
Lunges	Side lunges	Add jump	Doubles (with optional 180°)	Repeaters (in 3s or 5s)	On the spot
Mambo	Mambo	Add jump	Add pivot	Double time	On the spot, circle
March	March	Jog	High knee runs	Sprints	Any direction
Pendulum	—	Pendulum	Doubles	Syncopated (single, single-double time and hold)	On the spot
Ponies	—	Ponies	Travelling	180° or 360°	On the spot, forward and backward, circle
Rocking Horse	Rocking Horse (knee lift or hamstring curl)	Add jump —	Doubles —	Power —	On the spot —
Scoops	Scoops	Add hop	Add double leg jump	—	Forward and backward, diagonal
Side steps	Single side step	Ponies	Tap behind	Doubles	Sideways, diagonal
Spotty dogs	Spotty dogs	Add jump	Doubles	Add knee tuck	On the spot
Squat	Squat	Add jump	Power jump	Spider runs	On the spot, forward and backward
Twists	—	Twists	Doubles	Ski jumps	On the spot, forward and backward
Windmill	Windmill	Add jump	Double time	—	Sideways

CHAPTER SUMMARY

- Exercise to music classes can provide improvements in any of the five components of fitness, as well as posture, co-ordination and music appreciation, at the same time as being social.

- The warm-up consists of mobilization, pulse-raising and pre-aerobic stretches. Moves are low-impact in nature and progressively build the heart rate.

- Pre-aerobic stretches can be static or dynamic in nature but should retain the heart rate.

- The aerobic curve consists of the aerobic build-up, peak and build-down. Moves increase in intensity, and possibly impact, up to the peak and then reduce in intensity ready for the floorwork.

- The muscular strength and endurance section targets additional muscle groups that may not have been overloaded during the aerobics section, or it focuses on muscles that need additional strength to improve posture. The repetitions should reflect whether muscles are trained for strength or endurance. The selection of muscles worked should be balanced.

- The cool-down contains the flexibility, relaxation and revitalizer components.

- Music speed is measured in the number of beats in any minute (bpm). These beats are then arranged into phrases of usually 8, 16 or 32 counts.

- Some pieces of music can have errant 2,4 or 6 beats. These are known as bridges and can make choreography difficult.

- Recommended music speeds range from 128–160 bpm dependent on the style of the class and the ability level of the participants.

- Choreography is simply the moves you string together to make a routine. Most routines fit into a 32 count phrase of the music.

- To add variety to any move consider varying its timing, adding repeaters, impact, arm patterns, different directions and alternative rhythms.

- Choreography can be structured to a piece of music in several different ways: verse and chorus, add-on or combination add-on.

Step aerobics

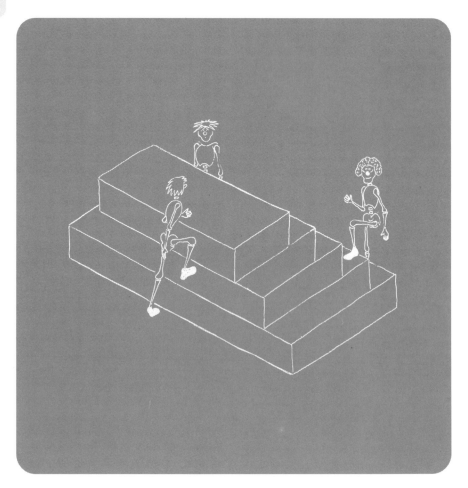

CHAPTER SUMMARY

- Exercise to music classes can provide improvements in any of the five components of fitness, as well as posture, co-ordination and music appreciation, at the same time as being social.

- The warm-up consists of mobilization, pulse-raising and pre-aerobic stretches. Moves are low-impact in nature and progressively build the heart rate.

- Pre-aerobic stretches can be static or dynamic in nature but should retain the heart rate.

- The aerobic curve consists of the aerobic build-up, peak and build-down. Moves increase in intensity, and possibly impact, up to the peak and then reduce in intensity ready for the floorwork.

- The muscular strength and endurance section targets additional muscle groups that may not have been overloaded during the aerobics section, or it focuses on muscles that need additional strength to improve posture. The repetitions should reflect whether muscles are trained for strength or endurance. The selection of muscles worked should be balanced.

- The cool-down contains the flexibility, relaxation and revitalizer components.

- Music speed is measured in the number of beats in any minute (bpm). These beats are then arranged into phrases of usually 8, 16 or 32 counts.

- Some pieces of music can have errant 2,4 or 6 beats. These are known as bridges and can make choreography difficult.

- Recommended music speeds range from 128–160 bpm dependent on the style of the class and the ability level of the participants.

- Choreography is simply the moves you string together to make a routine. Most routines fit into a 32 count phrase of the music.

- To add variety to any move consider varying its timing, adding repeaters, impact, arm patterns, different directions and alternative rhythms.

- Choreography can be structured to a piece of music in several different ways: verse and chorus, add-on or combination add-on.

Step aerobics

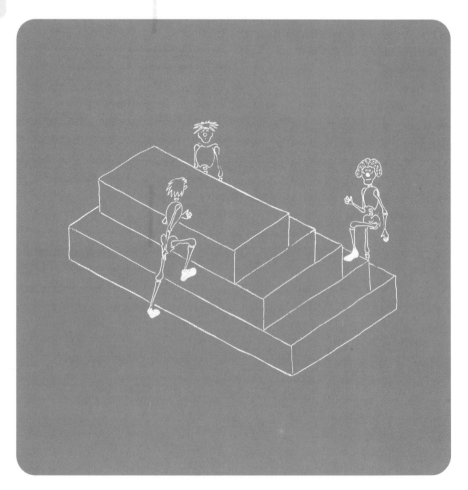

Topics to be covered in this chapter:

- The benefits of step
- The biomechanics of stepping
- Class design principles
- Different class formats
- Step choreography
- Stepping myths

Step aerobics originally began life on a milk crate and beam as part of **Gin Miller's** knee rehabilitation programme in the 1970s. The theory was that stepping up and down onto an object would strengthen the quadriceps and, therefore, support the knee joint. This concept then reached a wider audience during the 1980s when step revolutionized aerobic classes. Step classes are still going strong in many different formats. Step was introduced to add variety to the standard aerobics class and succeeded in enticing people into the studio who were not regular participants in aerobics classes.

Step's popularity stemmed from the fact that it was a low-impact class option, a novelty factor, and its versatility, which meant that it was introduced into circuits-style and body conditioning classes. It was also advertised as an excellent calorie and fat-burner.

Step has gained a reputation for causing injuries to the knee and lower back. These and other myths surrounding step can usually be linked to attendence in excessive number of classes per week, home video instruction leading to bad technique, or participants attempting classes unsuitable for them in terms of the complexity of the choreography or music speed. This chapter will consider the basic biomechanics of stepping and essential step technique, and will touch upon how you can vary your step class formats to reduce the risk of overuse injuries.

The benefits of step

The benefits of step are comparable to those cardiovascular improvements associated with aerobics classes or other forms of cardiovascular exercise. Studies have shown changes to participants' maximal oxygen consumption (VO_2 Max.), aerobic endurance and stamina levels. Other research has shown significant alterations to body composition, namely a lowering of body fat, and an increase in lean muscle mass. Your participants may be aware of the increased muscle tone they develop in the lower body muscle groups.

> *Improvements will only be seen if the intensity of the step class and choreography challenges the individual over and above what they are used to performing in their everyday life or in other exercise sessions.*

This concept revisits the training principles of **progressive overload** as discussed in Chapter 9. Progressive overload can be achieved by altering a variety of aspects of the step class.

This will involve a combination of the following:

- Use of longer levers (upper and lower body)
- More intense arm patterning
- Higher-impact, propulsive or power moves
- Travelling moves over and across the step and floor
- More complex foot choreography
- Introduction of intense aerobic and/or resistance intervals
- Increased speed of music (up to point where full range of movement can still be completed)

As with any other class format, consider changing only one factor at a time and always provide lower-intensity, low-impact and simpler options to accommodate all levels of ability in your classes.

Overall benefits are similar to any other exercise session, provided the content is varied and intensity sufficient:

- Improved posture
- Increased motor skills and co-ordination levels
- Increased aerobic capacity
- Increased anaerobic threshold (if intense intervals included within class)
- Increased muscle tone within the muscles of the lower body
- Improved flexibility (if included in class format)
- Assistance in weight maintenance
- Opportunity for social interaction

The biomechanics of stepping

Before we consider the basics of step posture and technique it is essential to consider the muscle groups that initiate the stepping action and the joints that allow this movement to occur. It is then worth spending time analysing the amount of repetitive stress that is placed through these joints.

The stepping action analysed

The prime movers involved in step include:

- gluteals
- quadriceps
- hamstrings
- adductors and abductors
- gastrocnemius
- soleus
- tibialis anterior

Remember, for a muscle to affect the movement of a joint it must cross the joint. More than one muscle can be responsible for the movement of a joint. Similarly, one muscle can cross two joints and be active for the entire movement. An example of this would be the hamstrings and quadriceps groups that affect both the hip and knee actions described in Table 13.1.

Table 13.1 Muscles involved in the stepping action

Joint	Joint action	Stepping phase	Muscle/muscle group
Hip	Flexion	Lifting leg to place onto step	Hip flexor group (including rectus femoris) Adductors
Hip	Extension	Planting lead foot to bring other leg onto step	Gluteal group Hamstrings Abductors
Knee	Flexion	Lifting leg to place onto step	Hamstrings Gastrocnemius
Knee	Extension	Planting lead foot to bring other leg onto step	Quadriceps
Ankle	Dorsiflexion	Lifting leg to place onto step	Anterior tibialis
Ankle	Plantar flexion	Planting lead foot to bring other leg onto step	Gastrocnemius Soleus

From this table it is easy to appreciate why step appeals to females who are concerned about muscle tone in the hip and thigh area. It is also important to appreciate that, as these muscle groups are active throughout the entire class, they will need stretching well both before and after the workout.

Impact forces when stepping

There are substantial impact and compression forces through the joints identified in Table 13.1, during the whole class. These forces are positive in that they will cause the muscles surrounding the joints and the bones making up these joints to become stronger. This adaptation is one of the goals of exercise. However, because of the repetitive nature of the stepping action, it is easy to veer into the arena of excessive impact and joint discomfort for those unused to stepping or regular activity. These forces can be minimized by adhering to correct step technique, stepping gently on and off the step and keeping all moves low-impact.

Excessive forces can occur if too many propulsive moves are strung together; if excessive repeater moves are linked together; if the step height is incorrect with respect to the height of the individual; and if moves are completed with poor step technique and body alignment.

Step height is the most basic way to alter the impact the lower body joints experience.

- When the step height is 4 inches the impact forces are around 1.75 times your body weight.
- With the step height up to 12 inches the forces escalate to around 2.25 times your body weight.
- If propulsion moves are added, the force on the feet is around 2.7 times the weight of the body.

If propulsions are added for more advanced participants, it is advisable that they are performed only onto the step, never off it. The impact forces if jumping off the step can be excessive, due to the drop involved. Alternatives should always be offered.

Stepping posture

Initially, it will be important to ensure that all participants demonstrate good lifting technique and posture when assembling and reassembling the step platform.

Lifting technique:

- Stand close to the object with a wide stance.
- Bend knees to go down to the object and keep a curve in the low back.
- Lean back to stay in balance and lift by extending the knees and the hips.
- Make the lift smooth and exhale as you lift the object.
- When upright pivot with the feet.
- Do not twist the back.

Posture check:

- Focus eyes forward with the neck in neutral alignment with the spine.
- Stand tall with the shoulders down and back.
- Chest should be lifted.
- Ensure the pelvis is in neutral alignment with the spine.
- Knees should be relaxed – not flexed or hyperextended.

Correct step technique

Step platform heights vary between 4 inches and 12 inches and usually increase in height by 2-inch increments if they are adjustable. Individuals will differ in terms of the step height that is correct for them, dependent on:

- their height
- their level of fitness
- familiarity with step
- the level of the class

It is your job, as the instructor, to ensure that every participant is stepping up on to a platform height suitable for them that will enable them to gain maximum benefit from the class with minimal injury risk.

Knee flexion test

A simple check can be made to determine if the step height is correct. Simply ask the individual to place a foot on top of the platform and look at the angle at the knee joint. This should never be less than 90°. If it is less than this, the individual should be advised to lower the platform by 2 inches (or 1 block) and look to increase intensity by one of the other methods listed earlier.

If in doubt over any beginner, always opt for the lower platform height, so that more of their concentration goes into the choreography.

Table 13.2 Essential step technique

Subject	Guidelines
Platform height	<ul><li>Always check the platform is secure before stepping.</li><li>Perform the knee flexion test to determine a suitable step height for each individual.</li><li>Encourage the de-conditioned and newcomers to perhaps use the base only.</li></ul>
Posture	<ul><li>Body weight is slightly forward onto the toes when on top of the step – lean from the ankles, not from the waist.</li><li>Adopt good posture, looking forward (try not to look down at the feet).</li><li>Hips, knees and ankles need to be in alignment.</li></ul>
Stepping up	<ul><li>When stepping up, contact the step with the heel first and roll forward onto the toe, placing the whole foot on the platform.</li><li>Step softly and quietly up and down to limit unnecessary impact.</li></ul>

Table 13.2 (*continued*)

Subject	Guidelines
Stepping down	• When stepping down from the step ensure you are close to the step (to reduce the risk of Achilles tendonitis) and roll from the toe through to the heel.
Leading leg	• Change the leading foot (the foot that begins the step pattern) after about 1 minute. The leading leg experiences more musculoskeletal stress than the non-leading leg.
Propulsive and pivotal moves	• If propulsive moves are involved, on landing, the knees need to be bent with feet flat on the step. • Any pivotal moves should occur with one foot leaving contact with the step to reduce the risk of twisting the knee.
Repeaters	• With repeater moves, ensure the supporting knee goes through the full range of motion without locking through full extension.
Arms	• Vary the arm patterns, ensuring a balance of low, mid and high arm patterns. Beware of overtiring the deltoid muscle.
Music	• Music speed is generally between 124–130 bpm.
Weights	• Not recommended. Light handweights do not significantly increase energy expenditure but do significantly increase potential injury and local fatigue in the shoulder area.

Class design principles

As expected, many of the class design principles will replicate those related to exercise to music. Usually the alterations for a step class involve utilizing the step within the basic component; the principles within each component stay the same. More time may be needed for your introduction for beginners and to run through the health and safety issues specific to step.

Step aerobics class overview

- Introduction to yourself, the venue, and class structure
- Warm-up (mobilization, first pulse-raiser and pre-workout stretches)
- Aerobic curve (build-up, peak and build-down)
- Muscular strength and endurance (MSE)
- Cool-down (flexibility, relaxation and revitalizer)
- Feedback from class

The warm-up phase (music speed: 128–136 bpm)

Mobilization

As with any class, this is the preparation phase, allowing the body and mind time to adjust to the demands of exercise and levels of co-ordination required. The core body temperature should rise slowly through rhythmical movements by the large muscle groups in the lower body. Those muscles in the upper body generally work through their range of movement, therefore, mobilizing each major joint thoroughly and reducing the risk of injury in later phases of the class when movements are faster and more energetic.

Pulse-raiser

The movements are a little bigger and more representative of the remainder of the class. In order to prepare the body for the vertical nature of step, it can be useful to practise marching on top of the step and off it in counts of 8 or maybe 4. Walking around the step allows participants to get used to the fact that an obstacle is in front of them. This can be a strange sensation for someone used only to aerobics. Generally, most work is done off the step, as the warm-up music speeds of between 128–136 bpm mean posture could be compromised for speed and heart rates would rise too dramatically if too much time is spent on the step. Certain step patterns can be introduced successfully at half-speed to prepare participants for the aerobic section. With beginners this can be an ideal time to practise the basic step at a slower speed and identify any postural and technique issues that need correction.

Pre-aerobic stretches

These remain important, as for any other class. Consider the main working muscles and focus on these. The main muscles that need stretching will be the quadriceps, hip flexors, hamstrings, adductors, abductors, gluteals, gastrocnemius and soleus.

The aerobic phase (music speed: 124–130 bpm)

Aerobic build-up

The intensity is gradually increased and routines are introduced at their lowest intensity and impact. The basic step is introduced and practised to ensure good technique. Changing feet is perfected and step names can be introduced.

Peak

The routines progress with arm patterns, travelling, propulsions and possibly power alternatives. Participants should aim to reach their target training zone during this phase. Low-impact options and alternatives should be given throughout.

Aerobic build-down

It is necessary to reduce the heart and breathing rates to their pre-exercise levels gradually. The step can still be used, but more floor patterns are used, similar to those of the pulse-raiser section. It is often a good idea to stretch the lower body muscle groups that will not be utilized during the floorwork component.

Muscular strength and endurance (music speed depends on the exercise)

The same exercises as performed in a normal aerobic class will apply. However, the step can be utilized as a prop for certain exercises. This is ideal for triceps dips, back extensions, incline or decline press-ups, and as a rest for the feet during abdominal work (to reduce the activity of the hip flexors).

The cool-down phase (music usually instrumental and relaxing)

Flexibility

Aim to increase flexibility in the remaining muscle groups not stretched post-aerobically and those worked during the MSE section. These may include: hamstrings, adductors, abductors, pectorals, triceps, abdominals and erector spinae.

The stretches within this section can be held anywhere between 10–30 seconds and beyond. Those held between 6–15 seconds are **maintenance** stretches. Muscles stretched in this way do not require additional flexibility and/or cannot be developmentally stretched.

Muscles that undergo maintenance stretching include:

- quadriceps
- abductors
- gluteals
- soleus
- abdominals
- upper back muscles (rhomboids and trapezius)
- deltoids
- triceps
- biceps

Other muscle stretches can be held for up to 30 seconds or longer. These are **developmental** stretches. This is when a muscle is taken to the point of tension, relaxed and then taken further, to increase the length and flexibility of the muscle. This will be applied to muscles that may be shorter due to daily activities, poor postural habits and the exercise type.

Muscles that may undergo developmental stretching include:

- hamstrings
- hip flexors
- adductors
- gastrocnemius
- erector spinae
- pectorals

Relaxation

This could take the format of a general body stretch with breathing prompts and imagery, a progressive relaxation routine, or simply suggesting participants adopt their most comfortable lying position, to empty their minds, breathe deeply and enjoy about 3 minutes of a chosen music track.

Revitalizer

Following the relaxation phase, it is important for you to know that each participant is awake and alert enough to leave the studio. This section is short and snappy, meant to wake everyone up, to increase their circulation and leave them on a happy note. The aim is not to raise pulse rates into their target training zones!

Different class formats

The step interval class

This class has many different formats and can involve a variety of equipment or none at all. Generally, the class is divided into sections of a number of minutes spent on the step, interspersed with exercises completed off the step. The intervals off the step could be aerobic in nature or more resistance-orientated using body weight, hand weights, bands, tubing or body bars. The intervals could last 1–10 minutes in an aerobic-based interval class.

The step circuit class

This format would generally consist of a number of different exercise stations. Each station would last anywhere from 30 seconds to 1 minute. This utilizes the standard circuit training principles and format, with the emphasis on the step as a prop.

The power step class

This utilizes propulsive moves to spice up the class and increase intensity. It is meant for the more advanced participants as there is greater force through the joints and greater need for stabilization and muscle control. The class format may be similar to a basic step class.

Tap-free step

This style of class does not necessarily abide by a set format or use specific intervals or choreography. Tap-free step has been developing popularity due to the simple fact that steps flow together and there is no need to change lead legs as these changes are programmed into the choreography. Although it may take you more time to plan your classes to make your choreography tap-free, it gives your participants one less thing to think about if they do not need to tap and change legs midway during the routine. It also means that there is less likelihood of leading leg imbalances when using this system.

Domino step

This is a great class concept that adds variety to an old routine with very little alteration and will keep your more advanced participants thinking and interested. The idea is that each participant in the class has the use of more than one step during the routine. Each person has what would be highlighted as their own step, but during the class will utilize their neighbour's step to either side and even behind and in front for certain moves. If designing this class, be aware that you will need to carefully space and arrange the steps at the start of the class and ensure that the step heights are identical within the same row if you are asking people to travel to them. This may involve moving a participant from their favourite spot, which could be unnerving for them. Finally, bear in mind that there need to be more steps than people, so this is an ideal format in classes with lower numbers.

Double trouble

This time the choreography involves two people using the same step at the same time. Usually, much of the routine will involve diagonal work, or maybe moves completed off the ends of the step. This can be a fun alternative and can encourage social interaction and correction of technique in their pairs.

Choreography

It is important, as with any class, to be able to progress the choreography on a regular basis, usually every 8–12 weeks, depending on the level and needs of the class. There needs to be a smooth transition between each step, assisted by good cueing skills. It is essential to practise the class well before delivering it to the unsuspecting participants.

Here are five key pointers on choreography that should be considered before planning any class:

1 Vary the movement patterns (both on the upper and lower body) to reduce unnecessary stress on any particular joint.

2 Try to change the leading leg regularly – no longer than 1 minute should be spent leading with one leg. Again there is additional musculoskeletal stress on the leading leg. (This does not apply with tap-free step.)

3 Arm patterns should only be added once participants are confident with the legs. Arm patterns should contain a mixture of low, mid- and high-range movements.

4 No hand-held weights should be encouraged, as the risk to the shoulder girdle outweighs the aerobic benefits obtained.

5 Progress all routines gradually after demonstrations and feedback from the class.

As with any other exercise to music class, choreography is generally built up to the music in phrases of 32 counts. Most choreography ideas within a class are adaptations of the basic step patterns given below.

A class can easily be built from this basic list of six moves by adding variety in terms of:

- Use of floor patterns
- Use of all sides of the step (front, sides and back)
- Directional changes (diagonals, over the top and across the step)
- Adding arm patterns
- Adding impact and power moves
- Utilizing rhythm and tempo changes
- Inserting interval sessions
- Changing music speed

The following are some of the most common moves to be found in step classes.

Basic step

If right (R) leg leading: R leg up; L leg up; R leg down; L leg down.

To change onto L leg leading, on the L leg down simply tap the L leg on the floor and step straight back onto the step with it.

This may take some time for absolute beginners to master. However, even with intermediates it is a useful prompt to say that if the choreography is getting the better of them or they wish to take a breather, this is an excellent step to return to regain their breath and co-ordination.

TEACHING POINTS

Heel contacts step first.
Place the full foot flat on the step.
Stay close to the step when stepping off.
Keep posture upright.
Tilt weight slightly forward from the ankles.

BEWARE!

Heel sliding off the step (damage to Achilles tendon).
Leaning backwards (stress on the lumbar vertebrae).
Locking the knees out (hyperextension).

Orientation: Facing front (narrow).

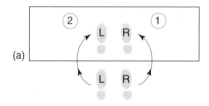

Variation: **V-step** – same foot sequencing, but when stepping up onto the step the legs go wide, to the edges of the step. When stepping off the legs return to the narrow position.

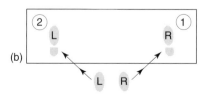

Horseshoe/turn step/half turn

If leading with the R leg, the R leg is nearest the platform with the body diagonal to the step, the R leg steps up and travels across the step. End sideways on to the step, facing the opposite direction, L leg nearest the step ready to return across the platform.

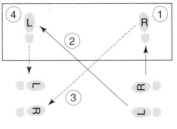

Feet facing towards the step

TEACHING POINTS

Place the whole foot on the step.
Ensure correct foot placement on the step to prevent twisting on the knee.
Always tap the foot as you complete the step, ready to begin again on the opposite leg.

Variation: **Reverse turn step** – the body facing away from the step. If the R leg leads the R leg steps up and across the step the L leg steps onto the other end of the step, the R leg steps off, followed by the L.

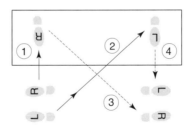

Feet facing away from the step

Over-the-top/windmill

With R leg leading and body facing sideways onto the step: R up; L up; R leg down; L leg down. Crossing from one side of the step to the other.

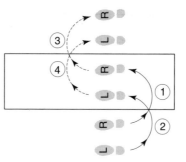

TEACHING POINTS

Step off the platform close to it.
Ensure heels contact the step as you travel across it.
Keep knees soft throughout.

Orientation: Can be done *lengthways* across the step:

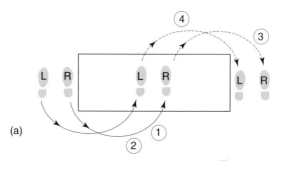

(a)

Can also be done *diagonally* across the step:

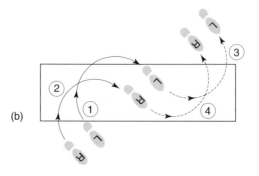

(b)

Variation: Can add propulsions as you cross the step.

Could add a pivot turn as you cross the step.

Lift step

Lifting the lower limb in relation to the lower body, e.g. knee lift; hamstring curl; abductor squeeze.

TEACHING POINTS

Maintain a lifted posture with weight gently forward.
Keep abdominals tight in support of the lower back.
Control the limb being lifted, do not use momentum.

Orientation: Facing front, on the diagonal or from the straddle position.

Variation: Add a propulsion or a power move.

Repeaters

A lift step on the non-weight-bearing leg is repeated up to 5 times consecutively (generally for either 3 or 5 repeaters). If there are more than 5 repetitions, there is stress on the supporting leg.

TEACHING POINTS

Keep the supporting leg soft.
Keep abdominals tight against the spine to minimize movement in the torso.
Limit the number of repetitions to 5.

Orientation: Facing the front, on the diagonal or from the straddle position.

Lunges

Starting from on top of the platform. If R leg leading: R leg extends to tap the floor with the toe (heel raised); R leg returns on top of the platform and weight shifts back onto it. L leg extends to tap the floor on the opposite side of the step.

TEACHING POINTS

Keep the heel raised off the floor on the extended leg.
When transferring weight to other leg, allow the whole body to rotate to prevent twisting of the knee.

Orientation:	Lunging off the back of the step facing the front.
	Lunging off the side of the step facing to the side.
Variation:	**Fast squats** – a squat off alternate sides of the step with a propulsion centrally in between.

There are then many ways to build upon these steps and provide choreography to fill any level and style of class.

Stepping myths

1. Step provides a more intense workout than aerobics classes/You need to be fitter to attend a step class than an aerobics class.

These claims are centred on the fact that, because the step height and music speed are set from the beginning of the class to the end, the pulse rate is maintained at a higher level throughout the hour than during an aerobics class of comparable duration. However, as with any class, there are ways to modify the intensity of any move. Arm patterns can be reduced or removed; step height can be reduced through removal of a platform; movements can be replicated off the step.

2. Step predominantly reduces fat around the buttocks and upper thigh area.

If this were true we would be able to spot reduce fat from any area of our body. This cannot be done. It is wrong to suggest that simply because we work a muscle, the fat overlying this area is more active. This is not so. Body fat will be lost from all over the body. If people notice changes to their lower body, it can usually be ascribed to an increase in muscle tone.

3. Step causes a large increase in calf strength and size.

Specific training will induce specific adaptations within the body. As we know, the prime movers involved in step training are the calf muscles. If the load upon the calf during a step class is in excess of the amount of work normally done on the calf, then changes will result. These changes will normally be seen as a definition of the muscle, and may be seen particularly within the first 12 weeks of regular training. There may be a *slight* increase in muscle size and strength. The changes will not continue at this rate, unless you continue to increase the load. To do this you would have to lift onto and off the step; i.e. by carrying weights or adding many propulsive moves.

4. Step causes knee injuries.

Experts are in agreement that step itself is not responsible for knee injuries. It is bad technique, excessive class attendance, and/or poor instructions that are responsible. Many of the injuries have occurred at home, while people have been following home video classes where there is no correction of incorrect technique.

5. Step is the best fat-burning class format.

Research has suggested that step has no advantage over other aerobic activities such as swimming, running, walking or other aerobic classes. Optimal fat burning is highly individual and dependent on many factors.

6. The faster the music speed the harder the workout.

This is not so. Once music speeds exceed 132 bpm, range of movement can be lost and there is a greater risk of injury as posture and technique compromise the lower back and knees.

Currently, following the incentive from the United States, step tape speeds have risen to 136 bpm. It is inadvisable to use these speeds, except with the most advanced of classes and even then the risks can outweigh the benefits. It may be more effective to introduce an intense interval.

7. The best way to increase exercise intensity is to increase the step height.

Not so – as described earlier there are many ways in which intensity can be increased. Always remember that knee flexion should not be less than 90° whatever the ability level of the individual.

CHAPTER SUMMARY

- The benefits of step can be equated to those of any other regular cardiovascular activity.

- All lower body muscles are active in moving the joints within the lower body and there is substantial impact and compression through these joints during a class.

- Step height varies within the range 4–12 inches. The higher the step the greater the impact forces through the joints. Adding propulsive and high-impact moves further increases the stress upon the joints.

- The correct step height for any individual can be determined through the knee flexion test plus their fitness level, competency at step and the level of the class.

- Correct step technique is essential to reduce risk of overuse, impact and twisting injuries. Incorrect technique can adversely effect the knees, lower back and Achilles tendon.

- The lead leg should be changed every minute (if choreography is not tap-free); pivot moves should involve one foot leaving contact with the step; no more than five repeaters should be successively done on one leg; avoid jumping down from the step; using hand weights is not recommended. →

- Different step class formats include: step intervals; step circuits; power step; tap-free step; domino step and double trouble.

- There are many myths still surrounding step training. All the basic principles of fitness apply to step as to any other form of cardiovascular activity. Adaptations within the body will only take place in relation to the amount of overload provided by the exercise. Intensity can be increased in a variety of ways. It is your role to decide which is the safest and most effective method for your class.

Aqua aerobics

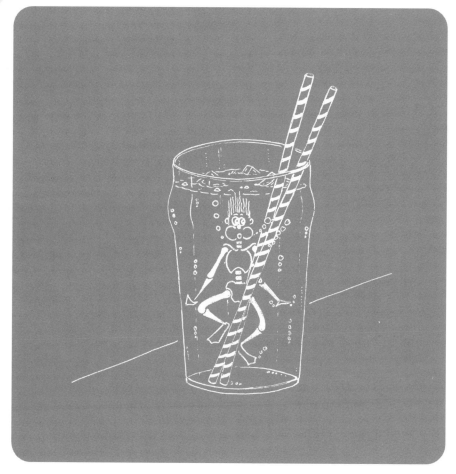

Topics to be covered in this chapter:

○ The benefits of aquatic exercise

○ The properties of water

○ Immersion theory

○ The facility

○ Class design principles

○ Aqua choreography

○ How to maximize your water workout

○ Teaching skills

○ Aquatic myths

Water is an excellent medium in which to train individuals and improve their fitness levels. Due to the natural properties of water each component of fitness can be improved. Water can be used for aerobic conditioning, muscular strength and muscular endurance training, flexibility and relaxation.

The nature of water allows individuals to benefit from low-impact to no-impact sessions. The use of equipment can further increase the ability to progressively overload the body both aerobically and in a resistance context.

Aquatic exercise has grown in popularity over the past decade, but still appears to appeal predominantly to those people who feel uncomfortable in the gym environment, or wish for a lower-intensity session. These and other myths surrounding aqua aerobics will be analysed and dispelled. An instructor with a thorough understanding of how to utilize the natural properties of water can provide a challenging workout for even the fittest of individuals. Your role will be to educate people to appreciate this and provide a variety of classes to appeal to a wide variety of participants.

Having completed your exercise to music qualification and become familiar with Chapter 12, you will have thoroughly understood class structuring, training principles of progression and adaptations, and appreciated the components of fitness that need to be trained. These will not be covered in this chapter. It will concentrate on the properties of water and how they affect your workout structure and teaching skills. You will soon realize that it is not effective to simply transfer your land aerobics class into the water!

The benefits of aquatic exercise

Water is often seen as a limiting medium, in the sense that cardiovascular and resistance gains cannot be realized easily, if at all. There are only a small percentage of our gym users and perhaps even land-based class participants who would consider using water as an exercise medium. These feelings are largely due to ignorance about the benefits that water has to offer and the fact that they may have witnessed a class that did not use the water to its best advantage.

Water is one of few environments that can adequately support any level of ability, co-ordination and confidence. The reasons for this are given below.

- It improves circulation and delivery of oxygen to the working muscles.
- The water is supportive and can therefore aid venous return (blood return to the heart), while preventing damaging falls if balance is in question.
- The density of the water provides resistance for the body to work against to improve muscle strength and endurance.
- Walking in water is an excellent way to improve the postural and stabilization muscles in the torso.
- The water temperature keeps participants cool; with the sweat dissipating in the water overheating is unlikely.
- Water can have a calming effect on many people. It is refreshing and allows a lot of fun to be had due to the nature of the exercises performed.
- It is a reduced-impact form of exercise that can be used for rehabilitation purposes or for those with chronic joint problems (such as arthritis).

Who benefits from aquatic exercise?

Although we have specified that aqua workouts are valuable to everyone, it is useful to highlight the benefits for certain specialist groups. It is valuable to stress these on promotional material. You may identify the need to put on specialist classes.

- Runners – needing to train for mileage but with reduced or no impact.
- Cross-trainers – water trains the entire body and offers variety.
- Rugby/football players – these frequently suffer contact-related injuries. Water can provide the supportive medium to enable them to maintain cardiovascular fitness through the rehabilitation period.
- Armed forces – as above, when stress injuries occur, cardiovascular fitness is maintained in water.
- Pregnant women – looking for ways to be weightless while maintaining their fitness.

- The injured – much rehabilitation work is done in water.
- Arthritis sufferers – water provides a rejuvenating workout, with excellent joint ROM opportunities.
- Larger individuals – who feel uncomfortable exercising on land.
- Individuals who dislike the hot and sweaty feeling of working out.
- Anyone wanting a challenge that is gentle on the body.
- Non-swimmers.

The properties of water

There are three properties of water that affect exercise within this medium:

- Buoyancy
- Resistance
- Pressure (hydrostatic)

Buoyancy

> Buoyancy is the degree to which the body floats upward when immersed in water.

As Archimedes discovered around 200 BC, when an object is placed in water, it displaces a volume of water equal to its own weight. The remaining water surrounding the object will then exert a pressure on the object, forcing it upwards towards the surface of the water.

The same thing happens when your participants enter the pool. They displace water equal to their own weight and are then subject to the pressure of the water surrounding them. How easily they resist this pressure is dependent on the following factors:

- Their centre of buoyancy (body composition of the individual)
- Gender
- The depth of the water
- The amount of air in the lungs

Centre of buoyancy

All individuals have a different centre of buoyancy that relates to their fat deposition (where fat is stored).

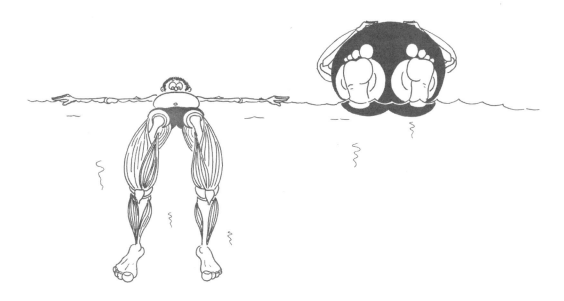

This will affect their workout in a number of ways:

- How their bodies naturally lie in the water
- The stability of their body in the water
- The speed at which the individual can move through the water
- The water depth at which the individual should aim to work within a class

 As lean muscle mass weighs more than body fat, those individuals who are lean, with a large percentage of muscle tissue, will be less buoyant and have a lower centre of buoyancy.

This can be appreciated when looking at competitive swimmers. There are very few of Afro-Caribbean origin because they genetically have a greater percentage of lean muscle mass. If placed into deep water they will lie a lot lower than those with a greater percentage of fat tissue. This means that those individuals with a lower centre of buoyancy will have to work harder to stay afloat during deep-water exercises. Their sculling technique will have to be very effective and they will expend more energy in doing so. Consider this when designing your resistance sections.

People who carry a greater percentage of body fat, will float more easily because their centre of buoyancy will be higher.

Consequently, if placed into deep water they will stay afloat with greater ease, but may have difficulty maintaining an upright position, if that is what is required. This is because, the higher the centre of buoyancy, the more the individual will be pushed horizontal by the pressure of the water. They will find it more difficult to move at speed through the water.

The following table summarizes the effects of the centre of buoyancy on general exercise capability within the water. It is worth remembering that, in addition to gender differences, there will also be body type differences between endomorphs, mesomorphs and ectomorphs.

Table 14.1 Effects of the centre of buoyancy

	High centre of buoyancy	Low centre of buoyancy
Gender differences	Females	Males
Body type differences	Endomorphs	Mesomorphs and ectomorphs
Position of the body within the water	Horizontal	Vertical
Stability of the body within the water	Poor	Good
Speed of movement through the water	Slow	Fast
Suggested water depth	Shallower	Deeper

If a male and a female both had the same high body fat level their centre of buoyancy would still be different due to gender differences. The female's centre of buoyancy would almost always be higher than the male's and the reasons for this are described in the next section.

Gender effects

As females genetically contain a greater percentage of fat than men, regardless of their muscle mass, women are generally more buoyant. Where the fat is stored on the body is also relevant. On women there will always be a higher percentage of fat stored around the chest, and almost always more around the hip and thigh region. The combined effect of these two storage areas will mean the female participant in your aqua classes will have a high centre of gravity. Water pressure will, therefore, force the female into a higher position out of the water, while making it easier for her to float, particularly on her back.

The male participant, if storing fat around the waist, as is characteristic, will have a lower centre of gravity that acts rather like a rubber ring. This will mean that he will stand fairly vertical in the water.

Water depth effects

If you have ever attended an aqua aerobics class in water up to your chest, you will appreciate that because you are very buoyant, it is difficult to control movements, work to music and travel with speed in any direction. If you work in water only up to your waist, movement becomes easier and buoyancy has less effect.

This difference is in part due to the fact that your lungs will act as a buoyancy aid when they are submersed. Normally, centre of buoyancy of an individual in water lies around the pelvic region, but when the lungs are submersed it moves towards the chest.

As water depth varies, the amount of impact and gravitational forces also varies significantly. It is this reduction in the forces of gravity that explains the difference between working in water and working on land.

- At waist depth 50 per cent of the gravitational forces exist.
- At chest depth only about 10 per cent of these forces exist.

Many individuals who attend water-based classes relish this feeling of weightlessness, particularly those who are in the later stages of pregnancy or suffering from joint pain. However, this effect needs to be balanced with the ability to work constructively in the water.

Resistance

Water is denser than air. Therefore, it exerts resistance to motion, increasing exercise intensity to compensate for the reduction to body weight (weightlessness).

As water has a greater density than air, movement performed in water encounters about 12 times more resistance than that done on land. Water resistance can also be affected by a variety of factors:

- Water depth
- Buoyancy of the individual
- Utilization of the eddy drag and turbulence within the water

Water depth

The deeper you are in the water the greater the resistance provided by the water. However, refer back to the centre of buoyancy issues to decide if the resistance provided by the water is effective for the individual or overpowering.

 The guide to an ideal depth is somewhere between chest and navel height, with the arms always worked underneath the water to maximize resistance.

There is little point in completing arm patterns above the water line, as there is only air and gravity to resist the movement.

Your participants' height is a factor to consider, if the water depth is not constant within the pool where you are teaching. If pool depth deepens from your front row backwards, then, ask your smaller participants to stay at the front to maximize their workout ability.

Eddy drag

Unlike swimming, exercising in water maximizes the resistance the body exerts through the water by creating:

- Eddy drag (turbulence)
- Opposition forces
- Inertia currents

When the body is in a vertical position there is a 75 per cent increase in the resistance over that exerted by the body when swimming.

When water is disturbed this causes **eddy drag** forces or **turbulence**. The water swirls against the walls of the pool and the people in it. This phenomenon affects the resistance that your participant works against. The more turbulence created by faster movements and arm patterns under the water, the greater the resistance will be. If your class size is large, there will also be greater turbulence within the pool as a whole, which will create a greater resistance for all participants.

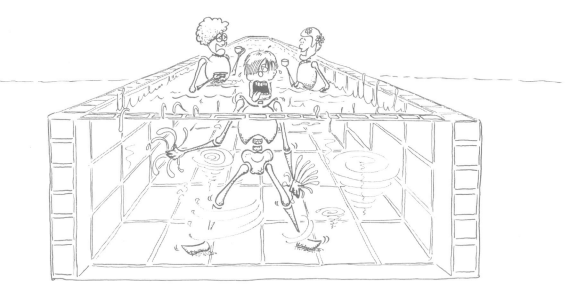

Once you have created turbulence and this is in a uniform direction, like stirring a cup of coffee clockwise, then there will a far greater amount of resistance opposing movement in the opposite direction, i.e. stirring the coffee anti-clockwise. It is wise to consider the turbulence you have set in motion with a particular move and what opposition there is to your next planned move. You need to provide your participants with enough time to change direction in aqua classes. You need to make sure too, that they have the strength to stabilize their torsos amidst this turbulence and then when trying to oppose the flow of water. You may find that some individuals need to increase their core stabilizing muscles (abdominals and lower back) before they can effectively and safely work out in water at these speeds.

The individual's position will affect the amount of turbulence and opposition forces they are subjected to.

The front line of your class will actually work harder as a result of them having to begin a move. These people initiate the turbulence and, as the water swirls around them, these eddy forces assist those behind, in the second row, in moving. This effect is often referred to as **'inertia currents'** and allows participants to cheat during the workout.

This is an excellent reason to change the direction of the class and your teaching position, so that every individual ends up on the front row at some stage of the workout.

This is partly why aquatic exercise is considered an easy option by many. If you relax your posture and muscles, it is easy for a person to move with the general direction of the class, and appear to be working. They will be enjoying the soothing and circulatory benefits of water, but few of the resistance benefits to be had. The idea is that each individual works against the water at all times, attempting to maintain an upright posture, with strong abdominal stability and low back support.

Water resistance also has two other effects on the ability of individuals to exercise:

- Movements cannot be done at speed
- Muscle contraction is altered

Movement speed

Due to the increased forces of resistance that oppose any movement, movements are done more slowly, both in the water by the participants and, as demonstrations, on the poolside by the instructor. If music is being used and worked to, this has to be of a slower tempo. This can vary between 100–136 bpm.

It is essential that, as the instructor, you demonstrate a speed of move that is achievable by the majority of your participants. If they see you moving too quickly on the poolside, they will attempt to replicate this speed in the water and will be demotivated if they are unsuccessful. This could also come across as ignorance on your part of how it feels to work out in water. Either way, your participants are less likely to return the following week.

The difference in muscle contraction

Due to the fact that there is a reduction in the effects of gravity within water, there is little opportunity for the muscles to contract eccentrically. In water, the muscles operate with a **dual concentric contraction** occurring in the muscle pair.

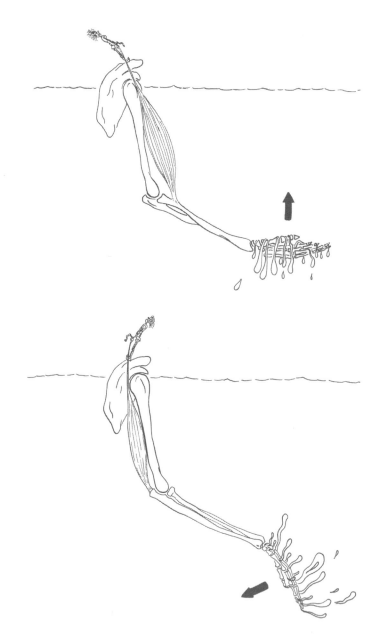

For example, when curling the leg into a hamstring curl, the hamstrings contract concentrically to bring the heel towards the bottom. When straightening the leg, the quadriceps also contract concentrically to return the leg to the start position. By contrast, on land this lengthening of the leg back to the start position would be assisted by gravity and the quadriceps would act as a brake and contract eccentrically.

Generally, when muscles are trained eccentrically, greater muscle soreness (delayed onset muscle soreness – DOMS) is felt for a day or two after the exercise session. As this work is reduced in the pool, less soreness may be felt. This is not an indication of less work having been done by class participants.

Hydrostatic pressure

> The pressure applied by water to a submerged object is called hydrostatic pressure. This pressure is exerted equally around the entire body when it is immersed in water.

It is hydrostatic pressure, coupled with the reduction in gravitational forces acting on an individual in the water, that creates differences in the way the circulation, lungs and kidneys operate when submersed in water.

Circulation

- Improvements in circulation that are found through water exercise can be ascribed to the fact that water has a massaging effect on the body and can assist the return of the blood to the heart.
- The actual muscle contraction process while exercising also assists this venous return. As the muscles contract they compress the blood vessels within the working muscles and force the blood along the vessel and back to the heart at a faster rate.
- There is less risk of blood pooling while exercising in water. This is due to the massaging effect detailed earlier and improved venous return in addition to the reduction of gravity when immersed.

Lung function

- The pressure of the water against the chest and lung region means that participants have to work harder to push the ribs out and up during inspiration to expand the lungs. In confirmation of this competitive swimmers score above average on the peak flow test that is a measure of lung function.
- Generally, pool environments are warm and humid. This can often be beneficial for asthmatics, provided that they do not have a problem with the pool chemicals.

Kidney function

When exercising on land, the functioning of the kidneys is reduced as blood is diverted to the working muscles away from this organ. In water, however, because of the increased venous return and blood supply to the abdomen, kidney function is maintained.

The physiological reason behind this phenomenon is too complex to go in to detail here. Briefly it is due to a hormone that is responsible for the production of urine controlling the body fluid levels and absorption of water. When an individual enters the pool they are subjected to the forces of hydrostatic pressure that increase venous return; this tricks the hormone into thinking the body's fluid levels have expanded. So while in the water the production of this diuretic hormone is decreased, which increases the production of urine. However, as soon as the body leaves the water, production of this hormone increases once again and this response disappears.

As added pressure on the kidneys causes them to produce more urine it is wise to inform your class of this, so that they prepare themselves. This has particular significance if teaching pre- and post-natal and seniors' aqua classes!

Water also affects other organs of the body, namely the heart. These effects are considered under the guise of the **immersion theory**.

The immersion theory

Heart rate drops in water, by about 10 beats per minute

This drop in heart rate, particularly evident in deep water, is due to the lower demands placed upon the cardiovascular system because of the reduced effects of gravity in water. Venous return is assisted by the massaging effects of the water and the muscular contraction. The body also has an increased ability to shed heat in water. This will keep the pulse rate lower during the entire workout.

If participants were to wear heart rate monitors and attempt to compare their heart rate levels to that of on-land training, this would be misleading. It is advisable to use the rating of perceived exertion (RPE) scale.

Blood pressure drops on entering the pool

There is some evidence to suggest that the diastolic pressure may decrease as an individual enters the pool. If this is the case then care needs to be taken with any participants with known low blood pressure or those recovering from a cardiac event. However, once the exercise begins, the blood pressure will rise as it does with any exercise.

However the research is inconclusive and further investigation is needed.

Circulation is improved

If more blood is circulating around the body at a faster rate, extra oxygen can be taken to the working muscles. This means that strenuous activity can be more easily achieved for a wider range of participants.

There is an increase in metabolism by 20 per cent

Despite the fact that there is an increase in venous return during exercise in water, the major organs of the body are functioning at a higher rate than they would during land-based exercise regimes.

Due to the fact that there is a larger volume of blood returning to the heart, the force of contraction within the cardiac muscle is greater, which leads to an increase in both stroke volume and cardiac output, as defined in Chapter 5.

As described earlier in this section, inspiration is now happening against a resistance and requires more effort on the part of the intercostal muscles than on land. This will increase the energy consumption of these inspiratory muscles.

In addition to these activities, the body may have to work harder to retain its core temperature if the class is taught in a cold pool. This too will increase the metabolic rate.

The facility

The overall structure of the class may resemble your average exercise to music land class. However, the length of time spent in certain sections will vary. Your main priority will be to keep your participants warm throughout the class. Static work needs to be avoided for periods longer than one minute at a time.

The pool

This may be of many shapes, sizes and depths, all of which can alter the structure and content of your classes.

Pool shapes

These could be square, rectangular, round, oblong or kidney-shaped. This will inevitably affect the choreography and available travelling space, along with safe class sizes.

Pool and class sizes

Always check the maximum number allowed into the pool at any time. Never exceed this value, for the safety of your participants and so as not to invalidate your insurance cover. Sometimes the number of participants alters the number of lifeguards needed on pools of certain sizes and you need to be aware of this and ensure the correct coverage is provided.

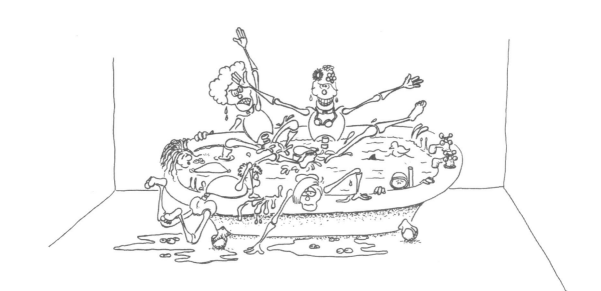

As the current law stands, with pools of less than 25m in length, there is no need for lifeguards to attend the poolside. However, it is strongly advisable to become qualified as a lifeguard. At the very least you need to have a current CPR certificate.

Pool depths

As mentioned before, the pool could be of a constant depth; the floor could slope towards a deep end or there could be shallow water at each end with deep water in the middle. Participants need to be made aware of the depth and where the slope begins. This is especially important if you have participants who are non-swimmers.

The pool depth should be clearly written on the pool side. Ideally, depths should be 3–4 feet and variable to accommodate all heights of people. If the water is of constant depth, this can make the intensity difficult for those participants who are small (as buoyancy increases). For those who are tall, underwater arm patterns will be difficult and their joints will undergo greater levels of impact with more of their body above water. As the instructor, you should make suggestions as to where each participant should stand to utilize the water resistance effectively, whilst not letting buoyancy take over.

Water quality

Water quality should be tested regularly by trained staff, this is generally done at four-hourly intervals by the pool or gym staff. They complete pool tests to monitor the levels of the disinfectant (chlorine, bromine or ozone) within the pool and the pH value of the water. Pollution within a pool can be a product of the bathers or of bacteria.

Within any pool, regardless of the origin water quality, every bather will add pollution to the water in the form of:

- Mucus
- Saliva
- Sweat
- Dead skin cells
- Body fat
- Urine
- Faecal matter
- Creams and lotions

If the water quality deteriorates and disinfection does not occur, numerous infections can result, including:

- Gastro-intestinal infections
- Skin rashes
- Ear inflammation
- Athlete's foot
- Verrucae
- Conjunctivitis

The water in the pool needs to be filtered and disinfected continually. The disinfectants most commonly used in pools include:

- Chlorine
- Bromine
- Ozone

If a pool contains ozone, it will also contain chlorine, but in a lower concentration. The presence of ozone makes the smaller quantities of chorine more effective.

Water temperature

Depending on whether your pool is based in a school, leisure centre or private health club, the temperature could vary within the range 28–34 degrees. These are considered to be 'neutral' temperatures. This means that within this range, the amount of heat lost to the water can equal the heat generated through the exercise. The temperature of the pool will very definitely affect the structure and format of your class.

DID YOU KNOW?

The conductivity of water is about 240 times greater than that of air. This means that the rate at which heat is lost from the body is a good deal quicker than on land. Heat is dissipated four times faster in water than in air.

It is advisable to check the temperature before you start the class. This is normally tested every four hours by the lifeguards or the gym team. These records can then be made available to you, if there is not a thermometer within the pool.

It is not only the pool water temperature that affects the comfort of your class members. The surrounding air temperature can fluctuate and will have an effect on how warm or cold the water feels to the participants. The effect of the surrounding air will depend on the depth to which they are submerged in the water.

If the surrounding air is cold, ask participants to submerge themselves more deeply in the water. If the reverse is true, ask them to move to shallower water, so less of their body is exposed to the water.

It will be irrelevant how interesting your choreography is, if your participants are shivering for the entire duration of the class.

The body has several mechanisms to draw upon in order to stay warm and preserve core body temperature. Shivering is one of these; blood vessel reaction is another. Blood vessels in the skin and in skeletal muscles can constrict strongly to create an outer shell that protects the body against greater heat loss. If muscles and nerves become cold, they react more slowly and produce movements of poor quality.

It is interesting to note that some areas of the body are particularly susceptible to heat loss. These include:

- Side of the chest
- Front of the neck (by the carotid artery)
- Groin
- Armpits
- Head

One solution to this would be to wear a cap and a 'chill-vest' or T-shirt. However, a way to reduce the effect is to splash pool water on these areas before entering the pool.

Factors that influence the rate or extent of core body temperature reduction include:

- Medications
- Tobacco/caffeine (vasoconstrictors)
- Alcohol (vasodilator)
- Immersion time and depth
- Poor nutrition/hunger
- Dehydration

- Fatigue
- Body fat levels
- Anaemia

Ensure, to the best of your ability, that there are no obvious draughts within the pool area. This wind chill factor can increase the heat loss by the processes of radiation, conduction, convection and evaporation.

 If the skin enters the pool already cold it is three times more sensitive to heat loss. So start warm and stay warm!

It may be as well to alert your participants to the fact that their appetite may also increase after a water class. Suggest they bring a healthy snack with them to eat on the way home otherwise a chocolate stop at the garage may be the result.

Class design principles

Class duration

Aqua aerobics classes normally last no longer than 45 minutes. This can be reduced to 30 minutes, while still providing an effective workout. Any longer than 45 minutes and body temperatures drop when tiredness sets in causing the class to do smaller movements.

The structure of the class is similar to that of the other exercise to music and step classes; it is the emphasis and time spent in each component that may differ.

Aqua aerobics class overview
- Introduction to yourself, the venue, and class structure.
- Warm-up (mobilization, first pulse-raiser and range of movement stretches).
- Aerobic curve (build-up, peak and build-down).
- Brief muscular strength and endurance (MSE).
- Cool-down (flexibility, relaxation and possibly a revitalizer).
- Feedback from class.

Class music

Some aqua classes are done without any music; some use only background music. Other instructors will choreograph their classes to a piece of music. This can feel strange initially, as people will move at different speeds in the water, due to their differing buoyancy levels. Your demonstrations, as the instructor, have to be done at half-speed. Generally, music speeds range between 100–136 bpm. On average, music speeds need to be about 10 bpm less than for the equivalent section on land.

It is best to mix fast tempo music (to increase resistance) with slower tempo tracks (that use longer levers and a greater range of movement). Ensure that you evenly distribute the stresses applied to the different joints and muscles of the body.

Common errors with music choice are:

- The music is too fast.
- The music is too repetitive, resulting in similar moves and muscle groups being overloaded.
- Music is selected without practising the routine in water first.

The stereo unit used varies considerably. Ideally, it should be battery-operated, but, if powered from the mains, the unit needs to be at least 1.5m away from the water's edge.

Typically, the acoustics in a pool area are not good, so you should ensure that your class can hear you at all times. Sometimes microphones can help this situation, but the output levels need to be closely monitored and you need to check that the class can hear you as you move around throughout the workout.

The warm-up

As with any class, the basis of the warm-up remains the same. The warm-up section in an average land-based aerobics class would contain:

- Mobilization
- Pulse-raiser
- Pre-aerobic stretches

These may be quite distinct sections. However, in an aqua class, these sections are combined to reduce the risk of participants getting too cold. Although the range of movement around a joint can often be larger in water it will need more time to complete each move. It is extremely difficult to maintain a static position for long in the water so joint isolation movements are not often performed.

Similarly, static stretches are not as effectively completed in water. Range of movement stretches are more useful. Beware of the temperature falling dramatically if many stretches are done consecutively. Attempt to keep the class moving between each stretch. It is essential that muscle temperature is effectively raised before stretching is attempted. It can be argued that the muscles, in general, are at less risk of injury in water. Therefore, stretching is not a great concern during this section of the class.

There is less injury risk because:

- Movement speeds are slower – risk of a muscle tearing is reduced.
- There is little potential to lose balance and fall as the water is supportive.
- Momentum forces that may cause a muscle to go beyond its normal range of movement are reduced.

Concentrate on stretching only those muscles that have not gone through their full range of motion during the pulse-raiser. If stretching the upper body, attempt to keep the legs moving.

The aerobic component

The main aim of this section is still to overload the cardiorespiratory system by providing a workout that is demanding for every individual in the class, encouraging them to work at levels above that usually needed for their everyday activity.

Overload in the water can be achieved by:

- Increasing the length of lever (but slowing music speed)
- Increasing the force applied through the water
- Increasing the speed of the movement performed
- Increasing the surface area of the limb applied to the water

Their target heart rate range would still be within the ACSM's (1990) recommended 60–90 per cent of their maximal heart rate. However, means of monitoring this may be limited in water.

As with any aerobics class there will be a mixture of low- and high-impact work, travelling moves off the spot, making use of forward, backward, diagonal, sideways and circular travel. Time has to be given for participants to complete the moves over slightly different periods. A holding pattern of a stationary jog may be ideal to allow the class to come back as a group before moving off the spot again.

Any choreography has to reflect an understanding of:

- Slower movement speeds
- The resistance of the water
- The difficulty of quick changes of direction
- Effects of turbulence and eddy drag forces
- Effects of reduced gravity on movement quality

The muscular strength and endurance component (MSE)

This section has less importance than in a land-based aerobics class. Due to the fact that the resistance in water is so much greater than air, many of the major muscles will have undergone endurance-type training throughout the aerobic component.

If this section is included in the class, it is necessary to understand that the way muscles contract in water is different and that the resistance offered by the water is different from that offered by air.

The three main types of muscle contractions are:

- **Isotonic** – A muscular contraction in which a constant load is moved through a range of motion of the involved joints. It is referred to as a dynamic contraction and encompasses both **concentric** and **eccentric** contractions.
- **Isometric** – A muscular contraction in which there is no change in the angle of the involved joints and little or no change in the length of the contracting muscle.
- **Isokinetic** – A muscle contraction through a range of motion at a constant muscle tension and velocity.

The isotonic contractions in water are dual concentric contractions. It is difficult to emphasize the eccentric phase with the reduction in the forces of gravity.

It can be appreciated that in water, isokinetic work can be done which would require specialist and expensive equipment if attempted on land. In a pool the water provides constant resistance and pressure throughout the range of movement of the joint.

To make effective use of strength gains, some individuals may need additional equipment. This will aim to increase the surface area of the limb being worked. This will be covered in a later chapter.

However, remember that any static work will cause a rapid drop in body temperature and enjoyment.

Any exercise suggested for this section should show appreciation of:

- The principle of overload
- The use of dual concentric contraction
- Equipment to increase the surface area to increase resistance

Flexibility section

Combination stretches are often used to limit the time spent in this section. The muscle and body temperature should remain elevated if this is done. While upper body stretches are performed the lower body needs to be kept moving. The use of floats may be needed to aid stability.

Relaxation

This can be done very effectively in water. Usually floats, woggles or flotation belts are used to increase the individual's buoyancy, allowing them to lie back and float completely relaxed.

Work can be done in pairs where one partner slowly pulls the other through the water. This increases the massaging and soothing effects of the water.

Alternative class formats

Aqua classes are advertised under a variety of different names. These are dependent on the target population, pool size and equipment available for use. Additionally, the depth of the water affects the activities possible. There are now specific courses and equipment for use in deep water. These utilize the additional buoyancy factors and absence of impact. Generally, the standard aerobic-style class in water can be expected when advertised under the following guises:

- Aqua aerobics
- Aqua fit
- Aqua dance
- Aqua splash
- Swim fit
- Water walking (good for postural and stabilization muscles)
- Water running (excellent for cross-training)
- Power aqua
- Aquatherapy (for rehabilitation purposes, arthritis sufferers, etc.)
- Pre-/post-natal aqua
- Aqua relax
- Aqua circuits
- Aqua intervals
- Aqua step
- Aqua step circuits
- Deep-water aqua

Deep-water aqua

In order to teach this well, additional considerations need to be taken into account:

1 The body has to remain vertical in the water. Neutral body alignment is essential throughout the class. This involves a process of re-education when in the water as the feet and ankles have lost contact with the pool floor.
2 There is less gravity affecting the body; the stabilization muscles determine if the body is vertical.
3 Flotation equipment is necessary.

4 Teaching skills need to be specific to the above factors. The class should begin with stationary exercises to establish vertical stabilization. This position may need to be returned to before challenging moves are introduced.

Aqua choreography

Many instructors believe that movement in water is limited compared with land-based class choreography. It is advisable to simplify the moves you use to make them strong and effective, however, this does not need to limit your creativity. Table 14.2 suggests some of the most commonly seen moves in current aqua classes. These moves are similar to those from land-based classes. However, there are many moves that can be taken from sporting disciplines and your imagination. Just get into the water and play!

Table 14.2 Choreography suggestions

Move	Low-impact	High-impact	Progressions	Alternative	Direction	Hand positions
Heel pumps	March	Jog	Sprint	⇒ Heel flicks ⇒ Twists	On the spot, forward, backward, 360° turns, circles around the pool	Fist on sprints; cups on travels
Heel digs	—	Jump heels	Front leg reaches	—	On the spot	Fists, cups
Alternate knee lifts	—	High knee runs	Tuck jumps	⇒ Frog jumps ⇒ Rocking horse	On the spot, 360° turns	Fist on high knee runs; cups on tuck and frog jumps
Side steps	Side squats	Side squat jump	Side leaps	—	On the spot, sideways, 360° turns	Slice or cup
Half jack	—	Full jack	Add tuck jump between each jack	Suspended deep water jack	On the spot, 360° turns	Slice or cup
Spotty dog	—	Alternate jump changes	Add tuck jump between leg changes	Suspended deep water leg changes	On the spot	Slice or cup

Remember that when teaching these moves from the poolside your demonstrations have to be slow but energetic. Your movement quality needs to be precise, particularly with reference to the hand positions. Ensure you use these demonstrations to good effect and learn rapidly how to conserve your own energy throughout the class while maintaining excellent class control and teaching skills.

How to maximize your water workout

Bearing in mind everything that has been said up until now, there are key ways in which you can maximize work done in water. As the instructor, you will need to inform your participants of these before and during the class.

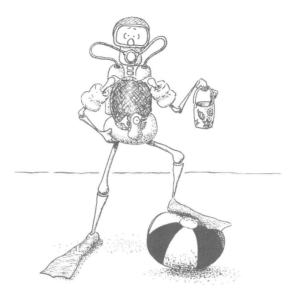

Everyone can benefit from the resistance provided by the water – however, it is easy to cheat and relax into the flow of water (turbulence) created by those around you.

Here are some essential points for participants to remember:

- Keep upright in the water with a strong posture (abdominals tight, back supported).
- Stand in water between waist and chest height (dependent on your buoyancy level and the content of the class).
- Work against the water at all times, not with it (use the water as if it is not there).
- Maximize the surface area of the hands as they work through the water (hands slightly cupped with fingers together).
- Increase speed of movement to increase resistance offered by the water.

Hand positions and movements

There are a number of basic positions that can alter the intensity of work done in the water. These offer variety to leg patterns, alter intensity and ensure that any one joint is not overstressed.

The slice

This is when the fingers are extended and together, the hand in line with the arm and wrist. This creates least resistance to the water and allows the upper body to recover, offers a lower-intensity option or allows concentration on fast work on the lower body, e.g. while doing a jumping jack.

The fist

This provides a moderate level of resistance as you present the surface area of the knuckles to the water. This works well with strong, powerful moves, usually done at speed, e.g. sprint run.

The cup

This provides most resistance for the upper body. This is best used when you wish to maximize work on the upper body, wish to increase intensity or need assistance or stability for a lower body move, e.g. while doing the twist.

The scull

This is a stabilizing move and is particularly useful when performing an exercise that requires the individual to remain on the spot, while concentrating work on the legs or abdominal area, e.g. abdominal flips.

Equipment

The aim in using equipment is not only to provide variety, but to maximize the three properties of water:

- Buoyancy
- Resistance
- Weight

This enables cardiovascular and muscular overload to be achievable for any individual.

The types of equipment currently available are:

- Floats and kickboards
- Swim buoys
- Mitts and gloves
- Woggles
- Dumb-bells
- Flotation belts
- Steps

Floats and kickboards

These aim to increase buoyancy or resistance and can preferentially train the upper or lower body. Made of foam, they are rigid squares or rectangles that vary in size and resistance or buoyancy.

Lower body emphasis – holding the float horizontally on top of the water you can kick the legs (front crawl or breaststroke-style). This can be repeated swimming on your back with the float placed behind the head or extended overhead.

Upper body emphasis – hold the float vertically beneath the surface of the water. It can then be pushed forward or down or around the body to strengthen the upper body muscles.

Swimbuoys

These increase the buoyancy of an individual as well as resistance through the water. Made of foam, they are moulded into a figure 8-shape, usually of a uniform size.

With one of these between the legs you can propel yourself forward or backwards through the water in a lying or more upright (seated) position.

Mitts and gloves

These increase resistance of the hands through the water by increasing the surface area of the limb. They are made of materials ranging from lycra to thick wetsuit material.

All the hand positions described above can be utilized with mitts to alter the resistance provided. Mitts also assist postural alignment as, when they are pushed down through the water, they provide a table of support for the body.

Woggles

These increase buoyancy and resistance. They are 4-inch cylinders of foam that can support the entire weight of the body or provide specific resistance for predominantly the upper body.

Dumb-bells

These add resistance to upper body movements and can replicate gym work and entice men into the class. They have a plastic core with foam heads that adds drag when moved under the water.

Flotation belts

These are designed to hold individuals at shoulder height in the water and so aid buoyancy. Upright posture is maintained and full ROM achieved in lower body.

Steps

These add variety and resistance and also impact as the body is lifted further out of the water. Ideally water depth should be such that when standing on the step the water comes midway up the forearms. Any deeper than this and overload is reduced.

Teaching skills

Although Chapter 15 is dedicated to the teaching and instructional skills needed by class teachers, this section highlights those skills that may be unique to the aqua environment or need emphasis.

Teaching position

To allow the class to see you at all times, you need to be situated on the poolside, out of the water. Only in this way can your posture be seen. Demonstrations need to be done slowly (half-speed). This can not only feel strange, but is extremely tiring!

If you have a chosen teaching position, consider placing a towel on the poolside to reduce the likelihood of you slipping.

If you change your teaching position do not be tempted to run as the poolside will inevitably be wet and slippery. Turn the class slowly to enable you to get there safely.

Instructor dress

Bear in mind that while your class is enjoying reduced-impact work in the water, you may be jumping around on a concrete floor. After several weeks your shins will complain about this. Wear trainers wherever possible, although some centres may have a no-shoe policy or request that you wear over-shoes but these can be slippery in themselves!

The other reduced-impact option is to use a rebounder on the poolside. If the centre does not possess one, this may be a piece of equipment that is worthwhile for you to purchase, especially if you are teaching a number of classes per week. However, it does limit the amount of travel you can demonstrate to your class.

Participant dress

Although the properties of water are supportive for the joints, this cannot be said for other areas of the body. Drag forces mean it is important for women to wear supportive bras under their swimming costumes, otherwise the ligaments supporting the chest can be affected as the turbulence of the water moves the chest.

Swimming costumes are generally worn, although general class wear is acceptable. The only issue here is that the chemicals in the pool may damage the material of these items.

As it is the speed and movement within the pool that increase intensity and provide overload, footwear is often worn. Pool floors are notoriously slippery and traction is difficult. There are now available trainers specifically designed for the pool; these being light and made of a synthetic substance that is less likely to be affected by the chemicals. However, a cheaper alternative is to wear a pair of ordinary socks. These allow sufficient traction on the pool floor to maximize travelling moves.

Observation

Your observation of the class will be made difficult due to the refraction of the water. Participants may look as though they are in the correct position, but your line of vision will be affected. This is particularly true when attempting to observe something like a gastrocnemius stretch. It is difficult to see if the leg is straight and if the heel is on the floor. Verbally, you need to be very clear about correct positioning, in addition to giving correct demonstrations on the poolside.

Rehydration

This is essential for both instructors and class participants. As the instructor, you will be exercising intensely in a very humid environment and will sweat profusely. You will also need to keep the vocal cords lubricated.

Class participants will be less aware of their fluid losses in water as their sweat will be dissipated in the water and they will need to be reminded to drink plenty during and after the class.

Aquatic myths

Generally these centre on one basic, prevalent and tenacious myth: that aqua classes are easy and are meant for the unfit, infirm and overweight. Here are the answers to the possible fallacies you will be come across as an aqua instructor.

1. Aqua classes are easier because you do not get as hot or sweat as much as in land-based sessions.

This is because sweat is dissipated in the water and heat loss is four times faster in a watery environment.

2. Water sessions are easier because your heart rate does not increase to the same extent as on-land classes.

Your resting heart rate is about 10 bpm lower in water due to the immersion factor, increased venous return, reduced forces of gravity and reduced core body temperature.

3. As there is no delayed onset muscle soreness (DOMS), exercise intensity must be lower than on land.

This absence of muscle soreness is due to the inability of the muscles to contract eccentrically in water. Water provides 12 times the resistance that air does, therefore, the potential can be greater in water.

4. Exercising in water encourages fat deposition and is no good for weight-loss purposes.

This fallacy grew up around a study of athletic female swimmers who trained in a cold pool. They found that, in relation to other athletes of the same calibre, the swimmers had higher body fat percentages. This was attributed to the low temperature of the pool meaning that the body had felt the need to retain fat for insulation purposes. This will not be a factor in any heated pool used for aqua classes!

CHAPTER SUMMARY

- Aqua aerobics is suitable for any individual of any level of experience, co-ordination and fitness level.

- The benefits of aqua aerobics are numerous and include lessened impact levels, increased support and resistance, improved circulation and excellent mobility and relaxation opportunities.

- The three properties of water are: buoyancy, resistance and hydrostatic pressure.

- Each of the properties of water needs to be understood and then utilized to maximize the effectiveness of water workouts.

- Buoyancy is affected by body composition, location of fat deposition, gender, depth of the water and the amount of the air in the lungs.

- An individual with a high centre of buoyancy will float easily, tend to lie more horizontal in the water and find it more difficult to stabilize their body position and travel with speed through the water. Females and endomorphs tend to fall into this category.

- An individual with a low centre of buoyancy will have a tendency to sink and lie vertical in the water. They will find it more difficult to complete deep water work without the use of flotation aids. They will be able to move through the water with speed. Males, mesomorphs and ectomorphs are typical examples. →

- Water provides a resistance to movement 12 times greater than that of air. Factors such as turbulence (eddy drag) and opposition will make quick changes in direction difficult.

- Inertia currents make it easier for the second row of a class to move against the water.

- Muscle contraction is dual concentric in nature. It is difficult to work the eccentric phase of an exercise due to lessened forces of gravity.

- Hydrostatic pressure improves circulation, increased resistance benefits breathing and kidney function.

- Immersion theory states that heart rate levels will be about 10 bpm lower in water, diastolic blood pressure may decrease and metabolism will rise by about 20 per cent.

- When designing your classes, pool shapes, size, depth and lifeguard cover need consideration.

- Water temperature should lie in the range 28–34°C to be neutral. Heat is dissipated four times more quickly in water than on land.

- Use of equipment in aqua classes adds either additional buoyancy, resistance or weight.

- Hand positions can also effectively alter the intensity of movements in water.

Teaching and instructional skills

CHAPTER
15

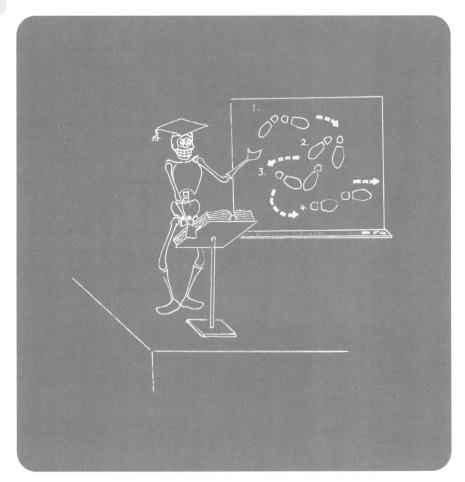

Topics to be covered in this chapter:

- The role of teaching skills
- How teaching skills affect performance
- Voice projection
- Defining advanced instruction skills
- Teaching skills for the class instructor
- Instructional skills for the gym instructor
- Combined instructor skills
- 30 tips to becoming an excellent class instructor
- 15 tips to becoming an excellent gym instructor

To be an instructor, you need to be able to programme activities for people that are safe and effective. To be an excellent instructor, there are many additional skills that can be brought to this role for the benefit and enjoyment of your clients. Some of these additional skills will need to be learnt and practised. The skills needed for the different roles of a gym instructor and class instructor have basic similarities. This chapter delves more deeply into the personal and interpersonal skills an instructor will need to develop and maintain in order to provide excellent customer service.

The role of teaching skills

The essential elements of any class or programme, regardless of level, are that it will be:

- Safe and effective
- Achievable
- Motivating
- Inspiring

For all of these elements to be present, the instructor will possess the following to some degree:

- Personality – and the ability to project this personality.
- Ability to motivate – knowledge of the different ways to motivate the class or individuals.

- Technical knowledge – of the body, exercise adaptation and progression, health and fitness and goal setting.
- A wide range of teaching and communication skills – to ensure that every individual enjoys any class or programme to the maximum.

How teaching skills affect performance

The class instructor

The skills needed by class instructors can be appreciated by comparing a newly qualified instructor with an international presenter. If the class format and choreography were identical, there would still be a large difference in the way the class was instructed. The way in which the moves were broken down and taught; the amount of personality projected would be different. This would lead to differences in the levels of motivation and, probably, the level of achievement by participants.

However, no matter how experienced the instructor, these skills, once acquired, should be practised and reviewed regularly, ideally by an external instructor. This ensures that they are improved and built upon continuously. Bad habits form easily.

The gym instructor

When in a gym environment it is also easy to detect experienced instructors. They usually contact more people in less time by spotting those individuals requiring help sooner and correcting them more quickly. While correcting any individual they keep their eyes and posture open to the rest of the gym and provide reassurance and greetings to other individuals in subtle ways whilst still in conversation.

Voice projection

At some stage in their career class instructors will experience problems with their voice. This may be as a result of continued teaching through a cold or flu or due to the lack of microphone facilities in a large studio or hall. All of us can probably name an instructor with this characteristic hoarse quality to their speech. A survey completed in 1996 suggested that up to 60 per cent of instructors suffered some form of voice problem. If left untreated, minor problems can deteriorate into a long-term issue. It is, therefore, essential to know how best to guard against potential problems and to deal with the situation if it arises.

How sound and speech are made

Speech is one of the most delicate and complex operations the body is capable of. There are literally hundreds of muscles in the lungs, throat and mouth that are responsible for producing the sound we know as speech. The entire respiratory system and the muscles from the abdomen to the nose co-operate to produce speech.

However, the most important of these are the:

- Larynx
- Tongue
- Lips
- Soft palate

The larynx

This is known as the **voice box** and contains the vocal cords. Situated at the top of the trachea (windpipe), it is covered by the epiglottis. This acts to close the trachea when food is swallowed, thus ensuring delivery down the oesophagus to the stomach and not into the lungs.

It is the vocal cords that vibrate to produce sound and speech. They act rather like a reed in a wind instrument; vibrating as air is passed over them. The throat, nose and mouth shape modifies the sound that is produced. The vocal cords are constructed of two ligaments, shaped like lips, which open and close as air is passed over them. The shape of the cords varies from a wide V when talking to a closed slit during swallowing.

To generate sound, air from the lungs is expelled over the vocal cords and through the larynx. This is known as phonation. The loudness of the sound made is dependent on how rapidly this air is expelled through the larynx. The pitch of a person's voice is dependent on the tension within the cords and length of time for which the air is expelled.

The general depth and timbre of a voice is down to the size of the nose, throat and mouth. This is why men have deeper voices, their larynx is larger and their vocal cords are slacker. The mouth and tongue then play a role in allowing us to differentiate between words.

Diaphragmatic breathing

The air that is passed over the vocal cords and through the larynx is produced in one of two areas:

- Stomach/diaphragm
- Chest/thoracic

If the air is generated in the chest/thoracic area voices tend to be of a higher pitch (generally associated with female voices). The voice is less supported in this situation and tends to have a weaker quality. This is more likely to become injured. Additionally neck tension can also build in an attempt to provide more air for longer sentences, to shout or to reach higher-pitched notes.

It is more useful and powerful if women can train themselves to breathe from their stomachs or diaphragms (as most men usually do). This allows their voices to be deeper, to be fully supported.

By standing up and placing a hand on your chest and one on your stomach you can easily check for this method of breathing. Breathing normally, you will either feel your shoulders rise first or your stomach lift first. If the chest and shoulders are moving first you are breathing from the thoracic region. Concentrate, keeping your hands in place, and focus on lifting the stomach hand first. This will take some time to feel comfortable and will need practice before it becomes second nature.

How to use the air generated from the diaphragm to best effect

The air we generate as instructors has to perform a number of important functions with clarity and at the same time. Generally, we are actively exercising and intent on supplying adequate oxygen to the working muscles. We also need to cue and communicate with our class at the same time. It is, therefore, essential that we develop the amount of breath that can be stored in the diaphragm and learn to control its release.

Intonation and diction

Having completed the diaphragmatic breathing exercises and having learned to control the release of air you can further add clarity to your voice by focusing on your intonation and diction. Practise saying letters and words in different voices:

- Tired voice
- Happy voice
- Angry voice
- Friendly voice

Consider different volumes available to each of these voices. The loudness of your voice when teaching can affect the motivation and enjoyment levels of your class. Too quiet and you will fail to motivate and cause frustration if people are straining to hear you. Too loud and this will be unpleasant.

Common vocal problems

These result from different issues, namely:

- Misuse – generally as a result of poor vocal technique.
- Abuse – resulting from dehydrating substances such as alcohol, caffeine or drugs or continued use during a bout of illness.
- Overuse – excessive use that does not allow time for adequate rest and recuperation.
- Illness – Commonly laryngitis, causing soreness and swelling. Severe sore throats and nodules may result if no rest is allowed during any illness affecting the throat.

How to reduce the risk of injury

As previously highlighted, the muscles and ligaments that support the action of speech need as much care and attention as we lavish on the other areas of our body. This means that before a period of prolonged use the vocal cords and surrounding tissue should be thoroughly and gradually warmed up and should be cooled down after use. Tension can remain in these tissues just as anywhere else.

Warm-up exercises

These include humming or singing before a class. Once muscles and ligaments of the larynx and vocal cords are warm you can then focus more on diction by repeating tongue-twisters or poems. Utilize the whole vocal range; vary the volume and speed of the words.

Cool-down exercises

Once again gently humming or singing will gradually relax the muscles and ligaments of the larynx and vocal cords.

Other methods of reducing injury risk

- Drink plenty of water.
- Avoid dehydrating substances (tea, coffee – caffeine; alcohol).
- Avoid whispering as this also dehydrates the vocal cords.
- Avoid smoking or smoky atmospheres.
- Improve your non-verbal cueing skills.
- Swallow in preference to clearing the throat (excessive phlegm can be reduced by cutting down the amount of dairy products eaten).
- Rest fully if a problem develops.

Microphone technique

Basic rules

- Do not shout. Talk into microphone normally.
- Still use diaphragmatic breathing and intonation.
- Position the microphone slightly above or below the mouth to prevent excessive whistling sounds and to prevent your mouth from being obscured by those who may use lip reading skills.

As with every other aspect of your class, you will need to practise using the mic to feel comfortable with it and to adjust the settings correctly.

Ensure the reverb knob on your stereo unit is turned down to zero and the volume of the microphone allows you to talk normally and be heard. This will be difficult for you to assess, as the sound of your voice through the mic will sound strange to you initially. Therefore, ask someone to stand in the centre of the studio and tell you if the volume is correct. Beware of standing directly in front of the speakers, as this will increase the feedback through the mic. Recognizable as a loud, high-pitched shriek that causes the entire class to wince!

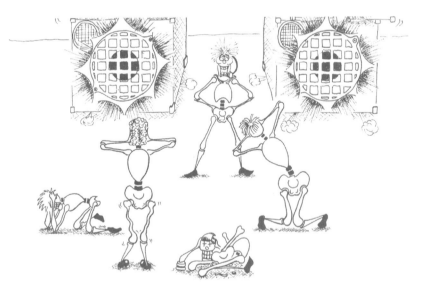

Women generally need less treble on the sound system and men will usually reduce the bass. Use a volume level and pitch of music that complements your vocal quality. Adjust the levels on the music first, then select your mic volumes. From this point on you should look to using the master control knobs to alter volumes throughout your class.

Defining advanced instruction skills

Advanced teaching skills are actually a combination of skills, which are developed and refined throughout an instructor's career.

Skills needed by gym and class instructors would incorporate:

- Rapport, communication and group interaction skills
- Observation and adjustment
- Motivational methods

If you acquire these skills it makes you look professional, improves participant adherence, increases the fun and enthusiasm and can decrease the risk of injuries.

Your reputation as a good instructor will be built from many aspects of your personality, image and basic teaching skills. It is these that your participants will comment and grade you upon. However, what makes an excellent instructor will be skills that your participants are generally unaware of and are unlikely to comment upon. They are often subtle skills that enhance participant enjoyment and develop your role as an instructor away from that of a performer.

Teaching skills for the class instructor

Those skills specific to class teaching would include:

- Musical interpretation
- Cueing techniques and demonstrations
- Class management and integration

Musical interpretation

Music appreciation has been covered earlier. It is worth reiterating that most choreography is built into blocks of 32 counts, each containing 4 phrases of 8 counts. There is an accent on the first beat of each phrase. Some more difficult music tracks may not be in such regular 32 count blocks. These errant 2, 4, 6 or 12 counts can produce a problem. The best way to 'bridge' these counts is to devise a simple holding pattern. More advanced choreography may cross-phrase, meaning the routine crosses over the 32-count phrasing and generally rejoins it later.

Other ways of interpreting music are to listen to and utilize the different beats within a phrase. Syncopated rhythms are used in jazz classes. This means moving on the half beat. Hip-hop classes make good use of pauses linked to double time moves. All these methods will add variety to any choreography.

Cueing technique and demonstration

Advance warning of changes in direction or movement patterns represents one of the most basic and necessary teaching skills. The amount of warning given depends on the speed of the cue, the type of class and the ability levels of the participants themselves. It is essential to cue to ensure movements are performed:

- With correct alignment
- With co-ordination
- At the correct time and with the rest of the class

Individuals pay attention in various ways, some people listen to instructions, and others only watch visual signals. Therefore, both of these techniques should be employed at all times.

It is a useful exercise to imagine you cannot speak and to cue your entire routine using arm patterns only. This will improve your visual signals considerably.

Verbal cueing techniques vary tremendously:

- Count down: 4–3–2–1–move
- Count down: 4–3–2–and–go
- Count up: 5–6–7–8–move
- Are we ready and – move

The speed of the cue will depend on instructor preference and the move that is being done at the time. For example, if the class is marching, this is a single-count move, with every foot strike representing one beat of the music. A fast count would suit this move. However, if they are doing a knee lift, this is a two-count move. A slow count would be more appropriate.

Class management and integration

You need to have control of the class at all times. This will be helped by accurate and advanced cueing techniques. A strong, well-projected voice assists authority. Cater for all individuals by offering alternatives and make people feel comfortable to adopt these. Ensure smooth transitions between different sections of the class.

Your teaching position is crucial, every participant should be able to see you at all times. This may mean you have to move to the back of the class, the sides, and even the centre. However, it is wise to inform your class when you are leaving the front and where you are going to, particularly if your class is large. It can be disconcerting for participants if you suddenly and unexpectedly move position. This is particularly off-putting for those individuals who rely on visual cueing techniques.

Instructional skills for the gym instructor

Possibly one of the greatest skills a gym instructor can develop is that of observation. Each individual within the gym environment could be doing a different exercise, each with its own technique. The gym instructor must therefore observe everyone and prioritize who needs help, correction or motivation first. Also, the approach to an individual will differ from that to a class. People attending a class know they are going to be instructed and corrected and are receptive to this. Those within a gym can be resistant to correction on occasions. This can be minimized by maintaining an open and welcoming posture, making all comments positive, and creating a rapport with the individual.

While talking to one person, the instructor needs to keep in view the rest of the gym to retain eye contact with other people. Contact should be encouraging and positive but brief and to the point, so that as many contacts are made as possible.

Combined instructor skills

These are the essential skills that are common to both class and gym instructors.

Rapport, communication and group interaction skills

Methods of communication should be tailored to each class or individual you instruct. Communication should begin the moment a participant enters the studio or gym and continue throughout.

Creating a rapport with individuals may involve humour, on unrelated topics to fitness. Communication is essential to pre-screen participants, to ensure everyone is working to their correct intensity and in giving feedback.

The social aspect of your classes or gym is important and you need to instigate interaction between the group before, during and after workouts. One way this may be done is through your choreography – getting the two halves of the class to face each other, partner work during the MSE or cool-down sections.

Within the gym you can encourage group inductions, introduce a new member to an existing one, create buddy (training partner) systems and set challenges and gym games, which involve group work of differing ability levels.

Observation and adjustment

All individuals should be observed at all times. This can be done most effectively if class sizes are controllable. Realistically, the maximum number of participants that can be effectively observed by one instructor is 25–30. Classes larger than this may need a spotter. This is a person who literally observes the participants' technique and is another demonstration body to ensure all participants can see the moves.

You will notice that more advanced instructors tend not to complete the entire class physically, but use improved communication and cueing skills to guide the class through the routine without their participation.

If you need to correct the technique or body position of any participant, the following procedure should be undertaken:

- Verbal reminder of correct technique to the class.
- A second verbal reminder, reworded – making eye contact with the individual, or standing closer to them.
- Individual verbal correction in positive tone of voice, not into the mic.
- Hands-on correction – only if permission has been asked and granted first!
- After class correction – speak to the individual concerned.

Within a gym, there is usually more than one instructor available at peak times to assist in correction, which can make it easier. However, some people can be resistant to correction, particularly if they are a regular exerciser and confidant of their abilities. It is still vital that you attempt to correct their posture and or exercise technique so that you can reduce the risk of injury, in addition to increasing the effectiveness of the exercise.

The way you approach someone within the gym is all-important. Your opening line should be chosen with care. Try to open with a positive. Consider the following method of correction but remember not to linger too long with one individual, as there will be many more people needing your help.

- Initially consider something the client is doing well and praise them.
- Ask the client what they want to achieve from the exercise.
- Ask them if you can make a suggestion.
- Alert them to the potential risks associated with adopting poor posture or incorrectly performing the exercise – make it specific to their mistake.
- Demonstrate or talk them through the correct technique.
- Ask them to try this.
- Reinforce specific teaching points and praise the client.
- Ask them if that feels more comfortable or better.
- If they have been unprepared to change technique, maybe introduce them to a different exercise that targets the same muscle group but may encourage better technique!

Motivational methods

Different things motivate people and therefore, different techniques need to be employed.

Motivational techniques can begin before the class or workout:

- As people enter, congratulate them on returning to the class or gym, or on finding the time or confidence to attend for the first time.
- Thank everyone for coming before a class starts.
- Once the class or workout has started, praise individuals for the speed with which they picked up a step/routine, their posture or technique.
- Comment on an individual's fitness level improvement, facial expression, outfit – the list could continue.
- After the class or workout, give feedback on an individual's performance and smile.
- Set short-term goals for each session.

The key is to get to know each person sufficiently to appreciate which of these comments would motivate them the most. In order for you to do this, you will have to know what the goals are for each person. Your comments will then attempt to reinforce behaviours that will allow them to achieve these.

As shown above, motivational techniques can be:

- verbal – words of praise, congratulation or compliments
- visual – eye contact, smile

These skills should be incorporated within a session, and will become second nature with practice and experience. Like routines, they need to be practised and appraised on a regular basis. An alternative to getting another instructor to appraise your teaching skills is to video one of your classes every so often. You can then sit at leisure and criticize yourself, writing down the positive and negative aspects of your teaching style. If you are unsure of your choreography, the teaching skills will disappear from your class as your mind is solely occupied with remembering the next step. Therefore, practice is the key.

With gym instructors you could suggest getting another instructor to rate your performance on the gym floor. For example, in terms of:

- How many people were spoken to within a specific time period
- How many non-verbal contacts were made
- If any individual was left struggling on a piece of equipment without being approached

30 TIPS TO BECOMING AN EXCELLENT CLASS INSTRUCTOR

Before the class:

1 Arrive early, look professional, sort tapes and microphone levels.

2 Bring your own towel and water bottle – be a role model.

3 Greet everyone as they enter the class.

4 Learn the names of all your participants as soon as possible.

5 Talk specifically to and individually screen all new participants.

As the class begins:

6 Introduce yourself, for the benefit of all newcomers.

7 Space out participants and ensure you can be seen by all.

8 Be prepared to deal with latecomers – speak to them and ensure they are warm.

9 Thank everyone for attending the class.

During the class:

10 Make eye contact with each participant.

11 Stay human throughout – introduce comments/questions/humour which are not fitness-related.

12 Ask open-ended questions to generate a class response.

13 Have verbal communication with each person once during the class.

14 Include educational information in every class.

15 Change your teaching position.

16 Communicate with individuals if you are leaving the front – this can unnerve them.

17 Feel comfortable to stop exercising yourself.

18 Avoid negative instruction – use positive cues.

19 Avoid repeating the same words or phrases throughout the class – they lose sincerity.

20 Compliment people on doing something right.

21 Smile.

22 Stay positive.

23 Avoid asking participants to smile – simply give them something to smile about.

24 Have a goal at the end of each session.

→

25 Thank everyone for attending and completing the class.

26 Communicate with anyone who leaves early – note, call, fax.

After the class:

27 Give individuals positive feedback.

28 Find out if they intend to return.

29 Find out individuals' fitness goals.

30 Accept feedback about your own performance.

15 TIPS TO BECOMING AN EXCELLENT GYM INSTRUCTOR

1 Visually greet every individual who enters the gym (smile, eye contact, wave)

2 Adopt a positive, open posture.

3 Verbally interact with every individual during their workout.

4 Use people's names whenever possible (look at their programme cards)

5 Be quick to correct poor technique.

6 Never stay on the same spot for more than a couple of minutes.

7 Cover the entire floor space, walking between machines, not on the perimeter of the gym.

8 Focus on speaking to the people you do not know, not just the ones you already know well.

9 Never stay more than a couple of minutes with each individual.

10 Attempt to book people in for a re-assessment.

11 Sell other services within the club – direct people to classes or the pool for variety.

12 Gather feedback about the club in general and pass this information on to the relevant people.

13 Compliment each individual on something – their physique, clothes, hair, trainers, etc.

14 Use a variety of motivational techniques, perhaps set session goals and coach them for 2 minutes.

15 Say goodbye to every individual as they leave the gym.

CHAPTER SUMMARY

- Any class or session you instruct must be: achievable, motivating, inspiring, safe and effective for all participants.

- As the instructor, you need to project your: personality, knowledge, motivation and excellent teaching skills.

- Projecting your voice effectively will increase the safety of your classes and enjoyment to be had by the participants.

- The volume, pitch, timbre and intonation of your voice need to be taken into account when teaching in a different venue or when using a different stereo and head mic system.

- Understanding how your vocal cords affect the above and the fact that they can be prone to injury should be essential for any instructor. Warm-up and cool-down exercises should be performed by instructors to safeguard their most valuable asset.

- Becoming familiar with your head mic and knowing how to use it effectively can improve the professionalism of your class and save your voice from overuse injuries.

- The basic teaching skills that need work are: musical interpretation, cueing, class management, rapport, observation and motivational methods.

- Your instruction begins before the class or workout and continues throughout and after.

Health and safety

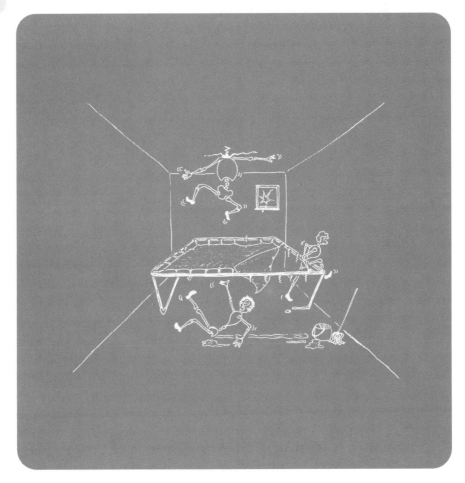

Topics to be covered in this chapter:

- ○ The instructor's role and responsibilities for health and safety in the workplace
- ○ The Health and Safety at Work Act (1974)
- ○ Safe working practices within the workplace
- ○ Essential health and safety legislation
- ○ Health and safety issues specific to the gym and class instructor
- ○ Essential site-specific health and safety checks

The purpose of this section is to raise awareness of prevalent health and safety issues within the leisure and health club setting. When assessing the risks associated with physical activity, the clients' safety is paramount.

Health and safety is becoming a growing concern for fitness instructors and centre managers due to the increased awareness of participants due to the increased number of law suits that relate to injuries in the health and fitness arena. The aim of this chapter is to make you aware of how to ensure your own safety, that of your colleagues and participants within the workplace. You should know the basics of emergency action procedures and the role you play in the treatment and reporting of common incidents you may encounter.

The instructor's role and responsibilities for health and safety in the workplace

It is any fitness instructor's job to ensure the health and safety of their participants. This is a field of training that is not emphasized sufficiently in many health clubs. When you begin to look into this area you realize just what a responsibility this is and the problems associated with neglecting this aspect of an individual's initial training, induction or professional development.

As with most fitness industry trends, the United Kingdom lags behind the United States in the arena of health and safety litigation. It is frighteningly common in the US for individuals to take their fitness instructors to court over an injury they have sustained, or claim to have sustained, while under their instruction, or lack of it! The number of such cases in Britain is climbing, as are the levels of compensation that are received if the plaintiff wins the case. It is, therefore, a topic that should be learnt and taken seriously.

When a person begins training with you and they are under your instruction they become your responsibility. Once the individual has set foot in your facility or turned up for their session they are in your hands, this applies, regardless of the environment in which you are training them. However, take some time to consider that some environments require additional insurance cover on your part, as they present higher risks. For instance, some health and leisure clubs will insure their instructors while they teach within the facility, but should the instructor set up a running or cycling club that takes them off-site and involves other equipment, separate insurance may be necessary. Insurance is essential in all of the following roles and environments:

- Full-time or part-time gym instructor within a health and fitness centre
- Full- or part-time fitness instructor within a health and fitness centre teaching circuit training, spin cycling or body pump
- Full- or part-time fitness instructor within a health and fitness centre leading power walking, running, rambling or cycling clubs outdoors
- Freelance class instructor teaching at a variety of venues
- Any instructor on poolside or teaching aqua classes
- Any instructor providing personal training services
- Any instructor providing nutritional advice

However, not to be forgotten is the duty of your employer to provide you with a safe working environment to aid this process. This is where it is necessary to introduce the bare essentials of the Health and Safety at Work Act and how it relates to your role and that of your employer.

Health and Safety at Work Act (1974)

The **Health and Safety at Work Act (1974)** is a landmark Act that extended employers' and employees' responsibilities for health and safety. It clearly lays down guidelines for implementing health and safety at many levels. The Act is known as an umbrella Act as it works with other legislation, in defining both what is needed and how to go about doing it.

In brief, the **Health and Safety at Work Act (1974)** places a duty of care onto the shoulders of **employers** which requires, as far as is reasonably practicable:

- Provision of a safe working environment.
- Safe use, handling, storing and transporting of articles and substances.
- Maintenance of a safe working environment, adequate facilities and arrangements for welfare at work.
- Provision of a written health and safety policy statement, which must be issued to employees, as must any revisions.
- Provision of information, instruction, training and supervision.
- Provision and maintenance of plant and systems of work that are safe and without risk to health.

Employees' duties are as follows:

- To take reasonable care of their own health and safety and that of others who may be affected by their acts and omissions.
- To co-operate with their employer.
- To use machinery, equipment, dangerous substances, transporting equipment and means of production or safety devices in accordance with their employer's training and instruction.
- To inform employers of any serious or immediate danger to health or shortcomings in the employer's arrangements for health and safety.

Safe working practices within the workplace

Any company that has five or more employees has to provide a written health and safety policy by law. This document should outline all the company's health and safety action plans. It is usually lengthy so there will often be a shortened version covering the salient areas specific to your job role. All such information should be read thoroughly and understood by you.

Employee induction

When joining a facility you should have an induction to the site. This should allow you to familiarize yourself with the building, systems and policies, and work colleagues. If it is unclear, question what your role would be in an emergency. Find out as much as possible about health and safety within the building and your role within it.

Ideally the induction should include:

- Information about the site's health and safety policies and procedures.
- Specific information on welfare issues (location of toilets, frequency and length of breaks and any additional hygiene issues).
- An introduction to the company's health and safety representative and your supervisor.

- Findings from any risk assessments.
- Verbal and written details on prohibition of any areas.
- Your responsibilities.
- Details on essential health and safety legislation (covered later in this chapter).

Once this material has been presented to you, you should sign to say that you have read and understood it.

Safe systems of work

A safe system of work is a working practice that has been instigated to ensure workplace tasks are done safely and efficiently. The site-competent person will have looked at all tasks carried out on site and worked out an optimally safe way of performing each one. For example they will have developed a safe way of vacuuming the motors inside the cowling of the treadmill. It is imperative that you are aware of the best way to proceed with any given task. If you are unsure, you ask.

Client screening

Screening guidelines are covered in depth in Chapter 8 but it is worth reiterating the importance of a thorough screening process for everyone who enters your facility. Although a screening form is not a legally binding document, even if the client has signed and dated it, it goes a long way to showing a court of law that you were attentive and attempting to tailor the exercise prescription to the client. The goal is to provide a safe and effective programme for all participants, whilst providing additional support for those who need to be supervised.

The essential aspects of this screening information are that:

- All information given to you verbally is noted in detail.
- Information is acted upon to ensure the safety of the client (via a referrals procedure).
- All information remains confidential.
- Records are kept in a locked room or cabinet.
- Regular updates are made to the information.
- Both you and the client sign and date the information sheet.

Essential health and safety legislation

There are many different aspects to this legislation, some of which may not be directly relevant to your centre or current job. The important fact is that you know the relevant and up-to-date legislation and act upon it at all times.

Reporting of Injuries, Diseases, and Dangerous Occurrences Regulations (1995) (RIDDOR)

The main factor here is to be aware of on-site reporting procedures for you and for others. There will be an accident book or forms kept at the main reception where any injury, accident, near-miss or disease resulting from work will be reported. Remember to record everything, even a minor cut!

Control of Substances Hazardous to Health (COSHH)

This relates to use of any chemicals on site. In the gym you may use strong cleansers, antibacterial substances, oils and sprays. If your site has a pool then you can be exposed to some extremely strong substances, such as chlorine.

The site-competent person will do a COSHH assessment to evaluate the risks of each chemical and try to make your contact with any of these chemicals as safe as possible. Ensure that you are fully knowledgeable about the chemicals you are in contact with in terms of what they are used for and what effects they may have on you. Ensure you are fully trained to deal safely with any chemical used at your facility.

Personal protective equipment (PPE)

If you are dealing with any hazardous chemicals, you will need to be physically protected from them, in addition to being armed with the knowledge of what effect they may have on you! For instance, if your facility has a pool, a common chemical used in this environment is chlorine. When handling this highly corrosive substance you should wear a full-length smock, gloves, goggles and face mask.

Any protective equipment in use should be regularly checked to ensure it is in good working order, stored in the correct environment and relevant to the task and chemical at hand.

Manual Handling Regulations (1997)

Due to the nature of the job of a fitness instructor, it is likely that you will be doing a lot of manual handling throughout the day. Your job will involve pulling, pushing, lifting and carrying. Consider yourself first and ensure that you do it safely.

The site-competent person should do an assessment of the manual handling tasks on site and, where possible, substitute or replace the task to reduce the possibility of orthopaedic injury. Make sure that you are aware of all necessary tasks especially those that need two people. Do not be tempted to go it alone.

First aid

Physical activity or exercise places stress on the body. This brings with it a certain degree of risk of an incident. When instructing in the fitness arena it is highly probable that, sooner or later, you will have to deal with a first aid event of some severity.

Initially, your job is one of prevention. You can reduce the risk of many accidents occurring by programming suitable exercises and levels of intensity for all your participants. By using keen observation skills when on the gym floor you can identify any symptoms of overexertion or illness.

However, even the most observant instructor can be party to an incident. It is therefore essential to be prepared with the necessary information to allow you to deal with the situation in the most professional and efficient way possible. This would involve knowing:

- Who the on site qualified first aiders are and how they can be found.
- The location and content of the nearest first aid box to your activity.
- The nearest telephone to your activity to call for help.
- How to operate the nearest telephone and who it will be connected to (reception or emergency services).
- What illnesses and injuries require the emergency services.
- The exact information the emergency services require if called to an incident.
- The reporting procedures that you must follow after attending to any first aid incident.

Evacuation procedures

Being prompt and positive in an emergency situation can save lives. Knowing the quickest route out of a building can save even more. Make sure you are familiar with the entire building you instruct in and know the procedures and your role, in the event of an evacuation due to fire or to a bomb threat.

Fire evacuation procedures

When evacuating a building you need to be aware of:

- The site emergency action plan.
- Possible warning signals; what the alarm sounds or, in some cases, what it looks like (lights will flash in areas where loud music is played).

- Location of the nearest exits from your teaching areas.
- Location of the breakpoints (fire alarm trigger points).
- Exact location of the meeting point.
- Location and appropriate use of each type of fire extinguisher.
- Location of all fire doors.
- General fire prevention practices.
- Your role in firefighting.

Bomb evacuation procedures

In some centres these may be identical to the above procedures. In others, there are specific alarm calls that relate to bombs and the meeting point is often as far as possible from any buildings and car parks. One of the biggest causes of injuries due to bomb explosions is the effect of the aftershock. Flying glass and objects within the surrounding area can cause as much injury as the explosion itself.

Health and safety issues specific to the gym and class instructor

In summary, whether you are employed or self-employed it pays to have knowledge of the basics of health and safety issues; otherwise you may find yourself in a situation where you are paying out to your clients.

If you fail to adhere to health and safety legislation *you* become **liable** or responsible for the consequences. You have a responsibility to your participants to know the capabilities and limitations of each of them and to recognize any problems they may be encountering.

Although it is difficult to prove that you were liable for a certain injury or problem you can further strengthen your position in the event of a court case. Generally, any court will consider two aspects about your instruction of and dealing with the client:

- Whether you provided a **standard of care** that is expected and up to current standards within the industry.
- Whether you were **negligent** in any respect in terms of failing to instruct correct technique, taking account of an injury or medical condition that would affect performance or in advocating contra-indicated practices or exercises.

A possible example of failure to show an appropriate standard of care may be the absence of any health screening and a standard programme being given to all members. There has been no attempt made here to take into account the needs of the individual. A further example would be the lack of any induction to show correct usage of the equipment, resulting in the individual using a piece of equipment unsuitable for their level of fitness and injuring themselves due to incorrect technique.

Negligence may be apparent if you complete a health screen on an individual who informs you of diagnosed coronary heart disease, but though you tick this positive response, you fail to refer for medical clearance and provide no adaptation to the programme in response to this condition. As a result, the high intensity of the aerobic work and the heavy nature of the resistance training triggers a cardiac event.

Completing all the recommended paperwork and fitness tests on an individual, followed by the design of an individualized plan and the completion of a one-on-one induction may not preclude the possibility of an accident. However, the individual involved would have a hard time proving you failed to show due care and attention and were negligent.

The following is a simple checklist to remind you of the areas of responsibility if you are instructing in either the gym or studio environment:

- Need for health screening.
- Possible case for fitness tests.
- Individualized gym programme prescription.
- Class choreography with adaptations to suit all ability levels.
- Gym inductions encouraging correct technique.
- Safe instruction skills (cueing, spotting and correction techniques).
- Excellent observation skills of active individuals.
- Full-time supervision of the environment.
- Regular maintenance checks on all equipment.
- Immediate reporting of faulty equipment.
- Regular checks for electrical safety.
- Ensuring that the exercising area is free of obstructions.
- Controlling the area to prevent maximum numbers being exceeded.
- Provision of water.
- Adequate ventilation of exercising area.
- Knowledge of first aiders and procedures.
- Knowledge of fire evacuation procedures.

Whatever the problem relating to health and safety, ignorance does not offer immunity from liability, so make sure you are aware of and up-to-date on all health and safety issues! The following questions within Table 16.1 may prompt you to check certain areas or help you to identify those that need attention in your centre.

Essential site-specific health and safety checks

Table 16.1 Site-specific health and safety checks

Entrance	Is it safe to get in and out of the gym? Are there any obstructions or foreseeable difficulties?
Emergency exit	Are the exits clearly labelled with the correct signage? Are the exits usable? Are there any obstructions?
Fire procedures	Is it obvious what to do in case of a fire? (signage, etc.) Is there adequate provision for dealing with fires?
First aid procedures	Is it obvious where the first aid supplies are? Are they suitable? Are there first aiders on shift? Where is the nearest phone?
Obstacles	Are there any obvious obstacles, barriers, protrusions that could cause an accident or damage in the future? Is the equipment set out so as not to cause problems to other users?
General housekeeping	What is the general housekeeping like? Suitable? Is the gym laid out for optimal use? Are exercise areas suitably compartmentalized?
Temperature	Is the temperature suitable for the activities taking place?
Lighting	Is there a good mix of natural and artificial light suitable for the activities?
Ventilation	Is there a good exchange of air within the area?
Maintenance procedures	How frequently is equipment checked? Is the equipment in good working order? Are there appropriate signs on equipment that is out of order? Make a visual check on all the equipment/Try it if you have time.
Electrical safety	Has any of the equipment been electrically tested? Do the electrical cables look suitable for use? Are there any trailing cables?
Water	Is there water available that is fit for drinking?
Signage	Are the signs around the gym suitable and sufficient? Are any additional signs needed?

CHAPTER SUMMARY

- The fitness instructor has an essential part to play in ensuring the health and safety of participants in their classes, just as an employer has the responsibility to its employees.

- The Health and Safety at Work Act (1974) has laid down clear guidelines for the employer and employee to follow.

- Every employee should undergo a full induction process that details all health and safety policies and safe systems of work. Any client of a fitness instructor should undergo a health screen and receive an individualized fitness programme. →

- RIDDOR stands for the Reporting of Injuries, Diseases and Dangerous Occurrences Regulations (1995) and stipulates that all major, minor and near-miss incidents should be recorded in detail.

- COSHH stands for the Control of Substances Hazardous to Health (1995). There should be detailed notes on the effects of each chemical in use and instructions on exactly how to handle them safely.

- PPE stands for Personal Protective Equipment, which should be worn at all times when handling chemicals.

- Manual Handling Regulations (1997) should be adhered to if you are required to move or lift any heavy objects in the course of your daily activities at work.

- Emergency action procedures should be known in the case of a first aid incident, fire or bomb threat. Know whom to inform, what role you play, and how to report the event later.

- It is essential that, as a fitness instructor, you are aware of the health and safety checks that need to be undertaken to ensure the safety of both yourself and your clients. It is your responsibility to report any problems that you detect during these regular checks.

- To reduce the likelihood of any court action always provide a high standard of care for your clients and when they exercise with you remain attentive and observant at all times.

Customer service

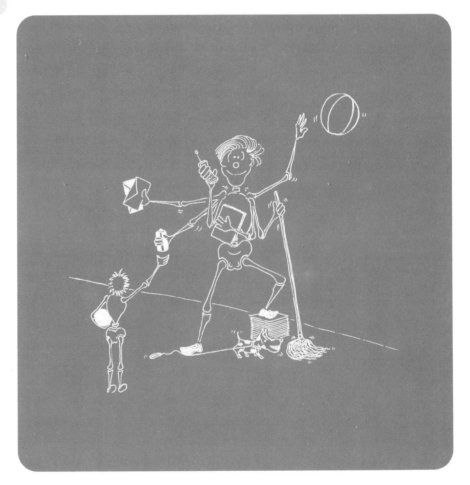

Topics to be covered:

○ Defining customer service

○ Providing good customer service

○ The elements that contribute to the service package

○ How to exceed expectations – that extra mile

The fitness industry is a service industry. The concept of what constitutes good, bad and excellent customer service should be thoroughly understood. Much of the knowledge we have on this subject has been gained from our counterparts in the United States. They still remain far ahead of us in this field and generally promote a better level of service than many clubs in the United Kingdom.

Unfortunately, customer service is often the final aspect to be considered by a class teacher, gym instructor or centre manager. We are often too concerned with the material aspects of a club or class to spend sufficient time ensuring the experience had by our customers reaches, or ideally, exceeds their expectations.

There is greater awareness nowadays of what constitutes good customer service. Additionally, our customers are more aware of what we should be providing and consequently have higher expectations and exercise their choice as to which club or class to attend. The winners are almost always those centres or instructors that provide better customer service than their competitors. Although a variety of factors initially attract an individual to a facility, it is how they feel and are treated by the staff at the centre that will affect the type of experience they have. In turn this will impact on member retention.

Defining customer service

For some individuals this chapter may simply represent what appears to be common sense. To others it is less natural and is more of a learned response.

In any service industry, the people buying your product keep your business alive. They are paying for you to provide them with a service, whether this is an aerobics class, a personalized gym programme or a health club that allows them simply to relax and take time out for themselves. Participants buying your product are likely to have different expectations of what they have bought, what they will experience and what they will ultimately achieve. It is your job to try to meet the needs of each and every one of these people, to the best of your ability.

It is wise at the start, to be precise in terms of what you are selling so that the customer knows what is being bought and what they may achieve. If people know what they are buying and come to you with similar expectations, your job will be easier. In the best scenario, you are providing the customer with what they want, because you have sold them what they were looking for. However, customer service does not stop there. This is when the fun begins.

Having bought your product, some individuals may not feel that they have got what they wanted, or may consider that it has failed to provide them with what they were looking for. In this instance it is your job to educate, motivate and/or pacify them in order to keep them as customers.

Inevitably in life, things do not always go as planned. Therefore, another essential skill encompassed within the realms of customer service is dealing quickly, effectively and courteously with the problems you encounter. Knowing your customers is the key, so that you can tailor your dealings with them, know when to apologize and what compensation to offer in difficult circumstances. Common problems involve the showers not working, the air-conditioning breaking down or no car park spaces being available at peak times.

You will quickly come to appreciate that you will spend much of your time dealing with issues that are not strictly within your job description and more often not within your power to correct! The most fundamental thing to understand is that if a member of a health club has a problem with any area of the club, then they will inform any member of staff and expect results. Even if you are off shift, on a break or a day off, the expectation will be the same and the issue should be politely and promptly dealt with.

Providing good customer service

A simple way in which this can be achieved is to give the customer what they want.

Herein lies your first problem – what do they want? Second problem, how are you going to find this out?

What the customer wants

If you begin asking people what they want from a club or class, you will soon realize that there are as many different answers as there are people. Hence, the reason why providing good customer service proves to be more problematic than you might have first thought.

The initial reality is that individuals will want something different from you, because their reasons for coming to you will be driven by very different forces. Everyone is motivated by different factors and will return to you for a multitude of different reasons. As their reasons for being with you are different, the image they have of you will also differ. They will notice different aspects about you, your class, and your club. Thus you have to be all things to all people.

People choose classes or clubs for a mixture of the following reasons:

- Location and convenience.
- Cost – either value for money or expensive to signify quality.
- Size – large can be a status symbol, small can be more personal.
- Opening hours and class times to suit lifestyles.
- Reputation and recommendation.
- Décor and quality and range of equipment.
- Range of products offered.
- Cleanliness.
- Personality of staff and personalized service.
- Social events.
- Directed by doctor or coerced by partner.

The service package

When looking to improve your levels of service you should consider the following:

- Your packaging
- Your product
- Your procedures
- Your people skills
- Your ability to identify problem areas
- Your willingness to learn from the past

Your packaging

It is useful to consider your product through the eyes of a stranger. Does it make an impact? If not, why not?

A recent example is the case of studio-based resistance classes, which have made a huge impact in the fitness industry. This has been due to many factors. One of the first reasons that springs to mind is their simplicity. Simple concepts work. People know what they are getting from these classes, there are no surprises. They claim to change your shape and have been successful in showing results in people over a relatively short space of time. In this way they have followed through on their promise.

Now consider your product and how you package it.

- How could more impact be made on your client base?
- How can you make people want to come to you?
- What advertising techniques do you use?
- Do you provide what you claim to?

This may relate to issues as wide-ranging as the wording of your posters and flyers or to the structure and decoration of the building where you instruct. Whatever it is, consider how to use it to its best advantage and market it as a positive feature to the customer.

Your product

You need to be aware of exactly what your product is. This should then prompt further questions to ask yourself:

- Is the product still valid?
- Have you kept up-to-date with current trends and thinking?
- Is your product suitable to your customer base?
- How can you improve your product?

The fact is that some customers will come purely because of your product. They will not place other aspects of customer service high on their list of priorities. So long as you provide them with the class, gym or club environment they want, they will be happy. These people can often be identified by the fact they arrive for your session, work out and leave. There is little interaction between them, with you or other members of staff, or with other participants.

For others, the product will be important, but there are other factors that rate as highly or higher than this. These people can often be found socializing before and after the class and talking to you about other issues aside from the content of your class, the quality of your gym equipment and the structure of the building.

Due to the ever-changing nature of the fitness world it is essential that all staff members keep up-to-date with developments in the industry, changes in thinking regarding the benefits or disadvantages in different methods of training and the use of different machines. Participants today are much more likely to know something about fitness and require education or answers to their questions, to dispel some of the more tenacious myths that they carry with them.

Your procedures

The emphasis should be on enabling the customer to go through the necessary procedures in the minimum amount of time, with the greatest efficiency. Procedures should not be adhered to because they make life easier for you or the management. Always remember you are in a service industry. Your work revolves around, and exists for the benefit of, your customers. However, procedures must be realistic for you to operate, being time-efficient and achievable.

There are many different factors to consider.

Entry procedures into your centre, club or gym

If membership cards are needed does this slow down a member's entry into the club? If payment is necessary for any activities consider how it can be made. Review the time it takes for a new member to enter the club, join and use your gym facility. Some centres enforce a variety of different appointments, screening sessions and inductions which can take several days to a couple of weeks to complete. Although this could be seen as thorough, it is also restrictive and quite possibly intimidating for the participant.

Entry procedure and control measure into classes

Individual entry into a class can also be a lengthy procedure. It is your responsibility to ensure the safety of all participants. This means they need to be screened and the maximum class numbers need to be adhered to. If tickets are collected this needs to be done efficiently in a way that allows you to identify quickly who may have either not booked or arrived last if the class is overfilled. If a booking system, cancellation policy and waiting list are implemented who will police them and how?

Screening process

Consider from the member's viewpoint when the screening process is best done and how the information is transferred to the relevant instructors. Remember, the information is confidential and needs to be kept under lock and key.

Latecomers will provide you with a challenge to these procedures. You can develop your own system for dealing with this situation. The very least which should be done is a verbal screening of the participant and close monitoring throughout the class.

Certain basic procedures in your centre or at your class will influence your customers. It is worth looking at the process of attending your class or gym from a stranger's viewpoint. Consider, step by step, the procedures you would have to go through. Sometimes it can appear as though you are deliberately trying to put people off coming to you!

Your people skills

The people employed within any facility are essential to its operation, regardless of the position they hold. They will spell success or failure for a company, whether they are situated on reception, the gym floor or within the changing rooms. Every member of staff has the potential to affect the experience of every client who walks through the door. We know that word of mouth referrals are the best and most cost-effective way of gaining new members. We should also be acutely aware that bad press travels far faster and to a wider audience and is remembered for a longer time. It is always easier to remember an experience of bad customer service. The chances are that it revolves around someone being uninterested, unhelpful or simply rude.

There are certain essential points to get across to any member of staff. Firstly, it is vital that all staff work as a team. Even if you are a freelance class instructor you are still part of the teaching team and you represent the club and what it stands for. It is ideal if there is teamwork across departments. This is particularly important between sales teams and gym instructors. Here lies the key to much member dissatisfaction. If someone is sold a membership based on the service provided in the gym, then this needs to be relayed to the gym team and the claims should represent a service that can be realistically provided.

Secondly, make sure that each member of staff knows the responsibility they have to their clients and the role that they play. Effectively, when you are in contact with members, on the gym floor, in the studio, in the car park, you are on stage. People enjoy positive contact with others, so it is inappropriate to let your clients know if you are depressed, angry or bored. They are at your class or facility to gain enjoyment. In this respect, you need to perform to the extent that you always appear happy and welcoming. The most essential aspect is that you seem genuine – possibly one of the hardest elements of customer service, particularly when you consider how tired you may be from working an early shift or teaching a number of classes in one day. If you can manage it you will come across as professional and your following will show their appreciation by loyally turning up to your classes.

However, a third point to make would be that within any company's customer service policy, there must be room for a staff member's personality to shine through, so long as limits are known.

Essential skills that are appreciated by participants include:

- being proactive about the members' needs
- being approachable
- being knowledgeable
- being willing to apologize and deal efficiently with problems

Human beings are weird and wonderful creatures. One of our traits is that we are heavily influenced by first impressions and usually make snap judgements about people and situations, perhaps within the first few seconds of meeting someone. It is vital, therefore, that you create an excellent impression within this time frame. Only certain things can be done effectively in such a short space of time. Consider what is feasible and aim to include these on greeting every customer.

Having successfully made it through these first harrowing seconds, you are now being judged in a slightly different way, but do not be fooled into thinking you are no longer being watched. Within these next few minutes, you should be seen to be efficient and attentive and to extend the qualities you displayed within the first few seconds into this longer time frame.

The last few seconds of your interaction with your customer are also vital and often overlooked. The likelihood is that it will be the contact at this stage which will encourage them to return to you and leave them feeling good for the rest of the day. They will be more forgiving over the first few seconds, if these final seconds are impressive.

Your ability to identify problem areas

Inevitably you will come across problems. Some you will solve easily and rapidly. Others may be ongoing problems that are being addressed. Others may present you with a situation that you cannot deal with alone. These may necessitate involvement of management or other agencies. Whatever the problem, try to know how you are going to deal with it before the occasion arises.

Initially, it is important to give your customers opportunities to feed back to you on anything relating to your role as instructor. This may be offered to them in a number of ways:

- Verbal feedback directly to you – but ensure you have a follow-up procedure in place. Do not just listen, smile and forget!
- Written feedback – either in the form of a comment card that is posted into a suggestion box or via a notebook that is laid out for clients near the exit or on reception.
- Questionnaire – the results of which will need to be fed back to clients.

When you receive a similar comment from a number of people you can be reasonably sure that you have identified a problem area. Have set procedures in place to efficiently follow up all feedback gained. This should be prompt – within 24 hours wherever possible – and recorded.

When dealing with complaints it is worth remembering three points:

1 Apologize – regardless of who is at fault. You are sorry that the situation has occurred at all. It helps to calm the customer.
2 Accept the customer's point of view – clarify the problem, ensure you understand the situation, thank the customer for taking the time to give you feedback. Inform them of what you intend to do and by when, or at least let them know when you intend to contact them again to tell them what has been actioned.
3 Act – if you yourself cannot directly take action, ensure you inform the person who can do so. Make sure that they then take the responsibility of keeping your customer informed. Check that your customer is happy with the outcome.

Your willingness to learn from the past

When successes occur make a note of them and build on them.

Identify:

- What was it that made it a success?
- Is it realistic to provide this all the time, considering time and available resources?

Many companies have customer service charters and handbooks and make claims based on these explicit promises. Customer service should not be one of the things you get right some of the time or nearly always. It has to be right each and every time without fail. Do not make promises that you cannot keep. If you do, your customers will rapidly lose faith in you and look elsewhere to take their business.

That extra mile

Providing good customer service means that you meet your clients' expectations. To provide **excellent** customer service you need to exceed their expectations. This can be done by reviewing all the above points and looking at ways in which you can feasibly go that extra mile. Go beyond the expected and provide a level of service that competitors do not offer. There is no set guideline for this; predominantly, this level of service needs to be tailored to individual situations. By knowing the expectations and motivations of each customer, you can tailor your service to exceed their expectations.

The opportunities for providing excellent service occur every day. Every contact you have with a client is an opportunity that should be seized and maximised.

CHAPTER SUMMARY

- Customer service consists of providing every customer with what they want.

- Good customer service meets the expectations of the customers; excellent customer service exceeds these expectations.

- When looking at customer service, you need to consider your product, people skills, procedures, packaging, managing problems and past successes.

- Your product needs to be valid, up-to-date, and relevant to your customers. It can always be improved.

- People skills need to be present at all times, but key times are the first few seconds, the 'middle minute' and the final few seconds. Key skills need to be demonstrated during these times.

- Your procedures should be efficient and customer-friendly. Imagine yourself as a customer – what procedures may present barriers to prevent people attending or having an enjoyable experience?

- The packaging of your product needs to be correct to create impact and attract the relevant customers.

- Problem-management is key to a positive experience for the customer. They need to feel their comments are valued; there are easy ways in which they can do so (verbally and in written form).

- All complaints need to be handled promptly and efficiently. You should always apologize, accept and act on every suggestion.

Promoting physical activity

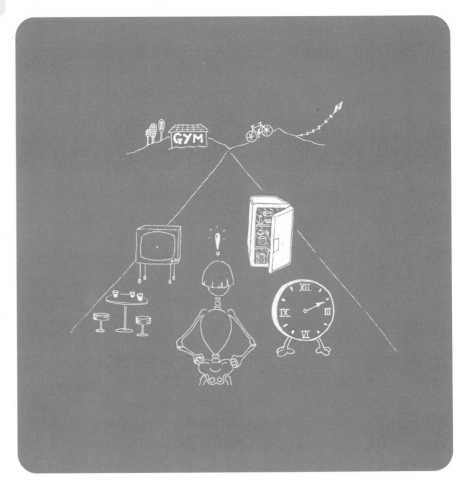

Topics to be covered in this chapter:

- Why promote regular physical activity?
- Reasons for inactivity
- Barriers to exercise
- Lifecycle influences
- Motivational methods
- The role of the instructor

The major health studies that have been completed over the past decade have concurred that less than 20 per cent of Britain's population are regularly active. The **Health of the Nation Report (1994)** raised awareness of the increasingly sedentary nature of the population and designated physical activity as a priority area. This chapter will consider why people remain so consistently inactive, despite their knowledge about the benefits of regular activity. Since changes over the lifecycle alter priorities, perceptions and motivation levels, it is beneficial to discuss these areas within this chapter.

Your role as a fitness instructor means that you are responsible for motivating people, many of whom are inactive, to be proactive about their health. In order for you to do this, you need to appreciate what barriers are currently preventing these individuals from being active. These barriers could be physical in nature or psychological; stemming from their perception of physical activity and exercise. Ideally, you should consider what factors affect these and what part you can play in shaping these perceptions.

Although an in-depth discussion of how to increase participant adherence is beyond the scope of this chapter, the role of the instructor will be outlined. By the end of the chapter you should have a greater understanding of the variety of individuals you will encounter at your centre and will be better prepared to develop an individualized action plan. Always remember, for someone to incorporate physical activity into their life is a major lifestyle change. With any such change, it will take time to develop confidence and physical activity should never be considered as separate from the other lifestyle issues that may need attention.

Why promote regular physical activity?

The **Health Education Symposium (1994)** was set up to develop a national strategy for promoting physical activity for England while the **ACSM (July 1998)** published the Health-related Fitness Guidelines that outlined the amount of activity necessary to make positive improvements to health and reduce risk of developing CHD, diabetes, obesity and other debilitating conditions.

This Health Education Symposium (1994) included a team of 45 experts in central and local government, the public health sector, health, sport, leisure and environmental management and research bodies. The objective was to develop a strategy with the aims of:

- reducing the percentage of the population who are sedentary
- increasing the percentage of the population engaged in regular moderately intense activity
- increasing the percentage of the population engaged in vigorous activity

An increasing percentage of our inactive population is classified as sedentary and obese. The government is keen to address this issue due to the increasing pressure on the health service.

The many different hypokinetic diseases discussed in Chapter 1 are costing millions of pounds every year to treat and rehabilitate. Physical activity and exercise are known to have a positive effect on an increasing number of medical conditions, ranging from coronary heart disease to depression.

Both the physiological adaptations and the psychological effects of exercise are responsible for the improvements in these medical conditions. Identifying exactly how much the physiological and psychological elements contribute to these conditions remains the subject of much research and controversy. For instance, we know that the structural changes that occur within the cardiovascular system as a result of exercise play an undeniably major role in preventing and treating individuals with coronary heart disease. In the case of someone diagnosed with cancer, however, the mechanisms are not fully understood and it is possible that the positive psychological outlook that an active patient develops may have a greater effect than physiological changes could account for.

Reasons for inactivity

Over the past 20 years, since the aerobics revolution was established in America at the Coopers Institute, we as a nation have been bombarded with information on how to stay active, fit and healthy. There has been a dramatic increase in the number of fitness and diet-related books, in addition to huge numbers of new magazines, telling us what to do and eat to optimize our health, fitness and quality of life.

There have been massive developments in the world of research, proving associations between lack of activity and a variety of cardiovascular, joint and bone conditions. Surveys have been completed that identify the fact that, as a population, we know what we should be doing to stay fit and healthy, but we are not acting on this knowledge. This reveals that human behaviour is not ruled by logic and is affected by a complex variety of factors. In order for us to encourage people to act on what they know they should be doing, we need to understand what triggers human behaviour and what factors, for the majority, mean that they do not adhere to a regular programme of activity.

The fact that people apparently ignore the information available to them about how exercise can improve health is not unlike the way they react to government health warnings on smoking. One suggestion is that they do not believe that the hypokinetic diseases that are linked to inactivity will affect them personally. If they believe that they are immune, then no amount of reiteration of the benefits of exercise will motivate them.

The outcome of the behaviour must be valued by the client

For most people exercise is a voluntary activity. It represents time out of their day, money out of their pockets and often constitutes an experience that takes them out of their comfort zone.

 In order for the activity to have more benefit than the costs attached to it, participants need to see the end result as significant and worthwhile.

Many people view exercise sessions as punishment. Others find that they have to sacrifice a more enjoyable and possibly unhealthy pastime to find the time for sessions. In order for individuals to adhere to a programme of activity they need to be definite about their goals and value the intended result.

The client must also believe that by completing the chosen activity, the desired result will be realized. They need to begin with a positive attitude and have the relevant education from you firstly to appreciate why the activity is appropriate, secondly how they progress to achieve the goal in the specified timeframe.

Goal setting

Before anyone can be expected to initiate an activity programme, it is essential to know what they intend to get from it. This overall goal is an important starting point. From this, you, as the instructor, need to clarify what exactly the individual expects to achieve and in what timeframe.

For instance, individuals often state that their fitness goal is to 'tone up'. It is essential that they define what they mean by this. For some it means building muscle, for others it may imply definition, for the rest it may mean a change in body composition that simply relates to a reduction in body fat.

Once the goal has been clarified, it is wise to ask them what they believe they need to do in order to achieve it. This will give you some indication of their knowledge base and their level of commitment.

Next, the timeframe needs to be considered. This will be dependent on the frequency, intensity and type of the client's chosen activity. It is vital that you are honest at this point.

Assuming that the goal is a long-term one and the timeframe is realistic, there is a need to develop some short- and medium-term goals. However motivated an individual is at the start of a programme, there will be times when this wanes or possibly disappears altogether. It is, therefore, wise to get them working towards a smaller but relevant goal that will make them appreciate the progress they have made to date. In order for this to be effective, you need to have an appreciation of what will be meaningful for the client at this stage.

Extrinsic versus intrinsic goals

Before you can successfully set goals and devise rewards, whether short-, medium- or long-term, you need to know if the individual is extrinsically or intrinsically motivated.

Individuals can be contracted to adopt a positive and healthy behaviour. For example, someone may agree to exercise three times a week for three months. At the end of this period if they have abided by the agreement they receive a reward. An extrinsic award may be in the shape of a T-shirt, money, vouchers for a beauty treatment or massage therapy – something that is valued by the client.

If rewards are intrinsic, they are internal. The person is motivated because of the positive way they feel during the session or by the increased energy reserves they have afterwards. It is common for a client to begin a programme needing extrinsic rewards and for their motivation to become intrinsic as time progresses as their feeling towards the sessions changes and the experience becomes more enjoyable and comfortable.

Social influences

No individual is immune to his or her environment. Therefore, we are all affected by the variety of social interactions we experience every day. These influences could come from very different areas of our lives:

- Family
- Work colleagues
- Friends
- Famous personalities

Ideally, find out how much support clients will receive from significant others. This can dramatically affect adherence levels. Partners can see exercise as taking time away from them and having a detrimental effect on the relationship. However, if you recruit support from others, it can increase motivation levels and the individual's enjoyment of the programme. If you clearly identify who this social influence is, then consider educating and involving them in the actual activity.

Barriers to exercise

Different people will have different reasons for not currently being active. An individual can list these reasons in order of importance for them. You should be able to determine exactly what may cause the individual to drop out during the early stages of a programme. As an instructor, empathizing with that individual's barrier may be difficult. What appears to be the most significant deterrent for them may appear to be totally inconsequential to you. However, do not fall into the trap of ignoring it. Your own values and beliefs should not be expressed at this point. Some of the factors that you comfortably associate with exercise, such as sweating, can outweigh the benefits of the activity for some. Consider this carefully and decide on an action plan and explain this to your client.

Remember to monitor an individual's progress through their programme, particularly at the beginning. Although you may have accounted for some of the obvious concerns and barriers the individuals have vocalized, there may be some surprises within the first few sessions.

Exercise places stress upon the body. This can be appreciated in the way the body temperature rises, sweating results and heart and breathing rates rise. To regular exercisers this stress is expected and easily tolerated. For someone new to activity, it can be very uncomfortable and sometimes frightening. How they deal with the stress of exercise may be predicted from how they deal with daily lifestyle hassles. This may be worth investigating before designing a programme.

There are different methods that can be employed in countering an adverse reaction to exercise:

- **Dissociation** – clients are taught to distract themselves from their activity. This may involve listening to music, reading a newspaper or magazine or simply learning the art of daydreaming.
- **Relaxation** – various methods may be employed both before and after the session to encourage the mind and body to relax. This may translate into a focus on positive aspects of the session while it is in progress.
- **Re-interpretation** – clients learn to think differently and positively about the sensations felt during the session. This may take some time to achieve and may involve the use of an exercise log where feelings are recorded and referred back to as a learning process.

Lifecycle influences

When people are prepared to be honest, they will give a variety of reasons for deciding to drop out of an activity programme. If you have completed an initial in-depth interview, you will be aware of which factors are the likeliest culprits to cause participant drop-out. We can appreciate the change in motivation levels as any exercise programme progresses. These changes will be linked to the comfort of the exercises, the amount of progress being made and the rewards participants receive during this process, whether intrinsic or extrinsic. Consider also that those individuals who drop out during the first week are going to quote the cause as being something very different from those who give up 6–12 months into a programme.

In addition to these factors you should consider the effect that the lifecycle has on participants' motivation levels and priorities. In general, we can consider the following different stages within the lifecycle that may need recognition.

Stage 1

This is considered to represent clients in their twenties and thirties. Across these decades, individuals are generally self-preoccupied and use exercise as a form of stress release, to improve their appearance, self-esteem and to control their weight. Therefore, you can expect their goals to reflect this. Usually their timeframes are short and they like to see results quickly. This may mean that you need to consider a variety of short-term goals to keep them motivated and active. Education is not always a priority, and, when given, should be a little at a time and specific to their goals. With this age-group limited emphasis may be placed on health gains and reducing risk of hypokinetic diseases.

Stage 2

This is usually apparent between the mid-thirties and the fifties. Lifestyle issues generally revolve around raising a family and dealing with work pressures. Although stress relief may be a goal of the activity programme, the health benefits and education will play a greater role and will become a more powerful motivator. There are likely to be conflicts on the priority list between lifestyle pressures and exercise needs. Goals will be more medium- and long-term, although short-term goals remain important.

Stage 3

In the sixties and seventies emphasis once again alters. Now participants' goals will be centred around maintaining what they may see to be their declining health. Due to an increased awareness of symptoms that confirm this, they may suffer from low self-esteem and lack confidence. They will enjoy the social interaction that accompanies activities and this aspect should be programmed in.

Motivational methods

Motivating some people at any point in time can be a difficult task. Motivating all of the people all of the time is a rare skill and one that has to be learnt. For you to be successful you will have different motivational methods for every individual, adapting these methods as participants progress through their training. No one motivational method will work all of the time.

Deciding what method will work with an individual may initially involve some trial and error. However, behind this there lies the knowledge that people have common needs; it is their priorities that differ. Initially, your own behaviour towards your client needs consideration, as this in itself can act as a deterrent or motivator.

- Make a good first impression with your greeting and presentation.
- Allow your client to tell their story while you listen.
- Using your body language and choice of words, make the interaction rewarding for the client.
- Try not to control the conversation or to impose your own viewpoint.
- Emphasize the importance of the client taking responsibility for their activity levels.

It is well known that the more involved the individual is in the design of their programme, the better their adherence levels.

People like recognition for the achievement of new skills, enjoy the social interaction and the approval that being active brings, in addition to the health benefits attached to this altered lifestyle.

The role of the instructor

Your role is diverse and draws on many areas of knowledge. Just as the priorities of your client will change through exercise, so will your methods of motivation as they get nearer to and achieve the goals they desire. Initially, the individual should guide you. Listen to their goals, their vision and their concerns. Identify their strengths, barriers, weaknesses and educational needs. Be clear, realistic and individual with each client. Set a mixture of short-, medium- and long-term goals.

Monitor the client's progress and adapt to all alterations, whether these are physiological or psychological in nature. Remember that what drives them is likely to be different from what motivates you. Similarly, their fears will differ and need attention. Beware of relating too many personal experiences, as your client may not be able to identify with the situation and feelings that were evoked.

Make sessions structured and flexible, but most importantly, enjoyable. If the fun element is missing, it will only be a short time before the costs of the sessions will outweigh the benefits and a participant's adherence will falter. Encourage back-up support from close friends, family members and partners wherever possible. Provide relevant education along the way and always impress on clients the need for regularity and continuity.

Stress that exercise does not need to involve visits to the gym, studio classes or any such structured, and intimidating, sessions. Help the client to understand that the initial level of activity may be low and needs to be progressed gradually. Make the distinction between training for fitness and health and, if necessary, lower the intensity accordingly until the individual is ready to move on. Great benefit can be gained from a brisk walk outdoors, doing gardening or housework. This can then fit in with a time-pressured lifestyle more easily. Walking the children to school is an excellent option. Encouraging family activities such as swimming or games in the park will allow clients to maximize their time and reduce the feeling that exercise takes them away from the family. It should also encourage the children to adopt an active lifestyle from an early point in their lives.

 Being regularly active is a major lifestyle change for some people. This means that it needs to operate in conjunction with other lifestyle activities, duties and pressures. The healthier their other lifestyle choices, the more effective the activity programme will prove to be.

CHAPTER SUMMARY

- Regular physical activity can reduce the incidence of, alleviate and possibly treat a wide variety of medical conditions including coronary heart disease, cancer, arthritis and depression.

- Around 80 per cent of our population are inactive, many of whom can be classified as sedentary and/or obese. These individuals recognize that they can improve their health through exercise but remain unmotivated to begin a regular programme of activity.

- These inactive individuals may remain so because they do not fully believe that they will succumb to the variety of conditions that exercise can treat or those symptoms it can alleviate. →

- For a person to commit to an exercise programme the benefits have to outweigh the costs. The outcome needs to be something they see as worthwhile.

- Once a client's long-term goal and their timeframe have been identified, short- and medium-term goals should be structured into the programme for motivational purposes.

- There are many different barriers to exercise that need identification so that an action plan can be developed.

- Encouraging a high level of social support and interaction surrounding activity sessions dramatically increases a participant's adherence level.

- Exercise is a stress on the human body. Certain individuals will react strongly to this stress and need to be either distracted or relaxed during the session or learn to reinterpret the sensations they feel when they are active.

- Different things motivate people at different stages of a training programme and during their lifecycle. Your role, as the instructor, is to recognize this and adapt methods accordingly.

- There are three lifecycle stages that have been identified that span the period from an individual's twenties through to their sixties and beyond.

- When rewarding participants for their achievements, ensure that the rewards are client specific. This needs awareness of whether clients are motivated by intrinsic or extrinsic rewards.

- Make the distinction between exercise for health or for fitness. Lower the intensity of sessions; incorporate everyday activities into the programme and gradually progress the individual when they are both physiologically and psychologically ready to do so.

- Remember that adopting a regular activity programme represents a significant lifestyle change and will take time and involve a learning process. Make sure it is compatible with the other aspects of an individual's life to ensure that it remains a long-term change.

Further reading

Alter, M. (1996) *Science of Flexibility*, 2nd edition, Human Kinetics, Leeds

—— (1998) *Sport Stretch*, 2nd edition, Human Kinetics, Leeds

A Step by Step Guide to COSSH Assessment (1997) Health and Safety Executive, London

Baum, G. (1991) *Aquaerobics*, Arrow Books, London

Bean, A. (1996) *The Complete Guide to Sports Nutrition*, 2nd edition, A and C Black, London

Blakey, P. (1992) *The Muscle Book*, Bibliotek Books Ltd, Stafford

Bompa, T. (1999) *Periodisation Training for Sports* (programmes for peak strength in 35 sports), Human Kinetics, Leeds

Bompa, T. and Cornacchia, L. (1998) *Serious Strength Training*, Human Kinetics, Leeds

Bouchard, C., Shephard, R. and Stephens, T. (1994) *Physical Activity, Fitness and Health* (International Proceedings and Consensus Statement), Human Kinetics, Leeds

Clarke, N. (1997) *Sports Nutrition Guidebook*, 2nd edition, Human Kinetics, Leeds

Floyd, R.T. and Thompson, C.W. (1998) *Manual of Structural Kinesiology* 13th edition, McGraw Hill, Singapore

Kapit, W., Macey, R.I. and Meisami, E. (1987) *The Physiology Colouring Book*, Harper and Row

Killoran, A.J., Fentam, P. and Caspersen, C. (1994) *Moving On – International Perspectives on Promoting Physical Activity*, Health Education Authority, London

McArdle, W., Katch, F. and Katch, V. (2000) *Essentials of Exercise Physiology*, 2nd edition, Lippincott Williams and Wilkins, Philadelphia

Neiman, D. (1998) *The Exercise–Health Connection*, Human Kinetics, Leeds

Radcliffe, J. and Farentinos, R. (1999) *High-Powered Plyometrics*, Human Kinetics, Leeds

Rejeski, W.J. and Kenney, E.A. (1998) *Fitness Motivation – Preventing Participant Dropout*, Human Kinetics, Leeds

The Chartered Institute of Environmental Health (1993) *Basic Health and Safety at Work*, Environmental Health Training Ltd

Useful addresses

Lifetime Health & Fitness
3 Berkeley Square
Bristol
BS8 1HL
Telephone: 0117 907 8200
Fax: 0117 907 8201
E-mail: info@lifetimehf.co.uk
Website: www.lifetimehf.co.uk

Accountants

Garry Taylor Accountants
Telephone: 01276 681661
Mobile: 07801 140561
E-mail: garrytaylor@btconnect.com
Website: www.gta-tax.co.uk

Houghton Stone
The Conifers
Filton Road
Hambrook
Bristol
BS16 1QG
Telephone: 0117 957 9000
Fax: 0117 957 9001
E-mail: info@houghtonstone.co.uk

Authorities, councils and societies

Arthritis Research Campaign
Copeman House
St Mary's Court
St Mary's Gate
Chesterfield
Derbyshire
S41 7TD
Telephone: 01246 558033
Fax: 01246 558007
Website: www.arc.org.uk

British Heart Foundation
14 Fitzhardinge Street
London
W1H 6DH
Telephone: 0207 935 0185
Fax: 0207 486 5820
Website: www.bhf.org.uk

National Osteoporosis Society
P.O. Box 10
Radstock
Bath
BA3 3YB
Telephone: 01761 471771
Fax: 01761 471104
E-mail: info@nos.org.uk
Website: www.nos.org.uk

Sport England
16 Upper Woburn Place
London
WC1H 0QP
Telephone: 0207 273 1500
Fax: 0207 383 5740
Website: www.english.sports.gov.uk

Diabetes UK
10 Queen Anne Street
London
W1G 9LH
Telephone: 0207 323 1531
Fax: 0207 637 3644
E-mail: info@diabetes.org.uk
Website: www.diabetes.org.uk

Awarding and governing bodies

FIA
5–11 Lavington Street
London
SE1 0NZ
Telephone: 0207 620 0700
Fax: 0207 620 0300
E-mail: info@fia.org.uk

OCR
Westwood Business Park
Coventry
CV4 8JQ
Telephone: 02476 470033
Fax: 02476 421944
E-mail: cib@ocr.org.uk
Website: www.ocr.org.uk

SPRITO
24 Stephenson Way
London
NW1 2HD
Telephone: 0207 388 7755
Fax: 0207 388 9733
E-mail: thento@sprito.org.uk
Website: www.sprito.org.uk

Music licensing and tape companies

Performing Rights Society
29–33 Berners Street
London
W1T 3AB
Telephone: 0207 580 5544
Fax: 0207 306 4050

Phonographic Performance Licence
1 Upper Danes Street
London
W1R 3HG
Telephone: 0207 534 1000
Fax: 0207 534 1111
Website: www.ppluk.com

Pure Energy Ltd
Hawthorne House
Fitzwilliam Street
Parkgate
Rotherham
South Yorkshire
S62 6EP
Telephone: 01709 710022
Fax: 01709 523141
E-mail: information@pureenergy.co.uk
Web site: www.pureenergy.co.uk
            www.gymtrax.co.uk

Telstar Fitness
113 London Road
E13 0DA
Telephone: 0990 134777
E-mail: telstar@fitpro.com

PPL-free tape companies:

Muscle Mixes Music
P.O. Box 1212
Melksham
Wiltshire
SN12 7TP
Telephone: 01225 700059
Fax: 01225 790745

Music Express tapes at:
Fitness Professionals Education Ltd
113 London Road
London
E13 0DA
Telephone: 0990 133 434
Fax: 0208 586 0685

Publishers

HSE Books
P.O. Box 1999
Sudbury
Suffolk
CO10 2WA
Telephone: 01787 881165

Fax: 01787 313995
E-mail: hsebooks@prolog.uk.com
Website: www.hsebooks.co.uk

HMSO Publications
HMSO Books
P.O. Box 276
London
SW8 5D1
Telephone: 0171 837 9090

Human Kinetics Europe Ltd
Units C2/C3
Wira Business Park
West Park
Ring Road
Leeds
LS16 6EB
Telephone: 0113 278 1708
Fax: 0113 278 1709
E-mail: custserv@hkeurope.com
Website: www.humankinetics.com

Teaching Insurance

Fitness Professionals
113 London Road
London
E13 0DA
Telephone: 0990 133 434
Fax: 0208 586 0685
E-mail: admin@fitpro.com
      Education@fitpro.com
Website: www.fitpro.com

Suggested subscriptions

Bodylife
Botany Barns
Barr's Lane
Knaphill
Woking
Surrey
GU21 2JW

Telephone: 01483 799669
Fax: 01483 486227
E-mail: office@bodylife.co.uk
Website: www.bodylife.co.uk

Leisure Opportunities
The Leisure Media Company Ltd
Portmill House
Portmill Lane
Hitchin
Herts
SG5 1DJ
Telephone: 01462 431385
Fax: 01462 433909
Website: www.leisureopportunities.co.uk

Equipment suppliers

Hydroactive
Steph Toogood
Bridgecourt House
Godshill
Ventnor
Isle of Wight
PO38 3JU
Telephone: 01983 840555
Fax: 01983 840522
E-mail: StephToo@aol.com

Physical Company
Cherry Cottage
Hedsor Road
Bourne End
Bucks
SL8 5DH
Telephone: 01628 520208
Fax: 01628 851249
E-mail: sales@physicalcompany.co.uk
Website: www.physicalcompany.co.uk

Proactive Health Ltd
Quarry Court
Bell Lane
Cassington
Oxon
OX8 1DS

Telephone: 01865 886300
Fax: 01865 886301
E-mail: info@proactive-health.co.uk
Website: www.proactive-health.co.uk

Sound Dynamics
Bridge Street
Belper
Derbyshire
DE56 1AY
Telephone: 01773 828486
Website: www.sound-dynamics.co.uk

Sound Guys Systems
23 The Parade
Colchester Road
Harold Park
Romford
Essex
RM3 OAQ
Telephone: 01708 379770
Fax: 01708 375940

Glossary of terms

Abduction	Movement of a limb or body part away from the mid-line of the body.
Achilles tendonitis	An inflammatory reaction in the achilles tendon and its sheath as a result of prolonged repeated loading.
Actin	The thin protein myofilament found within muscle.
Adaptation	A physiological change that takes place in response to a progressively increased training load.
Adduction	Movement of a limb or body part towards the mid-line of the body.
Adenosine diphosphate	A compound containing adenosine and two phosphate groups. Found within cells, it plays a vital role in energy transfer and the resynthesis of ATP.
Adenosine triphosphate (ATP)	A compound, known as the body's energy currency, made up of adenosine and three phosphate groups.
Adipose tissue	A fibrous connective tissue containing the fat storage cells known as adipocytes. Found underneath the skin and surrounding the internal organs.
Aerobic	Needing oxygen.
Agility	The ability to move nimbly and accurately.
Agonist (prime mover)	The main muscle or muscle group that contracts to cause movement at a joint.

Alveoli	Tiny air sacs that allow gaseous exchange to occur across their single-celled walls and those of the blood capillaries.
Amenorrhoea	A condition characterized by the lack of menstruation (periods).
Amino acids	Small organic compounds that contain an amino group (-NH2) and a carboxyl group (-COOH). These are the fundamental constituents of protein.
Anaerobic	Not needing oxygen
Anaerobic threshold	The point at which the body's ability to supply oxygen does not match demand and the energy systems operating work without oxygen.
Anatomical position	The standing position when the body is in neutral alignment. Weight is evenly distributed between the feet; arms are beside the body with palms facing forward.
Anatomy	The study of the structure of humans.
Angina	A pain in the chest brought on by exertion as the heart demands a greater blood supply than the blood vessels can provide.
Anorexia	Loss of appetite
Anorexia nervosa	A psychological illness that causes individuals to starve themselves via a variety of techniques.
Antagonist	A muscle whose action opposes that of another muscle known as the agonist or prime mover. As the agonist contracts the antagonist relaxes to allow smooth, precise movements to occur.
Anterior	Referring to the front of the body or, with reference to another object, 'in front'.
Aorta	The largest artery within the body. It originates from the left ventricle and gives rise to all other arteries.
Appendicular skeleton	The freely moveable section of the skeleton composed of the upper and lower limbs.
Arteries	The blood vessels that carry blood away from the heart under pressure. They have thick muscular walls.
Arterioles	The small branches of arteries that link arteries to the even smaller capillaries. The constriction and dilation of the arterioles has the greatest effect on blood flow and pressure.

Arthritis	A painful condition characterized by inflammation of one or more joints that limits the joint movement. The causes are numerous but the result is damage to the synovial membrane and/or cartilage within the affected joint.
Articular (hyaline) cartilage	The most common type of cartilage, bluish-white in colour, elastic in nature.
Asthma	A condition characterized by a shortness of breath and caused by a narrowing of the bronchial airways that may be triggered by an allergen, exercise or anxiety.
Atherosclerosis	A disease of the arteries characterized by fatty plaque deposits developing on the inner walls and obstructing the blood flow.
Atria	The two smaller superior receiving chambers of the heart.
Atrio-ventricular valve	The valve that lies between the atria and ventricles that ensures a one-way flow of blood from the atria to the ventricles in the heart.
Atrophy	The wasting away of muscle tissue due to disuse, ageing or disease that causes a reduction in size to the tissue.
Axial skeleton	The supportive section of the skeleton composed of the skull, vertebrae, sternum and rib cage.
Bicuspid valve	See definition of mitral valve.
Biomechanics	The study of mechanics as it relates to the function and structure of the body.
Bipennate	(Relating to a muscle) characterized by fibres that travel in two directions and have a high contraction speed.
Blood pressure	The pressure of blood on the walls of the arteries.
Blood vessels	The network of arteries, arterioles, capillaries, venules and veins that carry blood around the body.
Body composition	The ratio of fat tissue to fat-free mass in any individual.
Bone density	The weight and strength of a bone that affects its ability to withstand stress. The higher the bone density the less likely the bone will fracture when a load is applied to it. Cardiovascular impact work and resistance training can increase bone density.

Bronchi	The air passages that transport the air from the trachea into the bronchioles. The walls of these airways contain cartilage and mucus glands.
Bronchioles	A subdivision of the bronchial tree, these are the smaller airways that link the bronchi with the alveoli. The walls of these airways do not contain cartilage and mucus glands.
Calcification	The deposition of calcium salts in tissue, that occurs through the ossification process.
Calcium	The mineral found in bones and teeth and essential for muscle contraction. Dairy products and fresh green vegetables are sources of calcium.
Calisthenics	Movements or exercises designed to increase strength and flexibility without the use of equipment.
Calorie	The unit used to measure the energy contained within foods. A unit of heat equal to the amount of heat required to raise the temperature of 1 gram of water by 1°C.
Cancer	A malignant tumour that is formed from the abnormal and uncontrolled division of cells which then invades and destroys surrounding tissues.
Capillaries	The smallest blood vessels that form a network around the tissues of the body and allow for gaseous exchange to occur across their thin (one-cell thick) membrane. They are supplied with blood from the arterioles and drained by the venules.
Carbohydrates	An array of compounds ranging from simple sugars to starches that contain carbon, hydrogen and oxygen.
Carbon dioxide	A colourless, odourless and poisonous gas that is breathed in from the atmosphere in small amounts and breathed out in larger quantities as it is a by-product of many metabolic reactions.
Cardiac output (CO)	The amount of blood pumped out of the heart in any one minute. Measured in litres (l).
Cardiac muscle	The specialized muscle found only in the heart that is intrinsically innervated by a pacemaker.
Cardiopulmonary resuscitation (CPR)	The process of breathing oxygen into a casualty in order to keep their blood and tissues oxygenated if they are not breathing.

Cardiovascular fitness	The ability of the heart and lungs to deliver an adequate supply of oxygen to the working muscles.
Cardiovascular system	The heart and all the connected blood vessels known as the circulatory system. It is differentiated into the systemic and pulmonary circulations.
Cartilage	The dense semi-opaque or grey connective tissue that can withstand pressure. There are three separate types of cartilage found in different areas of the body: hyaline, elastic and fibrocartilage.
Cervical vertebrae	The seven bones making up the neck region of the spine.
Cholera	An acute bacterial infection of the small intestine. It is contracted from food or water contaminated by faeces from an individual already suffering from the disease. The symptoms include severe vomiting and diarrhoea that leads to dehydration.
Cholesterol	A fat-like steroid alcohol made by the liver that can accumulate and narrow the diameter of the arteries.
Choreography	A sequence of steps linked together to form a routine.
Circumduction	Motion that in 3D terms would make a cone shape. A sequential combination of flexion, abduction, extension and adduction.
Collagen	A relatively inelastic but strong protein that makes up the white fibrous connective tissue found in tendons. Also located in skin, bone and cartilage.
Compact (cortical) bone	The hard outer layer of bone tissue.
Concentric (positive phase)	The positive phase of an exercise that causes a muscle to shorten under contraction while the angle of the joint is decreased whilst working in the opposite direction to gravity.
Constriction	A narrowing.
Contraction	The shortening of a muscle in response to a motor nerve impulse. The tension within the muscle can create movement or remain static to brace against a load.
Coronary heart disease	Degenerative disease of the heart and blood vessels.
Coccyx	The lowermost nine fused vertebrae of the backbone that represents the remains of a tail.

COSHH	Control of substances hazardous to health. This relates to the legislation that concerns the duties and responsibilities of employers and employees to ensure that hazardous substances are used safely within the workplace.
Cramp	A prolonged and painful contraction of a muscle. Possibly brought about by an imbalance of salts, fatigue, stress or poor posture.
Creatine phosphate (creatine phosphagen)	A high-energy compound that assists in the resynthesis of adenosine triphosphate from adenosine diphosphate by contributing its phosphate group.
Cross-bridges	The attachments that are made from myosin to actin myofilaments to allow contraction to occur.
Decalcification	Loss or removal of calcium from salts from the bone or teeth.
Defibrillation	Administration of a controlled electric shock to restore the normal heart rhythm following ventricular fibrillation.
Delayed onset muscle soreness (DOMS)	Discomfort felt within muscles that have been trained eccentrically. Soreness can last between 24–72 hours. May be due to micro muscle tears.
Depression (psychological)	A mental state characterized by excessive sadness. Activity levels can be agitated or lethargic.
Depression (kinesiological)	Moving to an inferior position.
Diabetes mellitus	A disorder affecting carbohydrate metabolism in which sugars are not utilized efficiently due to a lack of insulin or reduced activity of this hormone.
Diaphragm	A dome-shaped muscle lying underneath the rib cage that contracts and flattens to allow inspiration to occur.
Diaphysis	The shaft of the bone.
Diastole	The rest period between two contractions of the heart that allows the blood to refill the atria.
Diffusion	The movement of gases from regions where they are in high concentrations to regions of low concentration until equilibrium is reached.
Dilation	The enlargement or widening of a hollow organ.

Distal	Away from the mid-line of the body.
Diuretic	A drug that promotes the production of urine by increasing the excretion of salts and water by the kidneys.
Dorsal	Relating to the back.
Dorsiflexion	Moving the top of the foot towards the anterior tibialis.
Eccentric (negative phase)	The negative phase of an exercise that lengthens the muscle under contraction as the angle at the joint is increased whilst working in the same direction as gravity.
Eclampsia	A Greek word meaning 'like a flash of lightening'. It is a medical condition that can occur during pregnancy where the blood vessels within the uterus go into spasm. This reduces the blood flow to the foetus and can cause the mother to fit and enter a coma. It is usually preceded by a condition called pre-eclampsia, the only symptom of which is an elevation in blood pressure.
Ectomorph	The tall, thin, lean physique characteristic of long-distance runners.
Elastic cartilage	A connective tissue that consists mainly of elastic yellow fibres. Found in the outer ear.
Elastin	The protein that makes up the bulk of the elastic tissue fibres.
Elevation	Moving to a superior position.
Endomorph	The round-shouldered, thick-waisted, high-body-fat physique characteristic of wrestlers.
Energy	The ability to perform work.
Epiphysis	The end of a long bone.
Essential amino acids	Amino acids needed by the body for growth but that cannot be manufactured by the body. These are obtained from a variety of food sources.
Erythrocytes (red blood cells)	The red blood cells manufactured in the bone marrow that contain the oxygen-carrying pigment haemoglobin.
Eversion	Lifting the lateral edge of the foot. Turning the sole of the foot away from the mid-line.
Excretion	The removal of waste products of metabolism from the body.

Exercise	Any activity that results in physical exertion that is intended to maintain physical fitness.
Expiration (exhalation)	Breathing out. This is a passive process at rest but can be assisted by the intercostal and abdominal muscles during exercise.
Extension	Increasing the angle between two bones.
External rotation (outward lateral rotation)	A rotary movement around the longitudinal axis of a bone away from the mid-line of the body.
Fast-twitch fibres (Type 2)	The rapidly contracting muscle fibres responsible for anaerobic, explosive work. The fibres have a susceptibility to increase in diameter with training.
Fatty acids	These are organic acids that make up many of the body's lipids, like triglycerides. Some fatty acids are essential and cannot be manufactured by the body.
Fibre (dietary)	Food substances that cannot be broken down or absorbed by the body to produce energy but act as roughage to speed up the journey through the digestive system.
Fibrocartilage	A tough connective tissue mainly made of collagen. Found in intervertebral discs.
Fibrinogen	A substance found within the blood plasma that is responsible for blood clotting processes.
Fixator	The muscle or muscle group that contracts isometrically to fix a nearby joint to prevent unwanted movement.
Fixed joint	A joint where no movement is possible.
Flexibility	The range of movement that can be accomplished at any joint.
Flexion	Decreasing the angle between two bones.
Fracture threshold	The point at which the force applied to a bone is sufficient to break it.
Freely moveable (synovial) joint	Where two bones meet and movement is possible in a variety of planes. Characterized by a synovial membrane, fluid and joint capsule.
Fusiform (parallel)	(Relating to a muscle) characterized by long parallel fibres that allow fast contraction. Also described as spindle-shaped, tapering at both ends.

Gaseous exchange	The process that occurs between capillaries and the many tissues of the body allowing oxygen to be delivered and carbon dioxide to be taken away.
Genetics	The science of inheritance that considers the similarities and differences between parents and their offspring.
Gluconeogenesis	The process in which glucose is manufactured within the body from non-carbohydrate sources within the liver and kidneys.
Glucose	The simplest monosaccharide that is the principal sugar within the bloodstream and the only sugar that can be directly used by the brain tissue.
Glycerol	A clear viscous liquid that is the result of the hydrolysis (breakdown) of fat.
Glycogen	The stored form of glucose found in the liver and muscle tissue.
Glycolysis	The conversion of glucose into lactic acid, which is possible either with or without oxygen being present.
Golgi tendon organ	A sensory receptor located and activated within the tendon of a muscle that has been placed under great tension. Information is relayed to the central nervous system and the reflex response is to cause the muscle to relax to avoid injury.
Growth (epiphyseal) plate	The cartilage plate that separates the ends (epiphysis) of the bone from the shaft (diaphysis). This is where growth occurs. Once this plate ossifies growth is complete.
Growth spurt	An increase in the activity of the osteoblast cell activity that encourages new bone formation.
Haemoglobin	The iron-containing pigment found in red blood cells that are responsible for carrying the oxygen within the bloodstream.
Health	A state characterized by the absence of disease.
Health-related fitness	This represents the ability to perform daily activities with vigour and the demonstration of traits and capacities that are associated with a low risk of premature development of hypokinetic diseases.
Heart rate (HR)	The number of times that the heart beats in any one minute. Measured in beats per minute (bpm).

High-density lipoprotein (HDL)	A type of lipoprotein (fat transporter) within the blood. Considered to be the healthiest of the lipoproteins, with levels rising with regular exercise or activity programmes.
Holistic	An approach to fitness that involves consideration of the physical, mental and spiritual well-being of the individual.
Homeostasis	A state of equilibrium that the body attempts to maintain internally, despite the changes to the external environment.
Horizontal abduction	Movement of the humerus in the horizontal plane away from the mid-line of the body.
Horizontal adduction	Movement of the humerus in the horizontal plane towards the mid-line of the body.
Hormones	Substances released from organs and glands into the bloodstream that act as messengers to influence the structure or function of other organs and tissues.
Hyperextension	Increasing the angle between two bones beyond the anatomical position.
Hyperglycaemia	High blood sugar levels.
Hypertension	High blood pressure.
Hypertrophy	An increase in size of a tissue or organ, e.g. muscle size.
Hyperventilation	Breathing at a very rapid rate. This reduces the concentration of carbon dioxide within arterial blood. Symptoms include dizziness and chest cramps, with possible loss of consciousness if the condition persists.
Hypoglycaemia	Low blood sugar.
Hypokinetic	Low levels of movement.
Hypotension	Low blood pressure.
Immoveable (fixed or fibrous) joint	Where two bones meet and no movement is possible.
Immunity	The body's ability to defend itself against disease and infection.
Inferior	Below or lower than.
Influenza	A viral infection that affects the respiratory system and is highly contagious.

Inhibition	The prevention of activity or a reduction to the activity within a tissue or organ as a result of nervous communication.
Innervation	The nervous supply to a tissue or organ that is responsible for transmitting the sensory and motor nerve information.
Insertion	The point of attachment of a muscle that lies furthest away from the mid-line of the body and, when the muscle contracts, moves more than the point of origin.
Inspiration (inhalation)	The process of breathing in. This is an active process involving the diaphragm, intercostal and abdominal muscles.
Insulin	A hormone released from the pancreas into the bloodstream to lower blood glucose levels and which affects carbohydrate and fat metabolism.
Internal rotation (inward medial rotation)	Rotary movement around the longitudinal axis of a bone towards the mid-line of the body.
Intervertebral discs	The fibrocartilage between the vertebrae of the spine which absorbs impact forces and protects the spinal cord.
Intrapulmonic	Within the lungs.
Inversion	Lifting the medial border of the foot. Turning the sole of the foot towards the mid-line.
Involuntary	Without conscious control.
Ischaemia	An inadequate blood flow to a tissue or organ, usually as a result of an obstruction or narrowing of a blood vessel.
Isometric contraction	When tension is generated within a muscle without a change of length resulting.
Isotonic contraction	When tension is generated within a muscle and the muscle changes length by either shortening or lengthening.
Joint	The place where two bones meet whether or not movement is possible.
Kinesiology	The science of human movement. A combination of biomechanics, anatomy and physiology.
Kinetic energy	Energy that moves objects.

Kyphosis	A spinal posture characterized by an excessive curvature to the thoracic vertebrae.
Lactic acid	The compound that is formed within muscles as the end product of the partial breakdown of glucose through the lactic acid (intermediate) energy system.
Lateral	Away from the mid-line.
Lateral flexion	Moving a body part away from the mid-line with the angle at the moving joint becoming smaller.
Leucocytes (white blood cells)	Manufactured within the bone marrow, these cells are responsible for the body's defence system (immunity).
Ligament	A tough, white connective tissue that joins bone to bone.
Lipoprotein	A group of proteins found in the bloodstream that combine with fats to transport them to their destination. Cholesterol is transported in this way by the low-density lipoproteins.
Lordosis	A spinal posture characterized by an excessive curvature of the lumbar spine.
Low-density lipoprotein (LDL)	The lipoprotein within the bloodstream that is responsible for transporting cholesterol around the body.
Lumbar vertebrae	The largest five moveable bones of the spine, located between the thoracic and sacral vertebrae.
Macronutrient	A food substance that is needed in large amounts in an individual's diet on a daily basis, e.g. carbohydrates and proteins and fats.
Manual handling	The correct methods of lifting and carrying objects that ensure the safety of the lifter.
Maximum heart rate (MHR)	The maximum number of times an individual's heart can beat per minute when maximally stressed.
Maximal oxygen consumption (VO$_2$ Max.)	The maximum amount of oxygen that the lung, heart and muscles can take in, transport and utilize.
Medullary cavity	The central hollow cavity within a long bone.
Medial	Towards the mid-line.
Membrane	A thin layer of tissue that surrounds a tissue or organ that differentiates adjacent structures.

Menopause	A time in a woman's reproductive history when the ovary no longer produces an egg every four weeks. Menstruation stops as a result and the woman can no longer become pregnant.
Mesomorph	The athletic, broad-shouldered and low-body-fat physique characteristic of a competitive swimmer.
Metabolism	The sum of all the chemical reactions that take place in the body to keep it alive.
Microgram (µg)	One millionth of a gram.
Micronutrient	A food substance that is needed in an individual's diet in small quantities on a daily basis, e.g. vitamins and minerals.
Mid-line	A theoretical central line that divides the body into left and right sides.
Milligram (mg)	One thousandth of a gram.
Millilitre (ml)	One thousandth of a litre.
Mitochondria	The power houses of the muscle cells that enable oxygen to be processed and energy in the form of adenosine triphosphate to be produced.
Mitral (bicuspid) valve	A double-flapped valve that is found between the left atrium and ventricle to prevent the backward flow of blood.
Mobility	The ability of the joints to move freely through their natural range of movement.
Modelling	The process whereby bone is shaped specifically to fit its function through the activity of the bone cells osteoblasts and osteoclasts.
Molecule	The smallest chemical unit of matter that reveals characteristics of the substance of which it forms a part.
Monosaccharide	The simplest and smallest of the carbohydrate sugars that contains only one sugar unit, e.g. glucose.
Motor nerve	A nerve that transports a message from the central nervous system to a muscle to bring about movement.
Motor neuron	One of the units that make up the communication system from the brain to skeletal muscle.
Motor skills	The ability to co-ordinate muscle and movement patterns in a controlled and practised way.

Motor unit	A branch of the motor neuron and all of the muscle fibres it innervates.
Multipennate (convergent)	(Relating to a muscle) characterized by fibres that cover a large area and generate much force.
Muscle fibres	Muscle cells.
Muscular endurance	The number of repeated contractions that a muscle or muscle group can perform against a resistance without fatiguing; or the amount of time a contraction can be held without fatigue.
Muscle spindle	A sensory device lying parallel to and between the muscle fibres of striated muscle tissue. Responds to changes of length within the muscle and the speed at which the muscle is stretched.
Muscular strength	The maximum amount of force that a muscle or muscle group can develop during a single contraction.
Muscle tone	The normal state of a muscle when it is partially relaxed but contains a small amount of tension to enable it to react quickly to situations.
Myocardial infarction	The death of a section of the heart muscle due to a lack of blood supply caused by a blockage in a blood vessel supplying the muscle.
Myofibril	A bundle of contractile fibres within a muscle cell.
Myofilaments	The smallest protein component of muscle tissue that has the ability to contract and gives striated muscle its stripey appearance. Actin and myosin are myofilaments.
Myoglobin (myohaemoglobin)	The protein found in muscle tissue that is responsible for the uptake and storage of oxygen.
Myosin	The thick protein myofilament found in muscle.
Myotatic reflex (stretch reflex)	The unconscious and protective contraction of a muscle in response to it being lengthened at speed.
Neuromuscular (myoneural) junction	The meeting point between the nerve and the muscle fibre with which it communicates.
Neutral alignment	When the joints and body segments are balanced with an even distribution of weight between them.

Neutral spine	The correct positioning of the spine that maintains its natural curvature and allows the intervertebral discs to absorb impact most efficiently and the muscles around the spine to expend the least amount of energy.
Nutrient	A substance that must be consumed within the diet to provide energy or material for growth and bodily function. Nutrients include carbohydrates, fats, proteins, vitamins and minerals.
Obesity	A condition characterized by the excessive storage of body fat subcutaneously. Clinically, this is considered to be when fat storage is greater than 20 per cent in excess of the recommended value for an individual's height and weight.
Onset of blood lactic acid accumulation (VOBLA)	The point in time where the blood lactic acid levels begin to rise steeply in response to a high exercise intensity that becomes anaerobic in nature. The levels of lactic acid increase out of proportion to the increase in intensity level. This can signify an individual's anaerobic threshold.
Organic	(Relating to a chemical compound) Containing carbon.
Origin	The point of attachment of a muscle that is closest to the mid-line of the body and that remains relatively fixed when the muscle contracts.
Orthopaedic	The practice of correcting deformities caused by damage or disease to the bones and joints.
Ossification (osteogenesis/ calcification/ mineralization)	The process by which cartilage is hardened into bone by the addition of the minerals calcium and phosphorus. Bone growth is controlled by the osteoblasts.
Osteoblasts	The bone cells responsible for bone building, strengthening and repair.
Osteoclasts	The bone cells responsible for cleaning and breaking down old or damaged bone tissue.
Osteons	A group of bone cells that are structured into layers within compact bone tissue.
Osteoporosis	A disease characterized by a reduction in bone density to the point where the fracture threshold is greatly lowered.

Overload	Placing a load on the body that it is unaccustomed to, and which requires the body to adapt to deal with it.
Overtraining	Training that fails to allow sufficient time for the body to recover and rebuild itself between sessions. The symptoms are various but generally represent a decrease in the body's immune system.
Oxygen	An odourless, colourless gas that makes up a fifth of the gases present in our atmosphere.
Oxygen debt	A situation where oxygen demand has outweighed the body's ability to supply it. In exercise this usually occurs following an intense exercise bout and it is necessary to reduce intensity and breathe quickly to replenish the oxygen supplies.
Pacemaker	The control centre within the heart muscle that initiates the regular heart beat.
Peak bone mass	The maximal amount of bone density that can be achieved by any individual.
Periodization	A structured method of programming an individual's fitness goals that balances the volume and intensity of the sessions by splitting the training into short-, medium- and long-term goals known as cycles.
Periosteum	The fibrous sheath that covers all but the ends of the long bones.
Phospholipids	A lipid that incorporates a phosphate group as part of the molecule.
Phosphorus	A mineral found in bone.
Physical fitness	A set of attributes that people have or achieve that relates to their ability to perform physical activity.
Physiology	The study of the systems within the body.
Pilates	An exercise class that blends the Alexander technique and yoga, aimed at increasing the body's strength and flexibility with a focus on core strength.
Plantar flexion	Moving the sole of the foot downwards. Planting the ball of the foot towards the floor.
Plasma	The major straw-coloured component of blood that contains the dissolved hormones, salts, fats and sugars.

Platelets (thrombocytes)	Cell fragments that act as containers to transport substances to the sites of injury to aid the blood clotting process.
Plyometric	Relating to a training method that involves an eccentric action followed by a maximal concentric effort. This is seen in many jumping or bounding movements.
Polysaccharide	The most complex of the carbohydrates made up of many linked sugar molecules.
Posterior	Relating to the back or behind.
Potential energy	Stored energy.
Power	A combination of speed and strength.
Pre-fatigue	A resistance training method that involves working a muscle to fatigue in an isolation exercise before progressing into a compound exercise for a second set, e.g. leg extension exercise followed by a squat.
Pronation	Rotating the hand and wrist medially from the elbow.
Prone	Lying face downward.
Protraction (abduction)	The movement of the shoulder girdles away from each other and away from the mid-line of the body.
Proprioception	The ability of the body to determine the position of the limbs in space. Information is relayed via 'proprioceptors' that are sensors within the muscles, tendons and ligaments that detect movement.
Proximal	Near to.
Pulmonary artery	The large blood vessel responsible for transporting the deoxygenated blood from the right ventricle to the lungs to pick up oxygen.
Pulmonary circulation	The circulation that is served by the right side of the heart and responsible for delivering blood to the lung tissues.
Reciprocal innervation	A process that describes the way one muscle of a pair relaxes when the opposing muscle contracts.
Recruitment	The process of generating more muscle force by activating a greater number of muscle fibres to assist the action.
Relaxin	A hormone that circulates within the body during pregnancy that has the effect of loosening the ligaments.

Resting metabolic rate	The sum total of all the chemical reactions necessary to keep the body alive when at rest.
Residual volume	The amount of air that remains within the lungs after a maximal expiration.
Respiration	The process of gas exchange that occurs between the individual and their environment.
Retraction (adduction)	The movement of the shoulder girdles together towards the mid-line of the body.
Revitalizer	The final component of a class that aims to ensure all participants are awake, alert and co-ordinated before leaving the studio.
Risk assessment	An evaluation of the number and severity of risk factors affecting an environment or an individual.
Risk factor	An attribute, habit or environmental stress that increases the likelihood of an individual contracting a disease or becoming injured.
Rotation	Medial or lateral turning about the vertical axis of the bone.
Sacral vertebrae	The five fused vertebrae found between the lumbar vertebrae and the coccyx.
Sarcomere	The distance between one complete unit of actin and myosin arrangements. The smallest unit of contraction.
Scoliosis	A spinal posture characterized by an S-shape due to excessive sideways curvature to either the thoracic or lumbar spine or both.
Sedentary	Inactive.
Semi-lunar valve	Either of the two valves that are found at the origin of the aorta or the pulmonary artery. They ensure the one-way flow of blood out of the heart.
Semi-moveable (cartilaginous) joint	Where two bones meet and limited movement is possible.
Septum	A dividing wall between two anatomical structures.
Shin splints	A condition characterized by anterior lower leg pain, thought to be due to excessive impact, muscle imbalance and/or inflammation of the anterior tibialis periosteum.
Skeletal (striated) muscle	Any of the 600 or more stripey, voluntary muscles used to initiate movement.

Skeleton	The interconnected series of bones that gives us our structure, protects internal organs and provides the attachment site for muscles to evoke movement.
Sliding filament theory	The name given to the process of muscle contraction when actin is rowed past myosin as the muscle shortens in length.
Slow-twitch fibres (Type 1)	The slow contracting endurance fibres that respond to aerobic training.
Smooth muscle	The involuntary muscle found in blood vessels and the intestines.
Spasticity	Resistance to the passive movement of a limb, leading to unco-ordinated movement patterns.
Spinal cord	The bundles of nerve fibres that run up and down the length of the spine.
Spongy (cancellous or trabecular) bone	The inner, honeycomb-like bone tissue.
Sprain	An injury resulting from overstretching the ligament.
Stimulus	Something that affects the functioning and activity within a cell or tissue.
Strain	An injury to muscle tissue resulting from the muscle being overstretched or overworked.
Stress	The sum of all non-specific biological responses invoked by adverse external influences.
Stroke volume (SV)	The amount of blood pumped by the heart with each contraction. Measured in millilitres (ml).
Superior	Above.
Supination	Rotating the hand and wrist laterally from the elbow.
Supine	Lying face upward.
Synergist	A muscle or muscle group that assists the movement of the agonist (prime mover).
Synovial fluid (synovia)	The colourless viscous liquid found within synovial joints that allows the joints to move smoothly and with little friction.
Synovial joint (diarthrosis)	A freely moveable joint that contains a joint capsule linking the two bones that secretes the synovial fluid into the synovial cavity ensuring smooth joint movement.

Systemic circulation	The circulation that is served by the left side of the heart that pumps blood to the body tissues.
T'ai chi	A Chinese exercise discipline aimed at harmonizing the body and mind to raise energy levels. This is done through slow and focused movement patterns.
Tendon	A connective tissue that attaches muscle to bone.
Thoracic vertebrae	The 12 moveable vertebrae that lie between the cervical and lumbar vertebrae.
Tidal volume	The amount of air that passes through the lungs in one minute.
Tissue	A collection of cells that are specialized to perform a specific function.
Total lung volume	The maximum amount of air that can be contained within the lungs.
Trachea	The windpipe that conveys air from the larynx into the bronchi.
Tricuspid valve	The three-part valve found between the right atrium and ventricle to prevent the backflow of blood.
Triglycerides	The storage form of fat found in the blood stream and within adipose tissue.
Tuberculosis	A bacterial infection that causes tissue lesions.
Type A characteristics	Personality traits that include aggression, ambition and anxiety about time pressures. These characteristics are common in people suffering from coronary heart disease and can indicate the likelihood of developing the disease.
Voluntary	With conscious control.
Wellbeing	A feeling of contentment that signifies a balance between the body and mind.
Wellness	A state of complete physical, mental and social wellbeing and not merely the absence of disease or infirmity.
Unipennate	(Relating to a muscle) characterized by fibres that travel in one direction, the fibre length being shorter than those of the parallel muscles.
Valsalva manoevre	Exhalation against a closed glottis causing an increase in the intrathoracic pressure and blood pressure. Common during weight training when lifting heavy weights whilst holding your breath.

Veins	The blood vessels that take blood towards the heart. They contain valves to encourage blood flow in one direction only.
Vena cavae	The main two veins that carry deoxygenated blood back to the heart.
Ventilation rate	The number of breaths taken in any one minute.
Ventricles	The two larger inferior pumping chambers within the heart. The left ventricle is significantly larger than the right.
Venules	The smaller version of veins that link veins to capillaries.
Vital capacity	The maximum amount of air you can inhale and exhale in one breath.
Yoga	A system of exercise that focuses on body alignment and flexibility to increase energy levels and muscular strength.
Yo-yo dieting	An eating habit that involves an individual following a very low-calorie diet for a certain period of time that results in dramatic weight reduction. Afterwards normal or overeating patterns are resumed, which mean the weight is put back on. This cycle is then repeated many times.

References

Allied Dunbar National Fitness Survey: Main Findings (1982) Health Education Authority and Sports Council

American College of Sports Medicine Position Stand (1990) 'The recommended quantity and quality of exercise for developing and maintaining cardiorespiratory and muscular fitness in healthy adults', *Medicine and Science in Sports and Exercise*, **22**, 265–74

American College of Sports Medicine Position Stand (1993) 'Physical activity, physical fitness, and hypertension', *Medicine and Science in Sports and Exercise*, **25**, i–x

American College of Sports Medicine Position Stand (1998) 'The recommended quantity and quality of exercise for developing and maintaining cardiorespiratory and muscular fitness, and flexibility in healthy adults', *Medicine and Science in Sports and Exercise*, **30**, 975–91

American College of Sports Medicine (2000) *Guidelines for Exercise Testing and Prescription*, 6th Edition, Lippincott Williams & Wilkins, Philadelphia

Baechle, T. (1994) *Essentials of Strength Training and Conditioning*, Human Kinetics, Leeds

Borg, G. (1998) *Borg's Perceived Exertion and Pain Scale*, Champaign, IL; Human Kinetics, Leeds

Corbin, C.V. and Noble, L. (1980) 'Flexibility: a major component of physical fitness', *Journal of Physical Education and Recreation*, **51**(6), 23–24 and 57–60

Control of Substances Hazardous to Health (COSHH) Regulations (1995), HSE, Norwich

Health & Safety at Work Act (1974), HSE, Suffolk

Health Education Symposium (1994)

Manual Handling Regulations (1997), HSE, Suffolk

The Reporting of Injuries, Diseases and Dangerous Occurrences (RIDDOR) Regulations (1995), HSE, Norwich

The Health of the Nation: A Strategy for Health in England (1994)

Westcott, W.L. (1993) 'How many repetitions?', *Nautilus*, **2**(3): 6–7

Westcott, W.L. (1995) *Strength Fitness – Physiological principles and training techniques*, 4th Edition, Wm. C. Brown Publishers, Duboque, Iowa

Westcott, W.L. and Wayne, (1996) *Building Strength and Stamina*, Human Kinetics, Leeds

World Health Organisation (1984)

Index